Advances in Polymeric Nanomaterials for Biomedical Applications

Advances in Polymeric Nanomaterials for Biomedical Applications

Edited by

Anil Kumar Bajpai
Government Model Science College, Jabalpur, India
Rajesh Kumar Saini
Government Model Science College, Jabalpur, India

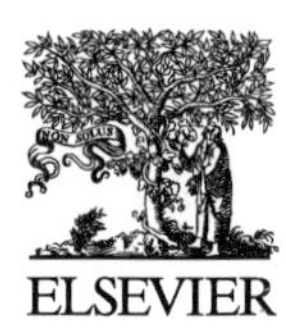

ELSEVIER

Elsevier
Radarweg 29, PO Box 211, 1000 AE Amsterdam, Netherlands
The Boulevard, Langford Lane, Kidlington, Oxford OX5 1GB, United Kingdom
50 Hampshire Street, 5th Floor, Cambridge, MA 02139, United States

British Library Cataloguing-in-Publication Data
A catalogue record for this book is available from the British Library

Library of Congress Cataloging-in-Publication Data
A catalog record for this book is available from the Library of Congress

ISBN: 978-0-12-814657-6

Publisher: Matthew Deans
Acquisitions Editor: Sabrina Webber
Editorial Project Manager: Lindsay Lawrence
Production Project Manager: Anitha Sivaraj
Cover Designer: Greg Harris

Typeset by MPS Limited, Chennai, India

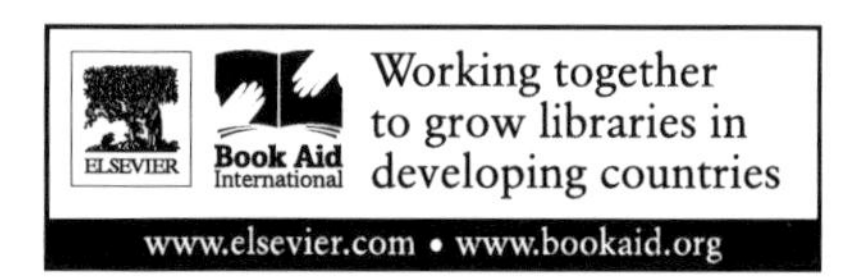

Contents

List of contributors

Naveed Ahmed
Department of Pharmacy, Quaid-i-Azam University, Islamabad, Pakistan

Gulsah Albayrak
Department of Medical Biology, Faculty of Medicine, Ufuk University, Ankara, Turkey

Narsireddy Amreddy
Department of Pathology, University of Oklahoma Health Sciences Center, Oklahoma City, OK, United States; Stephenson Cancer Center, University of Oklahoma Health Sciences Center, Oklahoma City, OK, United States

Falguni Baidya
Department of Pharmacology and Toxicology, National Institute of Pharmaceutical Education and Research (NIPER), Ahmedabad, Gandhinagar, India

Anil Kumar Bajpai
Government Model Science College, Jabalpur, India

Jaya Bajpai
Bose Memorial Research Laboratory, Department of Chemistry, Government Autonomous Science College, Jabalpur, India

Neha Bhatt
Department of Chemistry, Graphic Era Deemed to be University, Dehradun, India

Pallab Bhattacharya
Department of Pharmacology and Toxicology, National Institute of Pharmaceutical Education and Research (NIPER), Ahmedabad, Gandhinagar, India

Sarthak Bhattacharya
Department of Pharmaceutics and Pharmaceutical Technology, Shri R.D. Bhakt College of Pharmacy, Jalna, India; Dr. Babasaheb Ambedkar Marathwada University (BAMU), Aurangabad, India

Maria Bohra
Department of Pharmacology and Toxicology, National Institute of Pharmaceutical Education and Research (NIPER), Ahmedabad, Gandhinagar, India

Anupom Borah
Cellular and Molecular Neurobiology Laboratory, Department of Life Science and Bioinformatics, Assam University, Silchar, India

Iqra Chaudhery
Department of Pharmacy, Quaid-i-Azam University, Islamabad, Pakistan

Mahendran Chinnappan
Department of Pathology, University of Oklahoma Health Sciences Center, Oklahoma City, OK, United States; Stephenson Cancer Center, University of Oklahoma Health Sciences Center, Oklahoma City, OK, United States

Rashmi Choubey
Bose Memorial Research Laboratory, Department of Chemistry, Government Autonomous Science College, Jabalpur, India

Zeynep Cimen
Department of Chemistry, Polatlı Faculty of Arts and Sciences, Ankara Hacı Bayram Veli University, Ankara, Turkey

Aydan Dag
Department of Pharmaceutical Chemistry, Faculty of Pharmacy, Bezmialem Vakıf University, İstanbul, Turkey

Aishika Datta
Department of Pharmacology and Toxicology, National Institute of Pharmaceutical Education and Research (NIPER), Ahmedabad, Gandhinagar, India

Kunjan R. Dave
Department of Neurology, University of Miami Miller School of Medicine, Miami, FL, United States

Gokcen B. Demirel
Department of Chemistry, Polatlı Faculty of Arts and Sciences, Ankara Hacı Bayram Veli University, Ankara, Turkey

Fang Fang
Key Laboratory of Molecular Medicine and Biotherapy, School of Life Sciences, Beijing Institute of Technology, Beijing, P.R. China

Morteza Sasani Ghamsari
Photonics and Quantum Technologies Research School, Nuclear Science and Technology Research Institute, Tehran, Iran

Rekha Goswami
Department of Environmental Science, Graphic Era Hill University, Dehradun, India

Najam ul Hassan
Department of Pharmacy, Quaid-i-Azam University, Islamabad, Pakistan

Deepshikha Hazarika
Advanced Polymer and Nanomaterial Laboratory, Department of Chemical Sciences, Tezpur University, Tezpur, India

Priya Jagtap
Department of Pharmacology and Toxicology, National Institute of Pharmaceutical Education and Research (NIPER), Ahmedabad, Gandhinagar, India

Preeti Jain
Department of Chemistry, Medi-Caps University, Indore, India

Niranjan Karak
Advanced Polymer and Nanomaterial Laboratory, Department of Chemical Sciences, Tezpur University, Tezpur, India

Harpreet Kaur
Department of Pharmacology and Toxicology, National Institute of Pharmaceutical Education and Research (NIPER), Ahmedabad, Gandhinagar, India

Bridget La Prairie
Department of Chemical and Biological Engineering, The University of British Columbia, Vancouver, BC, Canada; School of Biomedical Engineering, The University of British Columbia, Vancouver, BC, Canada

Abhilasha Mishra
Department of Chemistry, Graphic Era Deemed to be University, Dehradun, India

Anupama Munshi
Stephenson Cancer Center, University of Oklahoma Health Sciences Center, Oklahoma City, OK, United States; Department of Radiation Oncology, University of Oklahoma Health Sciences Center, Oklahoma City, OK, United States

Siddarth Raghuvanshi
Department of Chemical and Biological Engineering, The University of British Columbia, Vancouver, BC, Canada

Sridaran Rajagopal
Department of Chemical and Biological Engineering, The University of British Columbia, Vancouver, BC, Canada; School of Biomedical Engineering, The University of British Columbia, Vancouver, BC, Canada; Department of Mechanical Engineering, The University of British Columbia, Vancouver, BC, Canada

Rajagopal Ramesh
Department of Pathology, University of Oklahoma Health Sciences Center, Oklahoma City, OK, United States; Stephenson Cancer Center, University of Oklahoma Health Sciences Center, Oklahoma City, OK, United States; Graduate Program in Biomedical Sciences, University of Oklahoma Health Sciences Center, Oklahoma City, OK, United States

Swapnil Raut
Department of Pharmacology and Toxicology, National Institute of Pharmaceutical Education and Research (NIPER), Ahmedabad, Gandhinagar, India

Rajesh Kumar Saini
Government Post Graduate College, Tikamgarh, India

Ankan Sarkar
Department of Pharmacology and Toxicology, National Institute of Pharmaceutical Education and Research (NIPER), Ahmedabad, Gandhinagar, India

Deepaneeta Sarmah
Department of Pharmacology and Toxicology, National Institute of Pharmaceutical Education and Research (NIPER), Ahmedabad, Gandhinagar, India

Birva Shah
Department of Pharmacology and Toxicology, National Institute of Pharmaceutical Education and Research (NIPER), Ahmedabad, Gandhinagar, India

Anamika Singh
Department of Chemistry, Medi-Caps University, Indore, India

Upasna Singh
Department of Pharmacology and Toxicology, National Institute of Pharmaceutical Education and Research (NIPER), Ahmedabad, Gandhinagar, India

Neha Sonker
Bose Memorial Research Laboratory, Department of Chemistry, Government Autonomous Science College, Jabalpur, India

Asim. ur.Rehman
Department of Pharmacy, Quaid-i-Azam University, Islamabad, Pakistan

Vikramaditya G. Yadav
Department of Chemical and Biological Engineering, The University of British Columbia, Vancouver, BC, Canada; School of Biomedical Engineering, The University of British Columbia, Vancouver, BC, Canada

Jinfeng Zhang
Key Laboratory of Molecular Medicine and Biotherapy, School of Life Sciences, Beijing Institute of Technology, Beijing, P.R. China

Mengjiao Zhou
School of Pharmacy, Nantong University, Nantong, P.R. China

Biographies

Brief Biodata

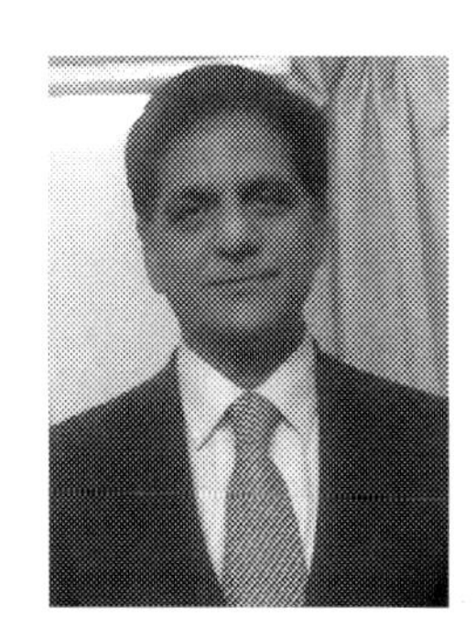

Name: Prof. Anil Kumar Bajpai

Prof. Anil Kumar Bajpai is currently working as Professor in Department of Chemistry, Government Model Science College, Jabalpur (M.P), India. Prof. Bajpai has been awarded with Ph.D. (Polymer Chemistry), D.Sc. from Rani Durgawati university, Jabalpur, India. Prof. Bajpai has expertise in synthesis and characterization of high performance smart materials for various industrial and biomedical applications such as tissue engineering, anti-cancer drug delivery, water purifications etc. He has 36 years of under graduate, post graduate and research experience. Prof. Bajpai has published more than 260 research Papers in reputed international journals (H-index 35), 25 chapters and 2 books published by international reputed publishers. Prof. Bajpai has completed many major projects of leading national funding agencies like Defense Research and Development Organization, Department of Science and Technology, University Grants Commission, Board of Research in Nuclear Sciences, and Department of Atomic Energy. He has one patent on water remediation in collaboration with DRDO, New Delhi, India.

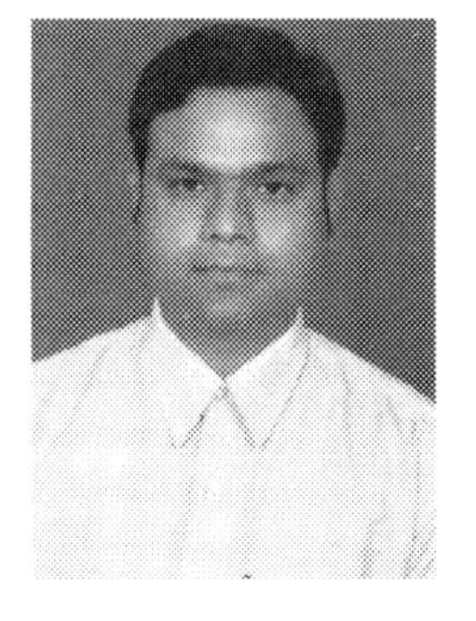

Dr. Rajesh Kumar Saini is currently working as an assistant professor in Chemistry, Department of Chemistry, Government Post Graduate College, Tikamgarh, India. Dr. Saini has expertise in synthesis and characterization of biomaterials for various applications such as bone substitutes, drug delivery through nano biomaterials and nanobiocomposites. He has worked as a coprincipal investigator in major research projects funded by premier national agencies. Dr. Saini has published more than 15 research papers in reputed international journals and 3 books, 20 chapters in international book published by international reputed publishers.

Contact: Dr. Rajesh Kumar Saini. E-mail: dr.sainichem@gmail.com; Mobile: 09753314507

Preface

The integration of polymer science and nanotechnology has emerged as one of the potential fields to find a wide spectrum of biomedical applications including the treatment of numerous complex diseases. The functional character of the macromolecular materials and unique properties of nanomaterials have made significant value addition in the properties of polymer nanomaterials and resulted in significant applications in medicine, pharmacy, and allied fields. Furthermore, the advantageous part of the polymers, that is their responsiveness to various stimuli, has radically changed the scenario of biomedical applications especially in drug delivery technology. The new and newer synthetic routes of fabricating various functional polymers and nanostructures have further widened the utility, acceptability, and performances of the end products in medicine and pharmacy.

The present book focuses on various aspects of polymer nanomaterials and their diversified applications in biomedical fields. This edited volume contains 13 chapters that cover different dimensions of biomaterials. Chapter 1, Fundamentals of Polymeric Nanostructured Materials, presents a brief account of various fundamental parts of polymeric nanostructured materials. Chapter 2, Synthesis of Polymer Nanomaterials, Mechanisms, and Their Structural Control, highlights synthesis and mechanisms of polymer nanomaterials and their structural control. Chapter 3, Polymeric Nanomaterials in Drug Delivery, describes the applications of polymer nanomaterials in drug delivery. Chapter 4, Nanostructures in Gene Delivery, presents an account of polymer nanostructures that are used in gene delivery. Chapter 5, Dendrimer-Based Nanoformulations as Drug Carriers for Cancer Treatment, discusses dendrimers-based nanoformulations that are helpful in the treatment of cancer. Chapter 6, Polymer Nanomaterials in Bioimaging, describes those polymer nanomaterials that are used in bioimaging. Chapter 7, Polymeric Nanoparticles Used in Tissue Engineering, speaks about polymer nanoparticles that are employed in tissue engineering. Chapter 8, Polymeric Nanomaterials as Broad-Spectrum Antimicrobial Compounds, tells about polymer nanomaterials that are used as antibacterial compounds. Chapter 9, Polymeric Nanomaterials for Targeting the Cellular Suborganelles, highlights those polymer nanomaterials used for targeting cellular suborganelles. Chapter 10, Polymeric Nanomaterials in Neuroscience, presents the utility of polymer nanomaterials in neuroscience. Chapter 11, Polymeric Nanomaterials for Ocular Drug Delivery, describes the role of polymer nanomaterials in ocular drug delivery. Chapter 12, Current and Future Challenges in Polymeric Nanomaterials for Biomedical Applications, analyzes current and future challenges in the area of polymer nanomaterials in biomedical applications.

We hope that this book will be helpful to medical practitioners, researchers working in biomedical and nanomaterials areas, pharmacy, and pharmacists working in Research and Development sections.

Anil Kumar Bajpai and Rajesh Kumar Saini
Government Model Science College, Jabalpur, India

CHAPTER

Fundamentals of polymeric nanostructured materials

1

Deepshikha Hazarika and Niranjan Karak

Advanced Polymer and Nanomaterial Laboratory, Department of Chemical Sciences, Tezpur University, Tezpur, India

1.1 Introduction

Nanotechnology is the combination of science and engineering related to develop materials, functional structures, and devices in the order of nanoscale region. It is one of the most interesting and active as well as important areas which have been rapidly growing in both academia and industries (Stander and Theodore, 2011). It deals with the design of nanoscale dimensional of particles and materials with amazing and fascinating properties which are not found in bulk materials. According to Drexler, "Nanotechnology is the principle of manipulation of the structure of matter at the molecular level. It entails the ability to build molecular systems with atom by atom precision yielding a variety of nanomachines (Waseem et al., 2012)." Materials which possess at least one dimension in nanometer range are known as nanomaterials. When two or more materials with dissimilar properties stay separate and distinctive on a macroscopic level with at least one of the phases possesses dimension in less than 100 nm, they are said to be nanocomposite (Stander and Theodore, 2011). Further, if the matrix is long-chain molecules with huge number of repeating units and reinforced by various kinds of nanoreinforcing agents, the nanocomposites are termed as polymer nanocomposites (Ray and Okamoto, 2003). Thus polymer nanocomposite is an intimate combination of polymers and nanomaterials where at least one phase lies in the nanometer range in the resulting material. The incorporation of nanomaterials into the polymer matrices not only improves their most of the properties including mechanical, gas barrier, thermal, biodegradability, flame retardant, magnetic, and optoelectronic of the pristine polymers but also inherently develops a new set of properties based on the used nanomaterials (Ray and Okamoto, 2003; DeLeon et al., 2012; De et al., 2015a,b; Rajabi et al., 2015). This is owing to the synergism of the features of the nanomaterials such as high surface area, excellent thermal stability, high surface reactivity, etc. with those of organic polymers including flexibility, good processability, etc. Further, high aspect ratio of the nanomaterials offers superior nanoreinforcement effect on the properties of the nanocomposites. In addition, size of the nanomaterials and the interface between

Advances in Polymeric Nanomaterials for Biomedical Applications. DOI: https://doi.org/10.1016/B978-0-12-814657-6.00002-1

the nanomaterials and the polymer matrices also remarkably influences the properties (DeLeon et al., 2012). The presence of nanomaterials changes the surface chemistry and modifies the physiochemical interactions which are directly linked to the performance characteristics of the resultant polymeric materials. Various critical factors like aspect ratio, surface chemistry, shape, and size of the nanomaterials help in tailoring such interactions and properties of the nanocomposites (Ray and Okamoto, 2003; DeLeon et al., 2012). It is believed that one of the major issues in preparing good polymer nanocomposites is the quality of dispersion of the nanoparticles in polymer matrices. Several interfaces can be observed depending on the size of the particles and dispersion, which can result in special properties (Liu et al., 2007). In literature, fabrication of different polymer nanocomposites are reported using various kinds of nanoparticles including zero, one, and two-dimensional nanomaterials and the research in this field is going on. The development of different types of polymer nanocomposites not only improved various properties but also produced multifunctional materials (Ray and Okamoto, 2003; Liu et al., 2007; DeLeon et al., 2012; Konwar and Karak, 2011). The applications of the nanocomposites are explored in the fields of catalysis, sensing, photonics, surface coatings, flame retardant materials, photocatalysis, smart materials, biomedical, energy storage, drug delivery, etc. (Liu et al., 2007; DeLeon et al., 2012; Konwar and Karak, 2011). Thus polymer nanocomposites have gained significant scientific and industrial attention or even develop multifunctional materials with unanticipated advanced properties.

1.2 Historical background

The research on nanostructured materials started about two decades ago however, until 1990s they did not achieve much importance (Gleiter, 1990). Michael Faraday reported the formation of colloidal gold nanoparticle, but the synthetic nanomaterials were developed much later in laboratories. Fumed and precipitated silica nanoparticles were industrially manufactured in early 1940s in Germany and the United states as the replacement of ultrafine carbon black for the reinforcement of silicone rubber. Hess and Parker in 1966 reported the stable and well dispersion of metallic cobalt nanoparticles with size less than 100 nm in polymer matrix (Hess and Parker, 1996). Polymer nanocomposite came to exist commercially as well as academically since the last part of 1980's though the term nanocomposite was first coined by Theng in 1970 (Theng and Walker, 1970). In the late 80s, Toyota research laboratories had reported nanoclay (layered-silicate)-based nylon-6 nanocomposites with significant improvement in mechanical properties and heat deflection temperature. These materials were commercialized as belt covers for Toyota cars (Kojima et al., 1993). In 1992 the term nanocomposite was universally accepted.

1.3 Classification of nanomaterials

Nanomaterials possess a huge surface area, high surface to mass ratio, and high aspect ratio. These unusual characteristics of the nanomaterials can remarkably affect the mechanical, physical, chemical, biological, electrical, etc. In case of nanomaterials, dimension is an important factor, and thus based on the number of dimensions, they can be classified into three different groups namely zero, one, and two dimensional, respectively (Fig. 1.1) (Fahlman, 2007).

1.3.1 Zero-dimensional nanomaterials

In this case, all the dimensions are within the nanoscale and mainly include nanoparticles, nanoclusters, and quantum dots (Tiwari et al., 2012). They can be amorphous, crystalline, ceramic, metallic, or polymeric. Metal nanoparticles (sulfur, silver, iron, gold, copper, etc.), metal oxides nanoparticles (ZnO, TiO_2, Fe_3O_4, CuO, SnO_2, SiO_2, etc.), and quantum dots [CdSe, carbon dot (CD), ZnS, CdS, etc.] are the examples of this class of nanoparticles (Fahlman, 2007). Different methods such as coprecipitation, hydrothermal, wet chemical reduction, sol–gel, microwave, sonochemical, reverse micelles, electrochemical, template synthesis, etc. are used for synthesis of these nanomaterials (Tiwari et al., 2012). The properties of these nanomaterials depend on various factors including size, shape, and distribution, which can be tuned by changing the reaction parameters. They are incorporated into various polymer matrices to improve some properties of pristine polymers and to achieve some interesting applications such as antimicrobial,

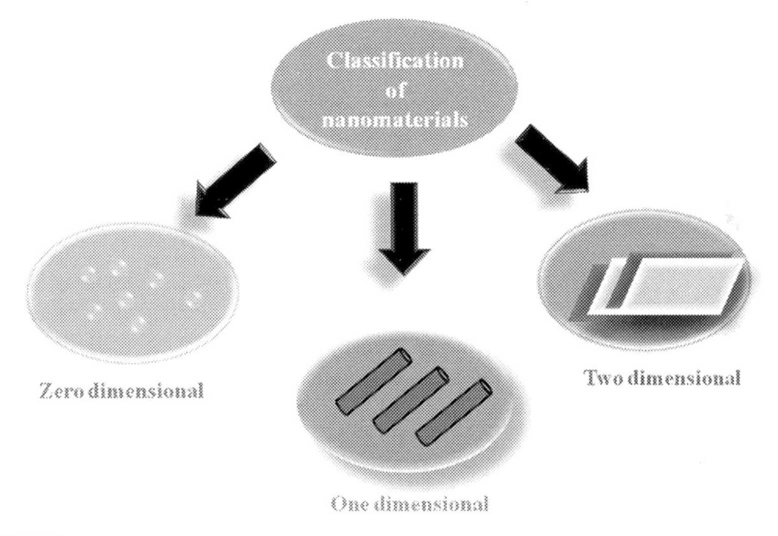

FIGURE 1.1

Classification of nanomaterials.

electronic, catalytic, optical, photonic, sensor, etc. (Tiwari et al., 2012). CD is the rising star of zero-dimensional carbon nanomaterials with less than 10 nm in size and is also a good alternative to traditional semiconducting quantum dots. It possesses favorable attributes like aqueous solubility, low toxicity, size- and wavelength-dependent photoluminescence (PL) properties, photostability, functionalizability, use of cheap and abundant raw materials, etc. (Yu et al., 2016). Further, polymer nanocomposites with quantum dots-based exhibited some exceptional applications including light-emitting diodes, solar cells, etc. (Mosconi et al., 2015).

1.3.2 One-dimensional nanomaterials

They have at least one dimension in nanoscale range and include nanotubes, nanowires, nanofibers, nanorods, etc. Some examples of this class of nanomaterials are single-walled carbon nanotubes, multiwalled carbon nanotubes (MWCNT), cellulose nanofibers, carbon nanofibers, polyaniline nanofiber (PANi), etc. (Coleman et al., 2006). CNT have an exceptional place due to their unique thermal, mechanical, electrical, chemical, etc. properties and found applications in numerous fields such as energy storage and conversion, drug delivery, sensors, etc. It possesses hollow tubular structures and composed of single and multiple numbers of sp^2-hybridized graphitic carbon layers (Spitalsky et al., 2010). Further, CNT are day by day becoming easier to prepare and incorporate into various polymer matrices including thermosets, thermoplastics, and conjugated polymers to fabricate CNT-based polymer nanocomposites (Ghosh and Karak, 2019). It is one of the foremost nanoreinforcing agents for the fabrication of nanocomposite owing to their small size and high aspect ratio as well as excellent properties, and research has been done for last two decades, and the research is still growing with the benefit of nanotechnology (Spitalsky et al., 2010). Cellulose nanofiber is a biopolymer which possesses a high strength and stiffness owing to the presence of extensive intermolecular or intramolecular hydrogen bonding (Goffin et al., 2012). In addition, PANi nanofibers have been used as a nanoreinforcing agent in different polymer matrices owing to their significantly improved processability, dispersability, mechanical performances, etc. (Razak et al., 2015). TiO_2 nanowire because of its favorable attributes like nontoxicity, good photoactivity, easily accessible, chemical durability, etc. has been widely used as a nanomaterial in the fields of photocatalysis, solar energy conversion, etc. (Wang et al., 2011).

1.3.3 Two-dimensional nanomaterials

In this case, two dimensions of the nanomaterials are in the nanoscale range and include nanotubes, nanofiber, whiskers, and nanorod. Some of the examples of this class are graphene oxide (GO), reduced graphene oxide (RGO), clay, etc. Clay usually consists of layered silicates or clay cominerals (aluminum phyllosilicates) including metal oxides like alkali metals, alkali earth metals, magnesium, etc. (Jin et al., 2018). The uniform dispersion of nanoclay in polymer matrices is a major problem due to the presence of strong interactions between the interlayers of clay sheets. Thus, clay particles are modified before incorporation into polymer matrices to resolve this problem. The spacing between the interlayers of nanoclay is increased during the modification by intercalation of grafting of hydrophobic functional groups, and such modified clay can be well dispersed in the polymer matrices (Cao et al., 2005). Further, carbon-based two-dimensional nanomaterials including graphene, GO, and RGO are extremely useful for fabrication of polymer nanocomposites (Ismail and Goh, 2018). Graphene has attracted significant interest owing to their outstanding mechanical, thermal, and electrical properties. It is a monolayer of sp^2-hybridized carbon atoms arranged in a two-dimensional lattice (Kim et al., 2010).

1.4 Different types of polymer nanocomposites

1.4.1 Polyurethane nanocomposites

Polyurethane is one of the multitalented high-performing polymers used in various fields like adhesives, coatings, foams, elastomers, etc. It possesses good chemical resistance, heat resistance, and mechanical and physical properties (Thakur and Karak, 2013). Further, incorporation of various nanoreinforcing agents such as GO, RGO, CD, CNT, metal oxide nanoparticles, etc. into polyurethane matrix showed enhancement in mechanical, thermal, chemical, etc. properties compared to the pristine polyurethane (Goffin et al., 2012; Ismail and Goh, 2018). The applications of such nanocomposites have been reported in various fields including catalysis, corrosion protection, textile, biomedical, etc. In literature, a wide variety of nanoreinforcing agents were used for the fabrication of polyurethane nanocomposite (Athanasopoulos et al., 2012; Gogoi et al., 2015; Duarah et al., 2016), and some of them are listed in Table 1.1.

1.4.2 Polyester nanocomposites

Polyesters are the most promising members owing to their fascinating attributes like biocompatibility, physical stability, ready availability, comparatively low cost, etc. Polyesters have broad spectrum of applications in the fields of surface coatings, biomedical, adhesives, paints, laminates, packagings, etc. (Kunduru et al., 2015). However, they suffer from inherent drawbacks like poor mechanical strength, low hardness, and weak alkali resistance which limit their applicability in many advanced fields. Thus the incorporation of nanomaterials into the polyester matrices not only addresses the above drawbacks but also imparts some exciting properties which widen the applicability of such resultant systems (Kim et al., 2008). Thus, the development of polyester nanocomposites, where at least one

Table 1.1 Properties and applications of polyurethane nanocomposites using different nanomaterials.

Nanocomposites	Properties and applications	References
Polyurethane/ MWCNT	Enhancement in mechanical and thermal properties. Further, the nanocomposite was used as a self-cleaning, self-healing, and antiicing material.	Goffin et al. (2012)
Waterborne polyurethane/ MWCNT	Increased surface hardness and wear resistance.	Athanasopoulos et al. (2012)
Waterborne polyurethane/CD	Enhancement in mechanical properties as well as biocompatible for in vitro adhesion and good cell viability.	Gogoi et al. (2015)
Polyurethane/ CD-Ag	Enhancement in mechanical and thermal properties. Further, it can be used as a biomaterial.	Duarah et al. (2016)
Polyurethane/ CD-ZnO	Enhancement in mechanical and thermal properties. It was also used as an efficient photocatalyst for removal of surfactants.	Duarah and Karak (2019)
Polyurethane/TiO_2	The nanocomposite exhibited excellent antibacterial activity against *Escherichia coli* and self-cleaning activity against stearic acid.	Charpentier et al. (2012)
Polyurethane/ZnO	The nanocomposite showed enhancement in tensile break strength and damping properties.	Guo et al. (2007)
Polyurethane/ sulfur-reduced RGO	Enhancement in mechanical, thermal, and flame retardant properties.	Thakur and Karak (2014)
Polyurethane/ cellulose	Nanocomposite with 30% cellulose content showed good shape memory effect, that is, high shape recovery ratio and high shape fixing, fast responsivity, and rapid water uptake behavior.	Wang et al. (2018)
Polyurethane/SiO_2	Increment in storage modulus, elongation at break, and tensile strength. The transparent nanocomposite is a promising material for high-performing water based UV curable coating.	Qiu et al. (2012)
Polyurethane/PANi	The nanocomposite was used as a strain sensing element in smart clothing as piezoresistivity of the resulting fiber was recognized in a high strain deformation range (up to 1500%).	Solouki et al. (2018)
Polyurethane/ RGO-TiO_2	Enhancement in mechanical properties and thermal properties as well as excellent shape recovery ratio and recovery rate. It also showed excellent self-cleaning activity for removal of methylene blue on exposure of sunlight.	Thakur and Karak (2015)

Table 1.2 Different polyester nanocomposites using various kinds of nanomaterials.

Nanocomposites	Properties and applications	References
Polyester/clay	Enhanced mechanical, thermal, and biodegradability behavior.	Cao et al. (2005)
Polyester/MWCNT	Viscosity of the nanocomposite increased confirmed the well dispersion of MWCNT in polyester matrix. It also showed en enhancement in crystallinity, tensile strength, impact strength, tensile modulus, and elongation at break.	Kim et al. (2008)
Polyester/ZnS	Exhibited interesting optical properties including good transmittance.	Zhao et al. (2007)
Waterborne polyester/ functionalized GO	Enhanced mechanical, thermal and biodegradable properties as well as used as a catalyst for Aza Michael addition reaction.	Hazarika et al. (2018)
Waterborne polyester/CD	Improved mechanical, thermal properties, and biodegradability behavior. It also exhibited photoluminescence properties as well as efficient self-cleaning activity and excellent transparency under visible light.	Hazarika and Karak (2016)
Polyester/ZnO	Enhancement in hardness and tensile strength.	Golgoon et al. (2017)
Waterborne polyester/CD@TiO_2	In addition to enhancement in mechanical and thermal properties, also showed some special properties like antiicing, antifogging, etc. Further, it was used as a membrane for oil–water separation.	Hazarika and Karak (2018)
Polyester/SiO_2	Improved tensile strength, impact strength, melting temperature, and crystallinity.	Ahmadizadegan et al. (2018)

phase must be in nanometer scale, is one of the most intelligent ways to enhance their performance and thus have attracted a great deal of attention from the material scientists and industrial community. In literature, different types of nanomaterials including zero-, one-, and two-dimensional are explored in polyester nanocomposites (Zhao et al., 2007; Hazarika et al., 2018; Hazarika and Karak, 2016), and the properties and applications of some of the polyester nanocomposites are listed in Table 1.2.

1.4.3 Epoxy nanocomposites

Epoxy is a vital engineered thermosetting polymeric material which finds various industrial applications such as coatings, aerospace, adhesive, electronic devices, marine systems, laminates, etc. (De and Karak, 2013). It possesses high thermal stability, Young's modulus, tensile strength, good thermal insulation, solvent resistance, etc. However, epoxy thermosets cannot address the advanced engineering applications due to high brittleness and lack of toughness (De et al., 2013). In order to address these drawbacks and to incorporate new sets of properties like optical, electrical conductivity, magnetic, anticorrosive, etc., different nanoreinforcing agents including graphene, iron oxide, nanoclay, carbon nanofiber, silica, PANi, zinc oxide, etc. are incorporated into the epoxy matrix to develop epoxy nanocomposites (Razaka et al., 2015; Tomic et al., 2016; Cha et al., 2019; Sadjadi and Farhadyar, 2009). Epoxy nanocomposites have achieved significant interest owing to their unique physico-chemical properties originating from the combined unique characteristics of the epoxy and the nanomaterials into one unit. Different types of epoxy nanocomposite and their properties and applications are given in Table 1.3.

Table 1.3 Different types of epoxy nanocomposites using various nanomaterials.

Nanomaterials	Properties and applications	References
PANi	Enhancement in mechanical and electrical properties.	Razaka et al. (2015)
Clay	Improvement in mechanical, thermal and fire resistance properties. The superiority of the corrosion resistance of the nanocomposite to the pristine one was confirmed from salt spray measurements.	Tomic et al. (2016)
CD	Increased in mechanical and thermal properties along with high transparency and fluorescent properties. Further, it can be used as a highly prospective material for bio-sealant applications as it exhibited good viability, proliferation, and spreading of skin fibroblasts and keratinocyte cell.	De et al. (2015a,b)
GO	GO remarkably enhanced barrier properties, adhesion to epoxy coatings, and corrosion resistance.	Rajabi et al. (2015)
Functionalized GO and CNT	Significantly increased fracture toughness, tensile strength, and Young's modulus.	Cha et al. (2019)
TiO_2	Enhanced the hydrophilicity with the loading of TiO_2 on the surface of the coatings.	Sadjadi and Farhadyar (2009)
CD	Nanocomposite showed improvement in mechanical and thermal properties.	De et al. (2013)
SiO_2	Used as a flame retardant material.	Gu et al. (2013)
Cellulose	Improved fracture toughness, flexural strength, impact toughness, and impact strength.	Tang and Weder (2010)
CuO/cellulose	Used as a high-performing biodegradable and antimicrobial scaffold material.	Barua et al. (2015)

1.4.4 Poly(esteramide) nanocomposites

Poly(esteramide) appears as an important family of biodegradable polymers. Aliphatic poly(esteramide)s are attractive materials for biomedical and environmental applications as they are highly biodegradable and have good processing and end use properties. They consist of both ester and amide linkages in their structures and show properties between those of polyamides and polyesters. Polyesters degrade through the cleavage of the ester linkages under physiological conditions and have better solubility in different organic solvents and flexibility than polyamides, whereas polyamides possesses better mechanical and thermal properties owing to the formation of strong hydrogen bonding between the amide linkages of individual chains (Winnacker and Rieger, 2016). However, they are resistant to degradation and often considered as nondegradable materials. Thus, the combination of ester and amide linkages in the same polymer can open opportunity in the design of new materials with various properties. Further, incorporation of different nanomaterials into the poly(esteramide) matrix enhanced their properties and also introduces some new properties to the pristine poly(esteramide) (Bhat and Ahmad, 2018; Pramanik et al., 2013; Irfan et al., 2019) and some of them are listed in Table 1.4.

1.4.5 Poly(methy methacrylate) nanocomposites

Poly(methy methacrylate) (PMMA) among the other available polymers is most commonly used in various applications owing to its optical clarity to visible light,

Table 1.4 Different poly(esteramide) nanocomposites with their properties and applications.

Nanomaterials	Properties and applications	References
SiO_2	Improved mechanical properties, hydrolysis rate of polyesteramide, and biodegradability behavior.	Liu et al. (2007)
TiO_2	Exhibited superior physic-mechanical, anticorrosive, and hydrophobic properties to pristine poly (esteramide).	Bhat and Ahmad (2018)
PANi	Enhanced impact resistance, elongation at break, tensile strength, scratch hardness, and decrease sheet resistance. The nanocomposite can be used as a potential antistatic material.	Pramanik et al. (2013)
RGO	Showed significantly improved bent test, scratch hardness, and impact resistance along with anticorrosive properties.	Irfan et al. (2019)
Clay	The nanocomposite can be used as a potential candidate in the area of environmentally benign waterborne protective coatings.	Zafar et al. (2015)
CD	Heterogeneous photocatalyst for green oxidation of benzyl alcohol to benzaldehyde in the presence of visible light.	Mosconi et al. (2015)

Table 1.5 Properties and applications of different PMMA nanocomposites.

Nanomaterials	Properties and applications	References
GO and GO-Fe_3O_4	Malachite green adsorption	Rajabia et al. (2019)
ZnO	Showed efficient photocatalytic activity for degradation of phenol and methylene blue on exposure of UV light.	Mauro et al. (2017)
Clay	Enhancement in Young's modulus, tensile strength, and hardness.	Kumar et al. (2015)
GO-TiO_2	Exhibited superior mechanical properties compared to pristine one and also used as a dental materials.	Alamgir et al. (2018)
Graphene	Gas-sensing application	Rattanabut et al. (2018)
SiO_2	Enhancement in surface hardness, scratch resistance, and thermal properties along with excellent transparency.	Abbas et al. (2018)
CD	Used for preparation of Ag nanoparticles	Mosconi et al. (2015)

chemical stability, high strength, good weather ability, low cost, exceptional dimensional stability, hydrophobicity, etc. It is a main member in the family of methacrylic esters and polyacrylic acid (Feuser et al., 2014). However, the applications of PMMA restricted due to its poor thermal stability, poor fatigue properties, low mechanical strength, and chemical degradation. Nanotechnology is executed in this field to address this problem and also to improve different properties of it. Different nanoreinforcing agents were incorporated into PMMA matrix to develop PMMA nanocomposites, and some of them are tabulated in Table 1.5.

1.5 Fabrication of the nanocomposites

The nanocomposites are fabricated by using different preparative techniques including solution, in situ polymerization, and melt mixing techniques (Fig. 1.2). A brief description of these methods is discussed below.

1.5.1 Solution technique

In this technique, nanomaterials are first swelled in an appropriate solvent/solvent mixture and dispersed into the host polymer solution with the help of mechanical shearing followed by ultrasonication. The remaining solvent is removed either by evaporation or precipitation of the nanomaterials dispersed polymer matrices from the homogeneous mixture. The resultant structure may be either intercalated or

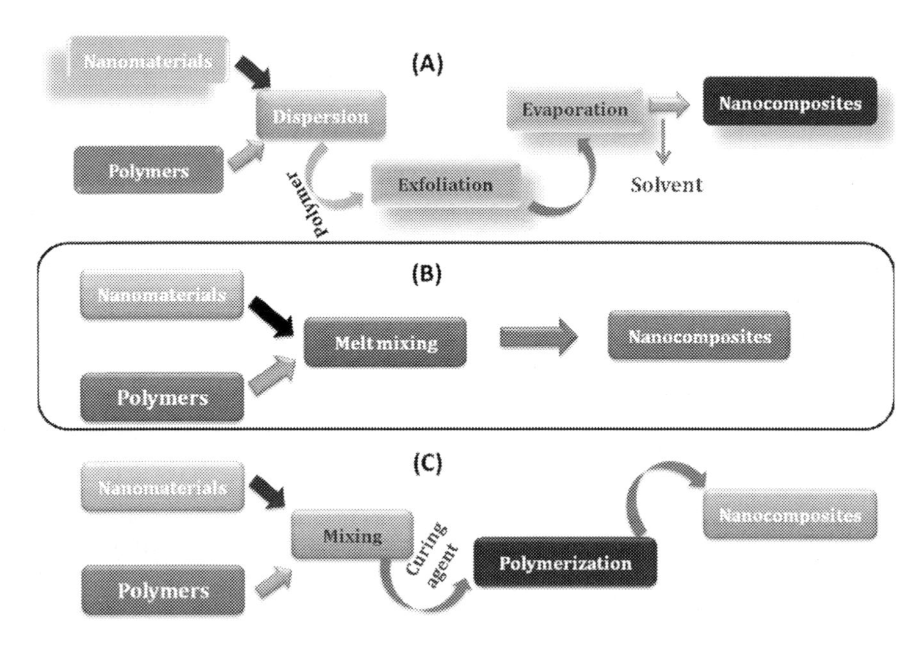

FIGURE 1.2

Fabrication of polymer nanocomposites by (A) solution, (B) melt mixing, and (C) in situ polymerization techniques.

exfoliated depending on the interactions between polymer and nanoreinforcing agents as well as degree of mixing. The entropy and enthalpy factors state the degree of intercalation of polymer into the nanomaterials. The internal energy determines the thermodynamic feasibility of the intercalation process as the overall change in entropy is negligible. This method is simple and normally only requires relatively low temperature as compared to melt compounding (Karak, 2019). During solvent evaporation or precipitation, if the nanomaterials do not reassemble or the polymer chains do not allow them to come closer, then the resultant composites will be exfoliated nanocomposites. In general, after solvent evaporation, the nanomaterials reassemble to reform the stack with polymer chains sandwiched in between and forming a well-ordered structure. In the intergallery space, the adsorbed polymer chains do not coil but remain in almost fully extended state. Thus generally an intercalated nanocomposite is formed after solvent evaporation. This method is good for the intercalation of polymers with little or no polarity into layered structures and facilitates production of thin films with polymer-oriented clay intercalated layers. Nevertheless, it is an attractive route for water soluble polymers, as water is used as solvent in that case. However, from industrial point of view, this method involves the abundant use of organic solvents, which is usually environmentally not acceptable as well as economically

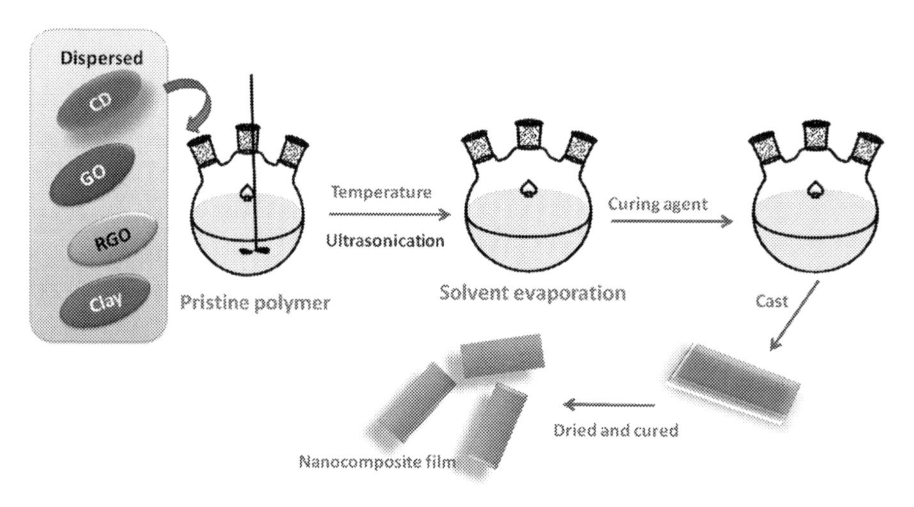

FIGURE 1.3

Fabrication of polymer nanocomposites with different nanomaterials by solution technique.

prohibitive. Some of the critical issues encountered in this technique are hazardous impacts, cost, and removal of the solvent. In literature, use of this technique for fabrication of various polymer nanocomposites was reported. Fig. 1.3 demonstrates the fabrication of epoxy nanocomposite using different nanomaterials through this technique.

1.5.2 In situ polymerization

This technique is used to create better interaction between polymer matrices and the nanomaterials. Further, it reduces or eliminates the use of solvent and decrease the energy required for the mixing process. This technique deals with the insertion of a polymeric precursor between the nanoreinforcing agents followed by dispersion and growth of the nanomaterials into the polymer matrices by polymerization process. For this, first nanomaterials are dispersed or swollen in a liquid monomer or prepolymer, subsequently forming polymeric chains in between the intercalated nanomaterials. In other words, the monomer molecules adsorb onto the surface of the nanomaterials followed by polymerization and thereby resulting in delamination of the nanomaterial agglomerates. The low viscosity of the monomers result in their high diffusivity into the nanomaterials which help in gaining uniform mixing of the two components, and favored formation of well-exfoliated nanocomposites be initiated by using catalyst, heat, initiator, or radiation (Hazarika and Karak, 2018). The polymeric chains start to grow during polymerization in the presence of nanomaterials which finally produced the exfoliated structure. This technique easily breaks the agglomerates using high shear force and helps to achieve more uniform dispersion of nanomaterials within

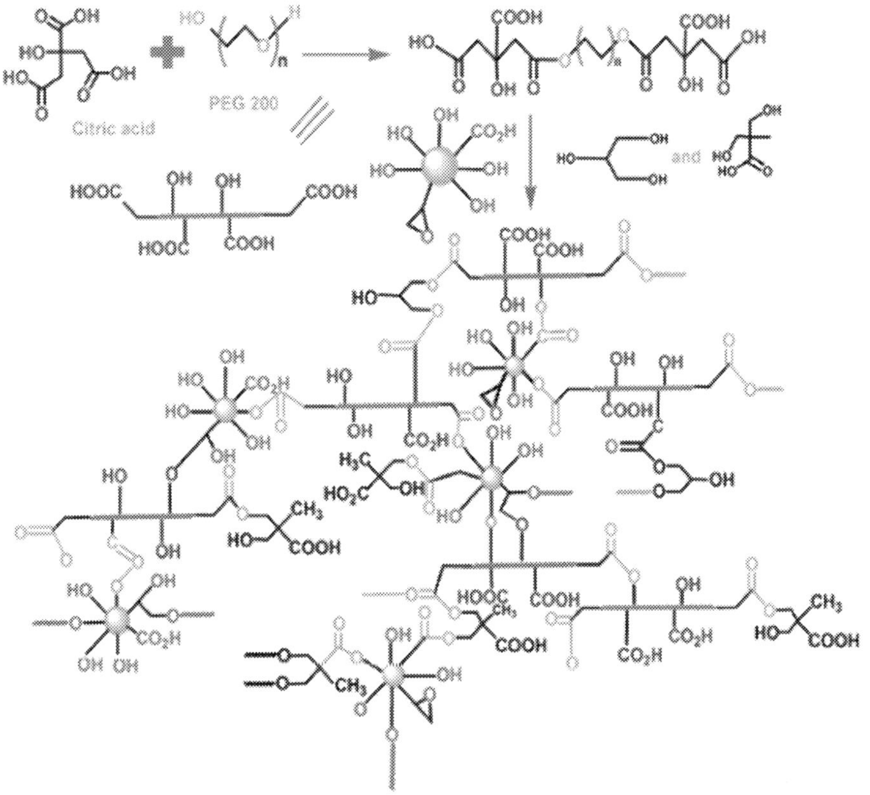

FIGURE 1.4

In situ fabrication of CD-based waterborne polyester nanocomposites. *CD*, carbon dot.

Source: Reproduced with permission from Hazarika, D., Karak, N., 2016. Biodegradable tough waterborne hyperbranched polyester/carbon dot nanocomposite: approach towards an eco-friendly material. Green Chem., 18, 5200–5211, Copyright@2016, The Royal Society of Chemistry.

the polymer matrices. The low viscosity of the monomers replicates the necessity of low energy for the mixing process. Stable polymer nanocomposites are formed by the presence of different secondary interactions. In case of resin, the nanomaterials not only assist in cross-linking reaction but may also influence the polymerization process. A schematic representation of in situ fabrication of waterborne hyperbranched polyester nanocomposite using CD as nanoreinforcing agent is shown in Fig. 1.4.

1.5.3 Melt mixing technique

In this technique, the polymer is heated above its softening temperature and mixed with the nanomaterials under a shearing force. Mixing can be done using screw intender, mixer, injection molding, rollers, etc. This process involves removing the use of toxic solvents entrapped in the solution technique and forms intercalated or partially exfoliated nanocomposites similar to in situ polymerization technique. In this case, there is loss of entropy related to the confinement of a polymer melt by the formation of nanocomposite, and entropy gain is related with the layer separation. This method may not be as resourceful as that of the solution and in situ technique and but can apply to produce nanocomposite using traditional polymer processing techniques like extrusion and injection molding in polymer processing industry. The melt mixing method may not be as resourceful as that of solution and in situ polymerization technique. However, polymer processing industries have applied this technique to fabricate polymer nanocomposites with the help of injection molding and extrusion. Further, the absence of solvent makes this process an economically feasible and environmentally benign process for industries (DeLeon et al., 2012). Thus, this method has adequate contribution for commercial development of polymer nanocomposites. A schematic representation of this technique is shown in Fig. 1.5.

Besides these, large varieties of other techniques are also are reported in literature for the fabrication of polymer nanocomposites which includes sol–gel process, template synthesis, cryogenic ball milling, thermal spraying process, plasma-induced polymerization, and so on. The cost and the challenge of attaining uniformly dispersed nanomaterials in the polymer matrix hinder the practical applicability of these techniques. However, to achieve the uniform distribution of the nanoparticles through these techniques is very difficult and thus they are usually not used (Karak, 2019).

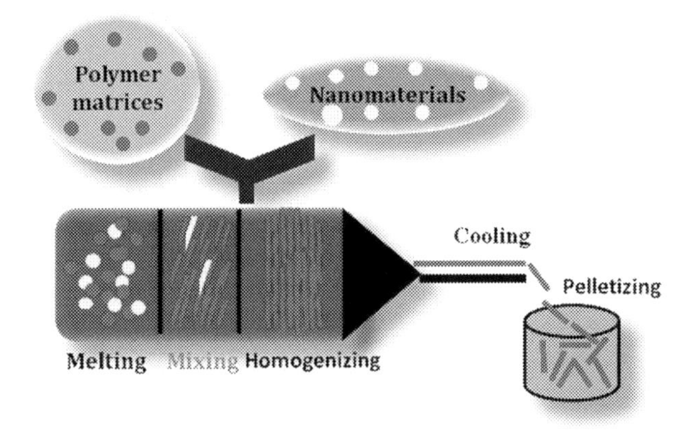

FIGURE 1.5

Schematic representation of twin screw extruder for melt mixing of nanomaterials with polymer matrices.

1.6 Characterization

Characterization is an important part of all investigations associated with materials. Different characterization techniques including spectroscopic, microscopic, diffraction, etc. are used for characterization of both the nanomaterials and the nanocomposites. The most widely used characterization tools are Fourier-transform infrared (FTIR) spectroscopy, UV-visible spectroscopy, X-ray diffractometer, Raman spectroscopy, transmission electron microscopy (TEM), scanning electron microscopy (SEM), atomic force microscopy (AFM), etc. A very brief description of these techniques is presented below.

1.6.1 UV-visible spectroscopy

It is one of the most regularly used simple and important techniques to characterize both the nanomaterials and the nanocomposites. Nanoparticles such as mainly semiconductor quantum dots and metal nanoparticles display surface plasma resonance bands at a particular UV region owing to the interaction between surface electrons of the nanoparticles and the UV radiation. This technique is further utilized to characterize other nanomaterials which have UV active functional groups that display a particular band in the UV-visible spectra owing to $\pi-\pi^*$ and $n-\pi^*$ transitions (Karak, 2017). This technique is also be utilized to detect the existence of a nanomaterial within the polymer nanocomposites. However, nature, position, and intensity of the peaks emerge differently with the loading of nanomaterials in polymer matrices. Further, the band gap of nanomaterials as well as nanocomposites can also be evaluated from the values of absorbance (Zhu et al., 2009a,b). In addition, the optical transmittance of both the polymers and their nanocomposites can be calculated by the help of this technique.

1.6.2 FTIR spectroscopy

It is an important and well known technique used for preliminary characterization of materials which provides information about the presence of various functional groups in nanomaterials (particularly nanoclay, CD, functionalized nanomaterials like functionalized CNT, GO, etc., and metal oxide nanoparticles) and the polymer nanocomposites (Ismail and Goh, 2018). In case of functionalized nanomaterials, the change in absorbance bands as well as disappearance of some characteristics bands confirms the functionalization. It is also possible to notice some physico-chemical interactions between the polymer matrices and the nanomaterials from the FTIR spectra of the polymer nanocomposites. The stretching bands of different functional groups of a nanomaterial are shifted to higher or lower values, or the percent of transmittance values are diminished due to these interactions (Bora et al., 2013).

1.6.3 Raman spectroscopy

The defects as well as photonic and electronic properties of both the nanomaterials and nanocomposites are studied using Raman spectroscopic technique. It is widely used for the characterization of various carbon-based nanomaterials including CD, GO, RGO, CNT, etc. and their nanocomposites (Mittal, 2007). This technique is highly responsive to the orientation, material crystallinity, and temperature. A laser in the UV, near infrared, or visible range is used as the light source in this technique, and it depends on the interaction of inelastic scattering of monochromatic light with materials. This technique is used for molecules without a dipole moment.

1.6.4 PL spectroscopy

PL spectroscopy is used to evaluate the optical properties of nanomaterials and polymer nanocomposites. The nanomaterials which are active in the UV-visible region and the fluorescent emission of them show excitation wavelength dependent behavior. Further, this technique together with UV-visible spectroscopy can be used to calculate the quantum yield of quantum dot (Yu et al., 2016). The yield is determined by a relative method using quinine sulfate with known quantum yield as the reference.

1.6.5 Dynamic light scattering

One of the important techniques used to understand the particle size distribution of the nanomaterials in colloidal suspensions or solution is dynamic light scattering. The dynamic diameter as well as change in size of the hydrated nanoparticles in aqueous medium with time is evaluated with the help of this technique. The average hydrodynamic diameter of the nanomaterials is evaluated by varying the intensity fluctuation of scattering light. As this process is fast and detection of dispersed phase is possible, thus it can monitor the real time variation of size. The measured size of the nanomaterials is larger than the size obtained from TEM analysis mainly because of the influence of Brownian motion. It is a nondestructive method, and it is possible to determine size of large quantity of particles simultaneously (Karak, 2019).

1.6.6 X-ray photoelectron spectroscopy

X-ray photoelectron spectroscopy (XPS) or electron spectroscopy for chemical analysis is a surface chemical analysis technique that provides information on surface elemental composition and oxidation state of the elements (Karak, 2019). The corresponding spectrum is obtained by determining the kinetic energy. The spectrum gives the number of escaping electrons from the surface and the binding energy. The binding energies depend on the oxidation state of the elements, and the values are different for specific groups and hence such elements can be distinguished from the XPS spectrum (Wang et al., 2014).

1.6.7 X-ray diffraction

It is also another important technique for the characterization of nanomaterials and polymeric nanocomposite. It gives information about crystal structure including degree of crystallinity, unit cell parameter, lattice constant, etc. The crystal structure of the nanomaterial can be recognized after determining the angles as well as intensities of the diffraction peaks. The formation of metal and metal oxide nanoparticles is established from their specific crystallographic peaks observed from X-ray diffraction (XRD) analysis. The crystal structure information of other nanomaterials like CNT, RGO, layered silicate, graphene, etc., and their corresponding nanocomposites can also be authenticated from this technique (Karak, 2019; Kalidindi et al., 2008). The intensity of the peaks of the nanoparticles is weakening after the fabrication of metal oxide or metal-based based-polymer nanocomposite due to the existence of various physical and chemical interactions between the polymer matrices and the nanomaterial. Further, interlayer spacing can also be evaluated using Bragg's equation, $2d\sin\theta = n\lambda$ (where d, n, θ, and λ are interlayer distance, the order of diffraction, diffraction angle, and wavelength of X-ray, respectively) from the shifting peak position (Karak, 2017; Karak, 2019). The nanomaterials can be identified by comparing the intensity values, and interplanar distances obtained from XRD data with the standard peaks using JCPDS files. Further, both small angle (less than 5 degrees) and wide angle (2–90 degrees) XRD techniques are used to achieve microstructural features of both the nanomaterials and the nanocomposites. Small angle XRD gives an idea about shape and size of the crystalline region, whereas information about the degree of crystallinity and nature of ordering arrangement can be achieved from wide angle XRD (Karak, 2019).

1.6.8 Scanning electron microscopy

The surface morphology as well as the dispersion of various nanomaterials within the polymer matrices can be visualized from the SEM. By scanning with focused electrons beam, it constructs the surface micrographs of the material. The atoms present in the material interact with the electrons which create different signals by emitting secondary electrons and they are detected by a detector. These secondary electrons give information on surface topography as well as phase composition of the materials (Vogel et al., 2004).

1.6.9 Transmission electron microscopy

It is the very important technique to visualize the actual structure of the nanomaterials and state of dispersion of them inside the polymer matrices. It is used to obtain the high-resolution imaging of nanomaterials. Further, it is used to verify the size and shape of the nanomaterials as well as to estimate the size distribution of the nanomaterials. It allows the transmission of beam of electrons through the ultrathin specimen that gives an internal structure of the material. Selected area electron diffraction provides information about the symmetry of the lattice, micro-diffraction patterns, interplanar distances, and crystal planes of the nanomaterials (Karak, 2019).

1.6.10 Atomic force microscopy

Similar to SEM, AFM can also provide information about the size, shape, distribution, surface roughness, surface area, and morphology of nanomaterials. The particle height and volume can be calculated from the three-dimensional images obtained from AFM. Further, oxide and electrically nonconducting surfaces can also be measured in aqueous fluids up to the subnanometer scale (Karak, 2019).

1.6.11 Energy dispersive X-ray spectroscopy

It is another commonly used tool for the elemental analysis and chemical characterization of the nanomaterials. The information on elemental composition including contents of carbon, oxygen, S, Si, N, P, etc. can be obtained from energy dispersive X-ray spectroscopy analysis. It is also most important to authenticate the presence of different metals in the case of metal oxide-based hybrid nanomaterials as well as in their nanocomposites.

1.6.12 Thermal analysis

The thermal properties of both the nanomaterials and the nanocomposites are studied using thermogravimetric analysis (TGA) as well as differential thermal analysis (DTA). TGA record the change in weight of the material as a function of either time or temperature, whereas DTA records the change in heat content, that is, measures the temperature difference between the reference and the sample. Further, the glass transition temperature (T_g) as well as melting temperature (T_m) of the materials is evaluated with the differential scanning calorimetry (Karak, 2019; Dai et al., 2015).

1.7 Properties

The remarkable enhancement in most of the properties of the pristine polymers as well as some special properties can also be achieved after fabrication of appropriate polymer nanocomposites. The extent of improvement is based on several factors like shape, size, aspect ratio, dispersion state as well as interfacial interactions of polymer matrices with the nanoreinforcing agents. Some of the significant properties of polymer nanocomposites are discussed here.

1.7.1 Physical

The incorporation of nanomaterials into the polymer matrices slightly changes the physical properties including solubility, density, crystallinity, etc. of the pristine polymers even though the properties remains almost similar to the pristine polymers in some cases. The polymer nanocomposites form stable dispersion in different solvents but they are not soluble in any solvent due to the interaction with nanomaterials most of them are insoluble. The enhancement in density for polymer nanocomposites is insignificant in almost all cases, so light weight feature of the polymers is retained after nanocomposite formation. The nanomaterials have little impact on crystallinity of polymer nanocomposites though in most of the cases the effect is less significant (Karak, 2019).

1.7.2 Rheological

Rheology is actually branch of physics which is used to study the deformation and flow of matter under the influence of an applied stress and conducted either by steady shear or dynamic oscillatory shear measurements. Thus study of rheological properties of polymers in the molten state is very useful to gain basic perceptive of the processability of the materials as these properties are strongly affected by the interfacial characteristics and structure of the materials (Tomic et al., 2016). Steady shear sweeps were utilized to explore the flow properties of polymers by determining the viscosity with increasing shear rate. Further, the variations of viscoelastic properties like storage and loss modulus demonstrate phase transition behavior upon fabrication of nanocomposites from liquid-like to solid-like (Hazarika and Karak, 2016). In addition, other factors such as complex viscosity, apparent viscosity, tanδ, yield stress, critical oscillatory stress, etc. of the nanocomposites can also be evaluated from rheological study. Rahmatpour studied the rheological properties of MWCNT-based waterborne polyurethane nanocomposites with the help of dynamic and steady shear measurements. They found that the nanocomposite exhibited non-Newtonnian and complex viscoelastic behavior upon higher loading of MWCNT. The dynamic behavior of the system changed from a polymer dispersion-like behavior to a solid-like behavior due to the presence of the functionalized CNTs (Rahmatpour et al., 2011). Chirayila et al. reported that the polyester/cellulose nanocomposites displayed two different regions shear thinning and Newtonian flow, whereas Newtonian behavior was observed in case of the epristine polyester (Chirayila et al., 2014). Authors reported that the shear thinning behavior of CD-based waterborne hyperbranched polyester (Hazarika and Karak, 2016).

1.7.3 Mechanical

The incorporation different types of nanoreinforcing agents such as clay, CD, GO, TiO_2, ZnO, MWCNT, RGO, g-C_3N_4, etc. with extremely huge surface area and high aspect ratio into polymer matrices significantly enhance the mechanical properties of the pristine polymers. The mechanical properties of the nanocomposites generally controlled by various factors including nature of the nanomaterials, properties of the matrices, chemistry of the polymer matrices, properties, and distribution of the nanomaterials as well as interfacial bonding and also the synthetic or processing methods. The most important requirement to achieve the desired mechanical properties is the uniform dispersion of the nanomaterials in the polymer matrices. Thus it is necessary to modify the surface of the nanomaterials to facilitate the better dispersion of the nanomaterials and to improve the interfacial interactions between the polymer matrices and the nanomaterials. In addition to the above factors, the geometrical confinement of polymeric chains also significantly influences the mechanical properties. The presence of hyperbranched architecture in the polymer nanocomposites resulted higher mechanical properties compared to the linear analog owing to the highly dense three-dimensional structure formed by the presence of large no of functional groups (Thakur and Karak, 2015). Many reports are available on enhancement in mechanical properties of various polymer nanocomposites on very loadings of different nanomaterials into the polymer matrices. Cha et al. reported the enhancement in tensile strength, Young's modulus, and fracture toughness of epoxy after incorporation of melamine functionalized CNT and graphene nanoplaetelets. Further, they also noticed that the functionalized nanomaterials exhibited higher enhancement mechanical properties compared to unfunctionalized one (Cha et al., 2019). The enhancement in breaking strain, breaking stress, and modulus of polyurethane was observed by Yadav and Cho after incorporation of functionalized graphene platelet into the matrix (Yadav and Cho, 2012). Many reports are also available from author's laboratory on enhancement in different mechanical properties including tensile strength, elongation at break, scratch hardness, impact resistance, toughness, and Young's modulus of pristine waterborne polyester, polyurethane, polyesteramide, epoxy etc. after incorporation of various nanomaterials like functionalized GO (Hazarika et al., 2018), CD@TiO_2 (Hazarika and Karak, 2018), CD (Gogoi et al., 2015), RGO@TiO_2 (Thakur and Karak, 2015), PANi (Pramanik et al., 2013), OMMT/CD/Cu_2O (De et al., 2015a,b), etc. The improvement in mechanical properties is because of the good interfacial interaction upon uniform dispersion of the nanomaterials in the polymer matrices. Further, there is also a possibility of direct linkages between various oxygenating groups of polymers and the nanomaterials physico-chemical interactions. This greatly enhances the compatibility of the nanomaterials with the polymer matrices. De et al. showed twofold enhancements in adhesive strength both for metal–metal and wood–wood after incorporation of neem oil modified organo-montmorillonite (OMMT) into epoxy matrix (De et al., 2015a,b). This improvement is because of the presence of highly polar nitrogen and oxygen containing functional groups of epoxy, clay, and the hardener, which help to produce strong interaction with the substrate. Further, the hypebranched architecture of the epoxy also helps to develop physical interlocking with the metal substrate.

1.7.4 Thermal

Thermal stability of the materials is the resistance of a material to decompose at elevated temperature. However, except the specially fabricated highly thermostable polymers, most of the pristine polymers possess poor thermal stability which can be enhanced by incorporating different kinds of nanomaterials into the polymer matrices. The presence of nanomaterials acts as heat insulators as well as mass transport barrier for generated volatile compounds during thermal decomposition process and thus increases the overall thermal stability and help in the generation of char after thermal decomposition. Further, they also confined the thermal motion of polymeric chains and delayed the release of volatile organic compounds (VOC) (Karak, 2009). The fabrication of polymer nanocomposites with various kinds of nanomaterials likes clay, RGO, CNT, GO, etc. enhanced the thermal properties and copious studies have been carried out on these. The incorporation of CD into waterborne polyester matrix showed enhancement of thermal degradation temperature from 234°C to 265°C (Hazarika and Karak, 2016). Further, Duarah et al. reported that the thermal degradation temperature increased 20°C after fabrication of polyurethane nanocomposite with CD-Ag (Duarah et al., 2016). Furthermore, the T_g of a polymer is usually affected by rigidity and flexibility of polymeric chains, and the addition of nanoreinforcing agents improves the T_g of pristine polymers as the rigidity of these nanomaterials restricted the mobility of the polymeric chains (Karak, 2017). Again, improvement in T_g of different polymers after formation of the nanocomposites was also reported in the literature. The shifting of T_g from 28°C to 208°C was reported on addition of GO (1–2 wt.%) in poly(butylene succinate) (Charlon et al., 2015). Further, the crystalline melting temperature of as well as total enthalpy of crystallization polymers is also improved after formation of the nanocomposites as the nanomaterials act as nucleating agent. Thakur and Karak reported that both T_g (20.3°C–22.3°C) and T_m (48.1°C–50.7°C) increased upon incorporation of 2 wt. % GO into polyurethane matrix. The small increment is due to the presence of GO, which may inflict restrictions on molecular mobility at earlier stages (Thakur and Karak, 2014).

1.7.5 Barrier

The barrier properties of polymers are also improved after incorporation of different types of nanomaterials into the polymer matrices. The nanomaterials with high aspect ratios provide very high surface areas, which hamper the diffusion pathways of different penetrating molecules. This can be described by the fact that the nanoreinforcing agents cause the tortuous diffusion paths for the gas molecules to follow, and hence, there is a reduction in diffusion rate (Sridhar et al., 2006). The rate of diffusion of a penetrating molecule further depends on the degree of dispersion of the nanomaterials. The high aspect ratio of two-dimensional nanomaterials usually reduces the gas permeability very effectively. Brule and Flat reported that the addition of exfoliated clay to polyamide 6/polyolefin blend improved the barrier to styrene permeation, and they observed that the blend nanocomposite showed better barrier than the control polyamide nanocomposite (Brule and Flat, 2006). Further, Ahmadizadegan *et al.* reported that addition of cellulose/silica into polyester matrix follows the gases permeability in the order of PO_2 (98%) > PCO_2 (88%) > PN_2 (58%) > PCH_4 (38%). The separation efficiency of carbon dioxide/nitrogen and carbon dioxide/methane gases was also improved after formation of the nanocomposite and the diffusion coefficients of gases enhanced with the increase in mass fraction of cellulose/silica in the membrane (Ahmadizadegan et al., 2018). Epoxy nanocomposite with 77% volume fraction of clay exhibited 2–3 times of magnitude of lower oxygen permeability than the pristine epoxy (Triantafyllidis et al., 2006).

1.7.6 Electrical

Electrical properties of polymers are usually related to dielectric and electrical conductivity. A good conductor is a material that allows the flow of current and the insulator is the material which opposes the current. Most of the pristine polymers act as insulators except the conducting one owing to the lack of ionic or electronic pathway and covalent nature of the polymers. The addition of different conducting nanomaterials into the polymer matrices introduces interesting electrical properties to the polymers. The incorporation of graphene sheet can offer percolated pathways for electron transfer in the nanocomposite, which makes the nanocomposite electrically conductive (Karak, 2019). Similar types of results can also be achieved by utilizing other carbon-based nanoreinforcing agents such as carbon nanofibers, CNT, graphene, etc. However, graphene allows the transition from insulator polymer to a conductor at significantly lower loading, compared to CNT. The electrical conductivity was enhanced from 3.32×10^{-9} to 2.05×10^{-3} S/cm by 5 wt.% graphene loading, which demonstrating about 10^6-fold enhancement. This progress can be ascribed to the formation of interrelated conducting networks produced by graphene nanosheets in the polyester matrix (Caradonna et al., 2019).

1.7.7 Flame retardancy

The flammability resistance of the pristine polymers also improved after addition of nanomaterials including nanofiber or nanoplatelets into the polymer matrices. The presence of nanomaterials slows down the decomposition and enhances the ignition temperature. Polymer nanocomposite with flame retardant property can inhibit, delay, or suppress the heating, decomposition or degradation, combustion with heat generation, and ignition flammable gases during the process of burning. The development of polymer nanocomposites with different nanomaterials such as GO, RGO, CNT, clay, carbon nanofiber, etc. improved the flame retardant property of pristine polymers. Generally, these nanomaterials decrease the maximum rate of heat release during burning and heating process as they formed nonflammable char (Karak, 2019). The char obstructs the fire from spreading by holding the structural integrity of the nanocomposites. Gu et al. reported that the functionalized silica/epoxy nanocomposites exhibited a better flame retardant performance than the unfunctionalized silica-based epoxy nanocomposites (Gu et al., 2013). Norouzian et al. observed that the addition of nanoclay reduced the burning time and the total heat evolved at flame out. The type of assembled clay structure (cluster, intercalated, or exfoliated) had a significant effect on the flame retardant property of the nanocomposite (Norouzian et al., 2012).

1.7.8 Optical

Polymer nanocomposites with optically active functional groups show different interesting optical properties including transparency, fluorescence, refractive index, luminescence, etc. based on the nanomaterials used. In most of the cases, the transparency of the polymer retained after formation of nanocomposite owing to the low scattering of light by the well-dispersed nanometer size particles as well as the presence of a very minute amount of nanomaterials. In literature, various nanomaterials were used to introduce interesting optical properties to the polymer nanocomposites which found enormous industrial applications. A transparent and luminescent CdSe quantum dot-based epoxy nanocomposite was developed by Zou et al. (2011), and ZnO-based light-emitting and transparent nanocomposite was reported by Yang et al. Zhao et al. (2007) reported that ZnS-based acrylated polyester nanocomposites with the transparency of >91% at the wavelength of 500 nm with different loadings of ZnS. From the authors' laboratory, CD and CD nanohybrid based transparent, light-emitting, and photoluminescent different polymer nanocomposites including epoxy, waterborne polyester and polyurethane have been reported (Gogoi et al., 2015; Hazarika and Karak, 2016; De et al., 2015a,b). Thus transparent and light-emitting polymer nanocomposites found potential applications in the field of optoelectronics.

1.7.9 Biological properties

The most vital biological properties of the polymer nanocomposites are biodegradability, biocompatibility, antibacterial activity, etc. The biodegradability of the polymeric material is essential and attractive attribute for the development of sustainable environment. The degradation of polymer waste is a serious issue and urgently need the development biodegradable polymers because of improper disposal of waste as well as extreme use of polymers with the rise of world population. The biodegradation of pristine polymers improved in some cases after incorporation of suitable nanomaterials into the polymer matrices. The rate of biodegradation usually depends on the presence of chemical linkages in the nanocomposites. Biodegradation usually involves four process namely absorption of water, oxidation and hydrolysis, formation of oligomeric fragments, and solubilization of these fragments by the microorganism present in the environment. Thus any factor which increases the hydrolysis tendency also improved the biodegradability behavior. Authors' group reported that the incorporation of CD and clay into polyester matrix increased the biodegradation rate with exposure time against both gram positive and negative bacterial strain. The presence of terminal hydroxyl groups in CD and clay may be responsible for this enhanced biodegradation behavior after nanocomposite formation (Hazarika and Karak, 2016; Konwar and Karak, 2011). The factor that enhances the hydrolysis propensity of polyester ultimately controls the degradation. Both CD and clay in the nanocomposite plays a catalytic role in the hydrolysis of ester groups. Further, the nanocomposites of polyester, polyurethane and polyamide are most studied biocompatible materials. Most metals and metal oxide nanoparticles synthesized through greener approach exhibited promising cell compatibility though they showed severe toxicity toward many cell lines. The toxicity of the material can be diminished by functionalization and incorporating into different polymer matrices. Further, the growth, adhesion, and proliferation of cells of polymer nanocomposites are found to be favorable for biocompatible materials. In addition, antimicrobial property of the polymer nanocomposites is very useful in the field of material sciences as well as biomedical research. The incorporation of different metal and metal oxide nanoparticles into various polymer matrices showed significant inhibitory effect against fungi and bacteria. Thakur and Karak reported that incorporation of sulfur-decorated RGO into polyurethane matrix showed antibacterial activity against *Staphylococcus aureus*, and *Bacillus subtilis* and antifungal activity against *Candida albicans* (Thakur and Karak, 2014). Epoxy nanocomposites with neem oil modified OMMT and OMMT-CD-reduced Cu_2O nanohybrid showed antibacterial activity against both Gram-negative and Gram-positive bacterial strains as well as antifungal activity (De et al., 2015a,b).

1.7.10 Smart and special properties

In addition to the above properties, the development of nanocomposite also displayed some smart and special properties. The ability of materials to sense and respond to external stimuli that allows these materials to alter their properties including shape, color, and electrical conductivity on exposure of temperature, pH, light, chemicals, or stimulation by an electric or magnetic field. This outstanding characteristic has significant scientific and technological importance as it truly the material "smart." The incorporation of various nanomaterials like GO, RGO, RGO/TiO_2, RGO-Ag, etc. into polyurethane materials showed both shape memory and self-healing behavior (Duarah et al., 2016). Shape memory materials are the materials which can able to fix their required temporary shape and return back to original shape with the external stimuli (heat, sunlight, UV light, magnetic field, electric field, microwave, etc.). Further, self-healing materials have the ability to heal by themselves in the presence of suitable stimulus. The incorporation of semiconducting nanomaterials like TiO_2, ZnO, quantum dot, etc. introduces self-cleaning property into the developed polymer nanocomposites. Self-cleaning polymeric materials keep their surface contaminant free in by superhydrophobic or superhydrophilic effects or by photocatalytic action.

Most interestingly, the addition of nanomaterials into the polymer matrices introduces some special properties like antifogging, antiicing, antireflecting, anticounterfeiting, oil–water separation, etc. A highly transparent antifogging films were reported on various substrates, including glass slides, silicon, copper, and PMMA, by spin-coating a mixture of poly(vinylpyrrolidone) and aminopropyl-functionalized nanoscale clay platelets. Further, the resulting nanocomposite films were superhydrophilic and showed more than 90% transmission of visible light as well as self-healing properties (England et al., 2016). MWCNT-reinforced polyurethane nanocomposite showed interesting self-healing, self-cleaning, and antiicing properties reported by Ghosh et al. (Ghosh and Karak, 2019). Further, waterborne polyester nanocomposite with CD@TiO_2 nanohybrid showed multifaceted properties including self-cleaning, antireflecting, antiicing, and anticounterfeiting. Further, this nanocomposite was used as a membrane for separation of oil and water from their mixture (Hazarika and Karak, 2018). Some of the special properties exhibited by different polymer nanocomposites are displayed in Fig. 1.6.

1.8 Applications

The remarkable enhancement in various desired properties of the polymer nanocomposites compared to pristine one makes them useful for wide range of applications in different fields including engineering, biomedical, automotive, electronics, agriculture, industrial, consumer, etc. Some of the applications of polymer nanocomposites are briefly discussed here.

1.8.1 Coatings and paints

Polymer nanocomposites found applications in the field of surface coatings and paints. The easy of processing and good flexibility of polymers along with hardness of the inorganic materials have been successfully applied on various substrates. Ag- and Cu-based epoxy nanocomposites are widely used in antimicrobial and antifouling surface coatings. Mohamadpour et al. developed a flexible and hard polyester coating and enhance the properties such as flexibility, scratch hardness, surface hardness, chemical resistance, and adhesion of the coating by

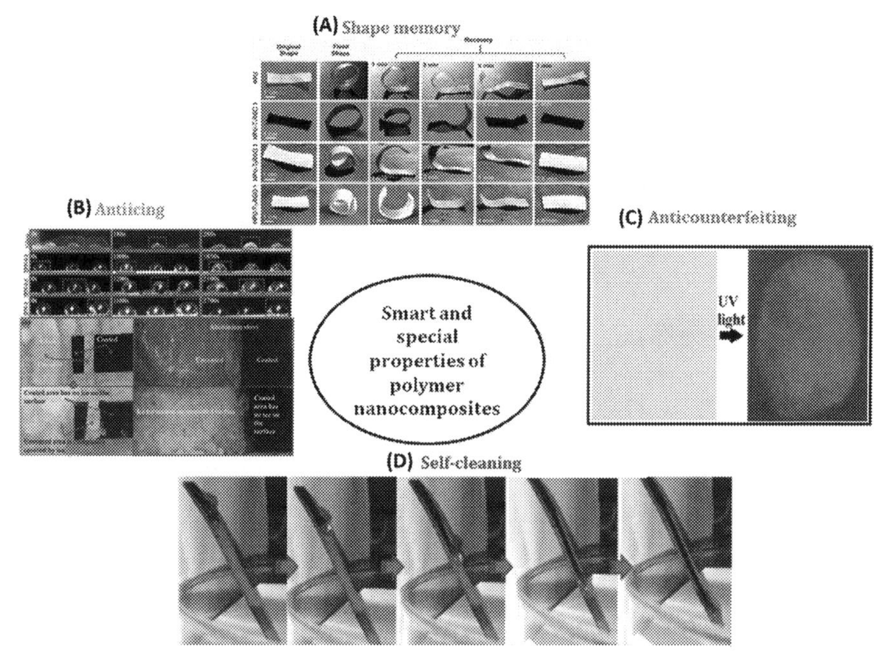

FIGURE 1.6

(A) Shape memory behavior of TiO_2-RGO based polyurethane nanocomposite, (B) antiicing property of MWCNT-reinforced interpenetrating polyurethane network, (C) anticounterfeiting property of epoxy/carbon oxide dot nanocomposite, and (D) self-cleaning activity of polyurethane nanocomposite.

(A) Reproduced from Thakur, S., Karak, N., 2015. Tuning of sunlight-induced self-cleaning and self-healing attributes of an elastomeric nanocomposite by judicious compositional variation of the TiO2-reduced graphene oxide. J. Mater. Chem. A, 3, 12334–12342, Copyright@2015, The Royal Society of Chemistry. (B) Reproduced from Ghosh, T., Karak, N., 2019. Multi-walled carbon nanotubes reinforced interpenetrating polymer network with ultrafast self-healing and anti-icing attributes. J. Colloid. Interface Sci., 540, 247–257, Copyright@2019, Elsevier Inc. (C) Reproduced with permission from De, B., Gupta, K., Mandal, M., Karak, N., 2015a. Biocide immobilized OMMT carbon dot reduced Cu2O nanohybrid/hyperbranched epoxy: mechanical, thermal, antimicrobial and optical properties. Mater. Sci. Eng., 56, 74–83; De, B., Kumar, M., Mandal, B.B., Karak, N., 2015b. An in situ prepared photoluminescent transparent biocompatible hyperbranched epoxy/carbon dot nanocomposite. RSC Adv., 5, 74692–74704, Copyright@2015, American Chemical Society. (D) Reproduced with permission from Ghosh, T., Karak, N., 2019. Multi-walled carbon nanotubes reinforced interpenetrating polymer network with ultrafast self-healing and anti-icing attributes. J. Colloid. Interface Sci., 540, 247–257, Copyright@2019, Elsevier Inc.

incorporating montmorillonite in the polyester matrix (Mohamadpour et al., 2011). Clay-based epoxy nanostructured coating on steel substrate was designed by Turri et al. and the scratch hardness of the nanocomposite was higher than the pristine one (Turri et al., 2010). These kinds of coatings are best candidates for various applications, such as construction, thermal barriers for aerospace applications, automobile, and pipe line coatings for marine applications, sometimes for decorative purpose, textiles, etc.

1.8.2 Biomedical

Polymer nanocomposites are broadly used in various biomedical applications including controlled drug delivery, tissue engineering, bone repair or replacement, dental applications, etc. Polymer nanocomposites should possess some criteria such as biodegradability, biocompatibility, good mechanical properties, etc. to be used in biomedical fields. Thus the proper choice of nanomaterials and polymer matrices are necessary for the fabrication of polymer nanocomposites for biomedical applications. The use of nanotechnology has been extended to biomedical areas such as fighting and preventing of diseases using atomic scale of functional materials. Metal nanoparticles such as Au and Ag owing are most extensively used as nanoreinforcing agents for fabrication of bionanocomposites as they possess strong antimicrobial activity. However, Ag nanoparticles are cytotoxic and embedding them in polymer matrices may reduce their cytotoxic effects. CD-Ag based polyurethane nanocomposite reported by Duarah et al. assisted the growth and proliferation of smooth muscle cells and endothelial cells which showed reduced platelet adhesion and also exhibited in vitro hemocompatibility of mammalian RBCs (Duarah et al., 2016). Das et al. reported that MWCNT-based polyurethane nanocomposite used as a bone tissue scaffold, and it exhibited safety potency as well as nontoxic characteristics confirmed from various biological tests (Das et al., 2013). Fig. 1.7 demonstrates no adverse effect on morphology of kidney, brain, heart, and liver after implantation of nanocomposite films within the rat.

Further, the nanocomposite exhibited antibacterial activity of against both Gram negative and Gram positive which is often responsible for biofilm formation. Barua et al. developed a bio-based hyperbranched epoxy nanocomposite using CuO-cellulose nanofiber and used as an implantable muscle tissue scaffold. The nanocomposite also exhibited biocompatibility activity and inhibitory effect against *Escherichia coli*, *Staphylococcus aureus*, and *Candida albicans*. This bio-based nanocomposite was used a biodegradable, high-performing, and antimicrobial scaffold material for reconstruction of muscle tissues (Barua et al., 2015). SiO_2-based PMMA nanocomposite was reported by Abbas et al. and observed that the in vivo drug release rate of aspirin increased with the loading of unmodified silica and decrease with surface-modified silica amount (Abbas et al., 2018).

1.8.3 Catalytic

Many polymer nanocomposites are gaining interest as heterogeneous and selective catalysts for different organic transformations owing to their high reactivity and huge surface area. The efficiency of such polymer-supported catalysts is also

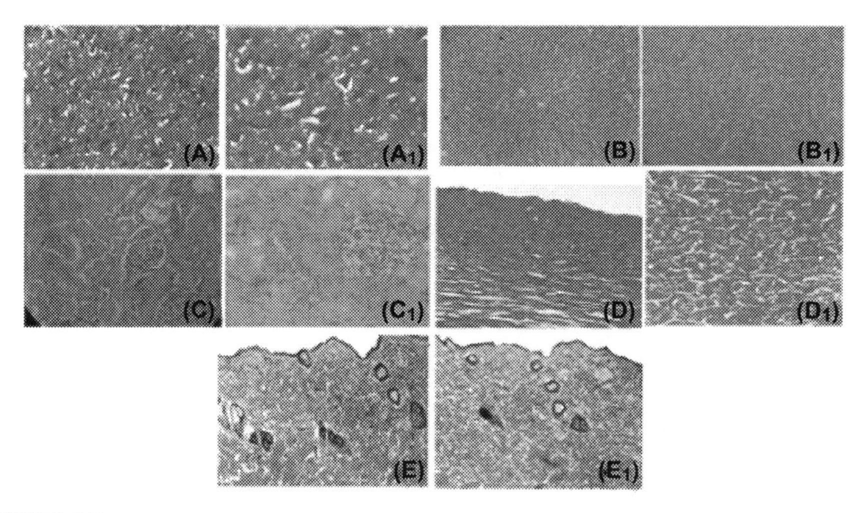

FIGURE 1.7

Representative histological sections of (A and A1) brain, (B and B1) liver, (C and C1) kidney, (D and D1) heart, and (E and E1) skin of Wistar rats implanted with polyurethane/MWCNT nanocomposite and pristine polyurethane.

Reproduced with permission from Das, B., Chattopadhaya, P., Mishara, D., Maiti, T.K., Maji, S., Narayan, R., et al., 2013. Nanocomposites of bio-derived hyperbranched polyurethane/functionalized MWCNT as non immunogenic, osteoconductive, biodegradable and biocompatible scaffold in bone tissue engineering. J. Mater. Chem. B., 1, 4115–4126, Copyright@2013, The Royal Society of Chemistry.

found to be better than the bare nanomaterials because of the uniform dispersion, stability, easy separation, reusability, storage ability, and increase of surface activity of nanomaterials in the polymer matrices. Table 1.6 demonstrates catalytic activity of some of the polymer nanocomposites for various organic transformation reactions.

Further, the photocatalytic effect of photoluminescenc polymer nanocomposites is found to more useful than that of bare nanophotocatalysts. Different types of highly efficient photocatalytic materials are reported in literature for purification of contaminated gases and water. The most widely used catalytic nanoparticles include metal nanoparticles (Fe, Cu, etc.), semiconducting materials (ZnO, TiO_2, CdS, etc.), and nanohybrids (RGO/TiO_2, Fe/Pd, CD/Ag, CD@TiO_2, Zn/Pd, etc.). They act as photocatalysts for removal of different types of organic pollutants like azo dye, polychlorinated biphenyls, halogenated aliphatics, nitroaromatics, etc. by photocatalytic degradation (Jumat et al., 2017; Zhu et al., 2009a,b). However, the use of aqueous suspensions restricts their wide applications because of the problem related to separation of fine particles and recycling of the catalyst. Incorporation of these nanomaterials into the different polymer matrices able to resolve this problem and also help in the prevention of agglomeration of nanoparticles as well as reduction of particle loss. In addition, polymer nanocomposite

Table 1.6 Catalytic applications of different polymer nanocomposites.

Nanocomposites	Catalytic reactions	References
Polyurethane/ Pd-Ag@CQD	Rapid ipso-hydroxylation mediated conversion of aryl boronic acids to phenol	Bayan and Karak (2018)
Waterborne polyester/ functionalized GO	Aza Michael addition reaction	Hazarika et al. (2018)
Waterborne polyurethane/CD	*Para* selective hydroxylation of substituted aromatic hydrocarbon	Das et al. (2017)
Waterborne polyester/ CD@TiO_2	Reduction of nitrophenol to aminophenol	Hazarika and Karak (2018)

Table 1.7 Different types of photocatalyst for removal of organic pollutants.

Photocatalysts	Organic pollutants	References
Polyaniline/TiO_2	Phenol	Jumat et al. (2017)
Waterborne polyester/CD	Formaldehyde and methylene blue	Hazarika and Karak (2016)
Polyurethane/ RGO-TiO_2	Methylene blue	Thakur and Karak (2015)
Chitosan/CdS	Congo red	Zhu et al. (2009a,b)
Waterborne polyester/ CD@TiO_2	Phenol, pesticide, mixed dye (methylene blue and methyl orange), bisphenol A, and methylene blue	Hazarika and Karak (2018)
Epoxy/CD-reduced Cu_2O	Pesticide	De et al. (2015a,b)
Polyurethane/ reduced CD-ZnO	Anionic surfactant contaminants (commercial detergents and dodecylbencene sulfonate)	Duarah and Karak (2019)

could also be used as benign alternatives for harmful materials, reducing the energy requirement and waste generation. Photocatalytic nanoparticles like TiO_2 have been widely used to produce photo-degradable polymers, which help to reduce emission of toxic byproducts during polymer incineration. In literature, many reports were available on photocatalytic activity of polymer nanocomposite. Table 1.7 summaries some of the polymer nanocomposites used for removal of different types of organic pollutants. Different polymer nanocomposites (polyurethane, epoxy, and waterborne polyester) fabricated in our laboratory using various nanomaterials (CD, RGO-TiO_2, CD@TiO_2, RCD, RCD/ZnO, etc.) exhibited photocatalytic activity against large variety of organic pollutants (Hazarika and Karak, 2016; Thakur and Karak, 2015; De et al., 2015a,b; Duarah and Karak, 2019).

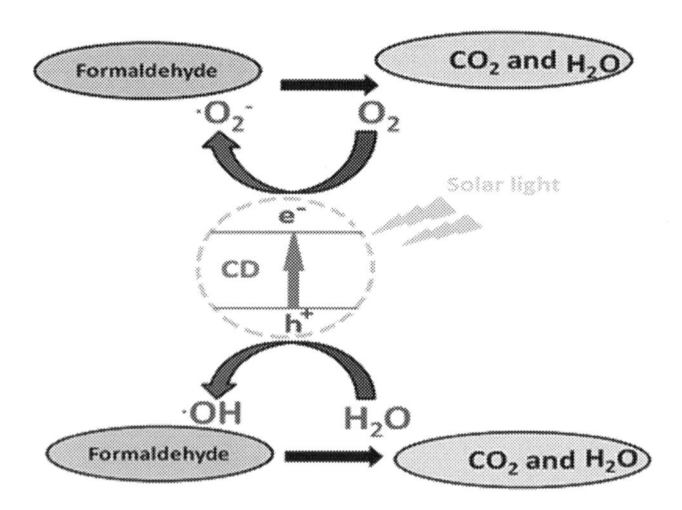

FIGURE 1.8

Mechanism of photocatalytic activity of waterborne polyester/CD nanocomposite.

Reproduced with permision from Hazarika, D., Karak, N., 2016. Biodegradable tough waterborne hyperbranched polyester/carbon dot nanocomposite: approach towards an eco-friendly material. Green Chem., 18, 5200–5211, Copyright@2016, The Royal Society of Chemistry.

A representative mechanistic scheme for degradation of formaldehyde in presence of sunlight by CD-based waterborne polyester nanocomposites is shown in Fig. 1.8.

1.9 Anticorrosion

Metals including magnesium, aluminum, steel, and their alloy are widely used in engineering and industrial structures owing to their high ductility and strength. However, significant losses have been caused by corrosion of these metals. Corrosion usually involves the oxidation of metals and reduction of oxygen, protons, and/or water has a key impact on economics of industrial applications. Thus protection of corrosion is an important issue especially in the modern metallic finishing industry (Shi et al., 2009). Conventional organic coatings such as vinyl, acrylic polyurethane, poly(vinyl butyral), etc. are usually used to protect the substrate from corrosion. These coatings provide a barrier blocking the passage of water and oxygen as well as enhance the resistance of ion movement at the metal/electrolyte interface. Further, the development of conducting polymer nanocomposites using PANi, polythiophene, epoxy, polypropylene, etc. enhance the corrosion protection of steel, iron, and other metal due to their superior performances in highly harsh environment and eco-friendly characteristic (Tomic et al., 2016;

Shi et al., 2009; Golgoon et al., 2017; Nguyen-Tri et al., 2018). Most interestingly, researchers are also tried to develop anticorrosive coating with self-healing properties, which shows potential to address the challenges existing in modern conventional coatings for example the susceptibility to cracks are difficult to detect and high cost associated with the maintenance.

1.9.1 Supercapacitor

Supercapacitor is an intermediate system between the battery and dielectric capacitor which plays very important role in electronic industry. Researchers are tried to develop economically feasible electrode materials with a high capacity of energy density and charge storage in the supercapacitor. The widely used materials for fabrication of supercapacitors are metal oxides, carbon, and conducting polymers. Among the carbon-based nanomaterials, graphene and CNT with extremely high surface area and excellent electrical conductivity have gained the attention of the scientific community for various applications. These materials are widely used as a substitute of metal oxide for the preparation of electrode of capacitors. The carbon-based nanomaterials-reinforced conducting polymer nanocomposites are regarded as a good substitute for the manufacturing of capacitors. They also act as the template for the electrosynthesis of conductive polymers and improve the dielectric conductivity as well as electron transportation of the device (Ebrahimi, 2012).

1.9.2 Sensors

There is a growing interest on the development of polymer nanocomposites for sensor applications. Polymers having conjugated double bonds for example polypyrole, PANi, polythiophene, etc. have been extremely used for the development of gas sensors. TA sensor is a transductor which senses or detect some features of the environment. It realizes events and offers a corresponding output usually as an optical or electrical signal. A biosensor is also an analytical device used for detection of an analyte that combines a biological component with a physicochemical detector gained importance in scientific community. There is a growing interest on the development of graphene-based polymer nanocomposites for sensor application for the unique property of graphene. The sensing behavior of metal-based polymer nanocomposite was studied for different biological applications. The sensing properties of them depend on chemical and structural changes occurred by incorporation of metal nanoparticles in polymer matrices as well as different electronic structures of the nanocomposites (Alshammari, 2018). The polymer matrices provide an appropriate electromagnetic and chemical environment for metal nanoparticles to interact with and detect chemical species. The proper design of strain sensors can also be effective factor to enhance sensing performance. Graphene-based nanocomposites are widely used for sensing applications as gases like NO_2, CO, NH_3, etc. are easily detected by graphene at very low pressure (Rattanabut et al., 2018). Engineering nanocomposite materials and improved device architecture could promote enhancements of gas-sensing properties as well as the range of sensing applications. A gas sensor based on graphene-based PMMA nanocomposite with rapid response and low detection limit of 200 ppm toward NO_2 under 5% strain has been reported in literature (Rattanabut et al., 2018). A highly sensitive aligned CNT-based epoxy nanocomposite sensor able to detect low-concentration NH_3 vapor of about tens ppm has also been reported (Sharma et al., 2014).

1.9.3 Light-emitting diode (LED)

Most interestingly quantum dot-based polymer nanocomposite can be used for emission of white light. Kwon et al. fabricated large-scale free standing films of PMMA with CD where PMMA not only provide mechanical support but also disperse CD to prevent solid state quenching (Kwon et al., 2013). They developed white LED which is consists of films as color converting phosphor and InGaN blue LED as illuminators (Fig. 1.9). This type of white light exhibited no temporal degradation in the emission spectrum under practical operation condition.

1.9.4 Superhydrophobic surface

The development superhydrophobic surfaces gained significant attention not only in scientific research but also in advanced technological applications owing to their unique structure and properties. They can be applied to various aspects such as antiicing, anticorrosion, oil–water separation, antifogging, stain resistant textile, self-cleaning, antifouling, solar cell, improved biocompatibility, self-cleaning, etc. (Das et al., 2018). Surfaces are considered as superhydrophobic

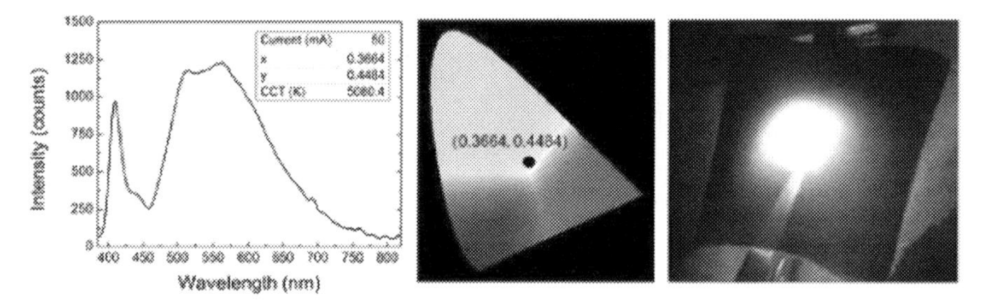

FIGURE 1.9

White light emission by a nanocomposite film and the corresponding emission spectrum.

Reproduced with permission from Kwon, W., Do, S., Lee, J., Hwang, S., Kim, J.K., Rhee, S.W., 2013. Freestanding luminescent films of nitrogen rich carbon nanodots toward large scale phosphor based white light emitting devices. Chem. Mater., 25, 1893–1899, Copyright@2013, American Chemical Society.

when the surfaces possess water contact angle greater than 150 degrees and angle of hysteresis less than 10 degrees. Various superhydrophobic coatings have been reported in literature using different kinds of materials (Ganesh et al., 2011). Further, incorporation of different nanoreinforcing agent into polymer matrices resulted nanofunctionalized superhydrophobic surfaces which can be designed for multifaceted applications. A superhydrophobic was developed by Cao et al. by incorporating organofluoro functionalized SiO_2 into photo cross-linked polyurethane and used the surfaces for preventing leakage in dental composite restoration (Cao et al., 2017). A superhydrophobic coating was designed by Zhu et al. using CNT through surface floatation method with good repairability and reusability (Zhu et al., 2014). Nonfluorinated zinc oxide-based PDMS nanocomposite coating with an oil-fouling resistant superhydrophobic property was reported by Zhang et al. (Zhang et al., 2017). The fabrication of some of the superhydrophobic surface reported in literature is shown in Fig. 1.10.

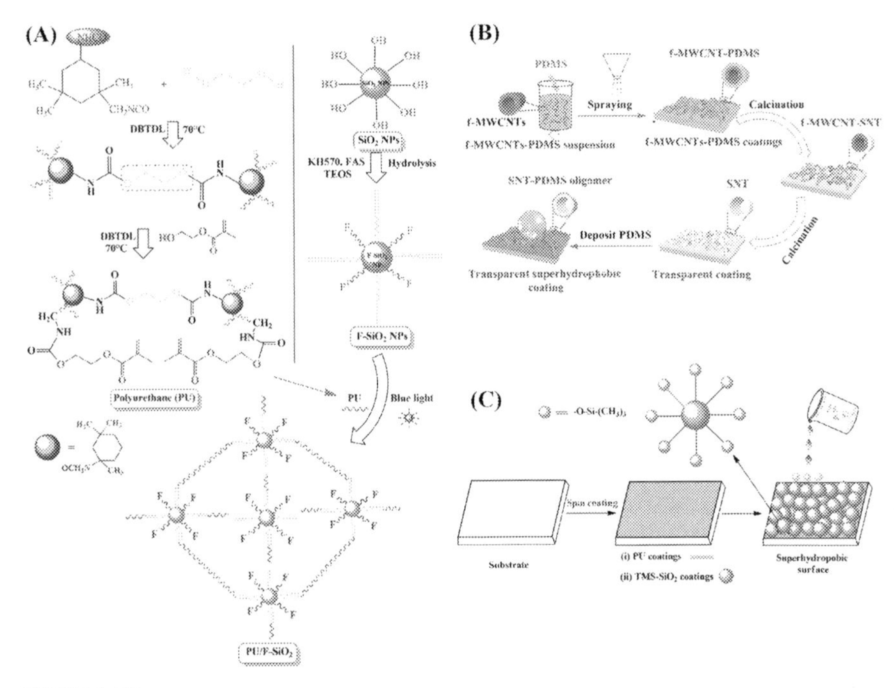

FIGURE 1.10

Fabrication of superhydrophobic (A) polyurethane/SiO_2, (B) PDMS/MWCNT, and (C) polyurethane/TMS-SiO_2.

Reproduced with permission from Das, S., Kumar, S., Samal, S.K., Mohanty, S., Nayak, S.K., 2018. A review on superhydrophobic polymer nanocoatings: recent development and applications. Ind. Eng. Chem. Res., 57, 2727–2745, Copyright@2018, American Chemical Society.

1.10 Conclusion and future scope

In this chapter, we tried to give a general idea about fabrication, characterization, and properties of polymer nanocomposites which are greatly affected by shape, size, and aspect ratio as well as interfacial interactions. Polymer nanocomposites are very significant in both academia and industry. Researchers paid attention on applications of polymer nanocomposite in many advanced fields including biomedical, photocatalysis, supercapacitor, sensors, etc. Polymer nanocomposites not only improve the properties of pristine polymers but also introduce many special properties into the bare polymer matrices. With the rapid development rate of nanotechnology, polymer nanocomposite becomes more functional and relatively cheaper materials. The applications of the polymer nanocomposites are expected to be board in future toward antireflecting, anticorrosion, drug delivery, antibacterial, self-cleaning, etc. However, in some cases, uniform dispersion of nanomaterials in the polymer matrices is a major problem which hampers their properties. This problem may be solved by use of some new advanced techniques or modification/functionalization of the nanomaterials before fabricating the polymer nanocomposites. In addition, large-scale production of polymer nanocomposite is also a main problem. Further, details study on effect of the size and shape on properties of the nanocomposites was lacked in literature. Most interestingly, the fabrication of waterborne superhydrophobic polymer nanocomposite has great advantages; however, work on this field is very rare and thus there is great scope in this field. Further, details study of some of the special properties like antiicing, antifogging, anticounterfeiting, of polymer nanocomposites are lacked. Further, from environment and economic point of view, the development of waterborne polymer nanocomposite plays an important role. Though there are few reports on waterborne polymer nanocomposites, the advanced applications of them are lacked in many cases, and thus there is scope for better understanding their exact structure as well as mechanism of their effect on properties and most importantly future commercial utilization.

References

Abbas, H., Iqbal, S., Ahmad, S., Arfin, N., 2018. Synthesis and characterization of poly (methylmethacrylate)-silica composites. Mater. Res. Express. 5, 085312.

Ahmadizadegan, H., Esmaielzadeh, S., Ranjbar, M., Marzban, Z., Ghavas, F., 2018. Synthesis and characterization of polyester bionanocomposite membrane with ultrasonic irradiation process for gas permeation and antibacterial activity. Ultrason. Sonochem. 41, 538–550.

Alamgir, M., Nayak, G.C., Mallick, A., Tiwari, S.K., Mondal, S., Gupta, M., 2018. Processing of PMMA nanocomposites containing biocompatible GO and TiO_2 nanomaterials. Mater. Manuf. Processes. 33, 1291–1298.

Alshammari, A.S., 2018. Carbon-based polymer nanocomposites for sensing applications. Carbon-Based Polymer Nanocomposites for Environmental and Energy Applications 331–360.

Athanasopoulos, N., Baltopoulos, A., Matzakou, M., Vavouliotis, A., 2012. Electrical conductivity of polyurethane/MWCNT nanocomposite foams. Polym. Compos. 33, 1302–1312.

Barua, S., Goigoi, B., Aidew, L., Buragohain, A.K., Chattopadhyay, P., Karak, N., 2015. Sustainable resource based hyperbranched epoxy nanocomposite as an infection resistant, biodegradable, implantable muscle scaffold. ACS Sustain. Chem. Eng. 3, 1136–1144.

Bayan, R., Karak, N., 2018. Hyperbranched polyurethane supported Pd-Ag@CQD nanocomposite: A high performing heterogenous catalyst. ChemistrySeclect 3, 11210–11218.

Bhat, S.I., Ahmad, S., 2018. Castor oil-TiO_2 hyperbranched poly(esteramide) nanocomposite: a sustainable, green precursor-based anticorrosive nanocomposite coatings. Prog. Org. Coat. 123, 326–336.

Bora, C., Gogoi, P., Baglari, S., Dolui, S.K., 2013. Preparation of polyester resin/graphene oxide nanocomposite with improved mechanical strength. J. Appl. Polym. Sci. 129, 3432–3438.

Brule, B., Flat, J.J., 2006. High barrier polyide/polyolefin/organoclay nanocomposites. Macromol. Symp. 233, 210–216.

Cao, X., Lee, L.J., Widya, T., Macosko, C., 2005. Polyurethane/clay nanocomposites foams: processing, structure and properties. Polymer 46, 775–783.

Cao, D., Zhang, Y., Li, Y., Shi, X., Gong, H., Feng, D., et al., 2017. Fabrication of superhydrophobic coating for preventing microleakage in a dental composite restoration. Mater. Sci. Eng. C 78, 333–340.

Caradonna, A., Badini, C., Padovano, E., Pietroluongo, M., 2019. Electriacal and the thermal conductivity of epoxy-carbon filler composite processed by calendaring. Materials 12, 1522.

Cha, J., Kim, J., Ryu, S., Hong, S.H., 2019. Comparision to mechanical properties of epoxy nanocomposites reinforced by functionalized carbon nanotubes and graphene nanoplatelets. Compos. Part. B: Eng. 162, 283–288.

Charlon, S., Follain, N., Chappey, C., Dargent, E., Soulestin, J., Scalvons, M., et al., 2015. Improvement of barrier properties of bio-based polyester nanocomposite membranes by water-assisted extrusion. J. Mem. Sci. 496, 185–198.

Charpentier, P.A., Burgess, K., Wang, L., Chowdhury, R.R., Lotus, A.F., Moula, G., 2012. Nano TiO_2/polyurethane composites for antibacterial and self cleaing coatings. Nanotechnology 23, 425206.

Chirayila, C.J., Mathewa, L., Hasaan, P.A., Mozetic, M., Thomas, S., 2014. Rheological behaviour of nanocellulose reinforced unsaturated polyester nanocomposites. Int. J. Biol. Macromolecules 274–281.

Coleman, J.N., Khan, U., Blau, W.J., Gun'ko, Y.K., 2006. Small but strong: a review of mechanical properties of carbon nanotubes-polymer composites. Carbon 44, 1624–1652.

Dai, J., Ma, S., Wu, Y., Han, L., Zhang, L., Zhua, J., et al., 2015. Polyesters derived from itaconic acid for the properties and bio-based content enhancement of soybean oil-based thermosets. Green Chem. 17, 2383–2392.

Das, B., Chattopadhaya, P., Mishara, D., Maiti, T.K., Maji, S., Narayan, R., et al., 2013. Nanocomposites of bio-derived hyperbranched polyurethane/functionalized MWCNT as non immunogenic, osteoconductive, biodegradable and biocompatible scaffold in bone tissue engineering. J. Mater. Chem. B 1, 4115–4126.

Das, V.K., Gogoi, S., Choudary, B.M., Karak, N., 2017. A promising catalyst for executive para hydroxylation of substituted aromatic hydrocarbons under UV light. Green Chem. 19, 4278–4283.

Das, S., Kumar, S., Samal, S.K., Mohanty, S., Nayak, S.K., 2018. A review on superhydrophobic polymer nanocoatings: recent development and applications. Ind. Eng. Chem. Res. 57, 2727–2745.

De, B., Voit, B., Karak, N., 2013. Transparent luminescent hyperbranched epoxy/carbon dot nanocomposite with outstanding toughness and ductility. ACS Appl. Mater. Interfaces 5, 10027–10034.

De, B., Gupta, K., Mandal, M., Karak, N., 2015a. Biocide immobilized OMMT carbon dot reduced Cu_2O nanohybrid/hyperbranched epoxy: mechanical, thermal, antimicrobial and optical properties. Mater. Sci. Eng. 56, 74–83.

De, B., Karak, N., 2013. Novel high performance tough hyperbranched epoxy by an $A_2 + B_3$ polycondensation reaction. J. Mater. Chem. A 1, 348–353.

De, B., Kumar, M., Mandal, B.B., Karak, N., 2015b. An *in situ* prepared photoluminescent transparent biocompatible hyperbranched epoxy/carbon dot nanocomposite. RSC Adv. 5, 74692–74704.

DeLeon, V.H., Nguyen, T.D., Nar, M., Souza, N.A., Golden, T.D., 2012. Polymer nanocomposites for improved drug delivery efficiency. Mater. Chem. Phys. 132, 409–415.

Duarah, R., Karak, N., 2019. Hyperbranched/reduced carbon dot-zinc oxide nanocomposite-mediated solar assisted photocatalytic degradation of organic contaminant: an approach towards environmental remediation. Chem. Eng. J. 370, 716–728.

Duarah, R., Singh, Y.P., Gupta, P., Mandal, B.B., Karak, N., 2016. High performance bio-based hyperbranched polyurethane/carbon dot-silver nanocomposite: a rapid self-expandable stent. Biofabrication 8, 045013.

Ebrahimi, F., 2012. Application of nanocomposites for supercapacitors: characteristics and properties. Nanocomposites—New Trends and Developments. InTech.

England, M.W., Urata, C., Dunderdale, G.J., Hozumi, A., 2016. Antifogging/self-healing properties of clay containing transparent nanocomposite thin films. ACS Appl. Mater. Interfaces 8, 4318–4322.

Fahlman, B.D., 2007. Material Chemistry, 2nd Ed. Springer, New York, Kindle edition.

Feuser, P.E., Gaspar, P.C., Junior, E.R., Silva, M.C.S., Nele, M., Sayer, C., et al., 2014. Synthesis and characterization of poly(methylmethacrylate) PMMA and evaluation of cytotoxicity for biomedical application. Macromol. Symp. 343, 65–69.

Ganesh, V.A., Raut, H.K., Nair, A.S., Ramakrishna, S.A., 2011. A review on self-cleaning coatings. J. Mater. Chem. 21, 16304–16322.

Ghosh, T., Karak, N., 2019. Multi-walled carbon nanotubes reinforced interpenetrating polymer network with ultrafast self-healing and anti-icing attributes. J. Colloid. Interface Sci. 540, 247–257.

Gleiter, H., 1990. Nanocrystalline materials. Prog. Mater. Sci. 33, 223–315.

Goffin, A.L., Habibi, Y., Raquez, J.M., Dubois, P., 2012. Polyester-grafted cellulose nanowhiskers: a new approach for tuning the microstructure of immiscible polyester blends. ACS Appl. Mater. Interfaces 4, 3364–3371.

Gogoi, S., Kumar, M., Mandal, B.B., Karak, N., 2015. High performance luminescent thermosetting waterborne polyurethane/carbon quantum dot nanocomposite with *in vitro* cytocompatibility. Compos. Sci. Technol. 118, 39–46.

Golgoon, A., Aliofkhazraei, M., Toorani, M., Moradi, M.H., Rouhaghdam, A.S., Asgari, M., 2017. Corrosion behavior of ZnO-polyester nanocomposite powder coating. Anticorr. Methods Mater. 64, 380–388.

Guo, C., Zheng, Z., Zhu, Q., Wang, X., 2007. Preparation and characterization of polyurethane/ZnO nanoparticle composites. Polym. Plast. Technol. Eng. 46, 10–12.

Gu, H., Guo, J., He, Q., Tadakamalla, S., Zhang, X., Yan, X., et al., 2013. Flame-retardant epoxy resin nanocomposites reinforced with polyaniline-stablized silica nanoparticles. Ind. Eng. Chem. Res. 52, 7718–7728.

Hazarika, D., Karak, N., 2016. Biodegradable tough waterborne hyperbranched polyester/carbon dot nanocomposite: approach towards an eco-friendly material. Green Chem. 18, 5200–5211.

Hazarika, D., Karak, N., 2018. Unprecedented influence of carbon dot@TiO_2 nanohybrid on multifaceted attributes of waterborne hyperbranched polyester nanocomposite. ACS Omega 3, 1757–1769.

Hazarika, D., Gupta, K., Karak, Mandal, M., Karak, N., 2018. High-performing biodegradable waterborne polyester/functionalized graphene oxide nanocomposites as an eco-friendly material. ACS Omega 3, 2292–2303.

Hess, P.H., Parker, P.H., 1996. Polymer for stabilization of colloidal cobalt species. J. Appl. Polym. Sci. 10, 1915–1926.

Irfan, M., Bhat, S.I., Ahmad, S., 2019. Waterborne reduced graphene oxide dispersed polyesteramide nanocomposites: an approach towards eco-friendly anticorrosive coatings. N. J. Chem. 43, 4706–4720.

Ismail, A.F., Goh, P.S., 2018. Carbon Based Polymer Nanocomposite for Energy and Environmental Applications, 1st Ed. Elsevier.

Jin, H., Guo, C., Liu, X., Liu, J., Vasileff, A., Jiao, Y., et al., 2018. Emerging two-dimensional nanomaterials for electrocatalysis. Chem. Rev. 118, 6337–6408.

Jumat, N.A., Wai, P.S., Juan, J.C., Basirun, W.F., 2017. Synthesis of polyaniline-TiO_2 nanocomposites and their application in photocatalytic degradation. Polym. Polym. Compos. 25, 507–514.

Kalidindi, S.B., Indirani, M., Jagirdar, B.R., 2008. First row transition metal ion-assisted ammonia-borane hydrolysis for hydrogen generation. Inorg. Chem. 47, 7424–7429.

Karak, N., 2009. Fundamentals of Polymers: Raw Materials to Finish Products. PHI Learning Private Ltd., New Delhi.

Karak, N., 2017. Biobased Smart Polyurethane Nanocomposites: From Synthesis to Applications. The Royal Society of Chemistry, Cambridge.

Karak, N., 2019. Fundamentals of nanomaterials and polymer nanocomposites. Nanomaterials and Polymer Nanocomposites. Elsevier.

Kim, J.Y., Han, S.I., Hong, S., 2008. Effect of modified carbon nanotube on the properties of aromatic polyester nanocomposites. Polymer 49, 3335–3345.

Kim, H., Abdala, A.A., Macosko, C.W., 2010. Graphene/polymer nanocomposites. Macromolecules 43, 6515–6530.

Kojima, Y., Usuki, A., Kawasumi, M., Okada, A., 1993. Mechanical properties of nylon 6-clay hybrid. J. Mater. Res. 8, 1185–1189.

Konwar, U., Karak, N., 2011. *Mesua ferrea* L. seed oil based highly branched environment friendly polyester resin/clay nanocomposites. J. Polym. Environ. 19, 90–99.

Kumar, M., Arun, S., Upadhyaya, P., Pugazhethi, G., 2015. Properties of PMMA/clay nanocomposites prepared using various compatibilizers. Int. J. Mech. Mater. Eng. 10, 7.

Kunduru, K.R., Basu, A., Zada, M.H., Domb, A.J., 2015. Castor oil-based biodegradable polyesters. Biomacromolecules 16, 2572–2587.

Kwon, W., Do, S., Lee, J., Hwang, S., Kim, J.K., Rhee, S.W., 2013. Freestanding luminescent films of nitrogen rich carbon nanodots toward large scale phosphor based white light emitting devices. Chem. Mater. 25, 1893–1899.

Liu, X., Zou, Y., Cao, G., Luo, D., 2007. The preparation and properties of biodegradable polyesteramide composites reinforced with nano-$CaCO_3$ and nano SiO_2. Mater. Lett. 61, 4216–4221.

Mauro, Ad, Cantarella, M., Nicotra, G., Pellegrino, G., Gulino, A., Brundo, M.V., et al., 2017. Novel synthesis of ZnO/PMMA nanocomposites for photocatalytic applications. Sci. Rep. 7, 40895.

Mittal, V., 2007. Characterization Technique for Polymer Nanocomposite. Wiley-VCH.

Mohamadpour, S., Pourabbas, B., Fabbri, P., 2011. Anti-scratch and adhesion properties of photo-curable polymer/clay nanocomposite coatings on methacrylate monomers. Sci. Iran. 18, 765–771.

Mosconi, D., Mazzier, D., Silvestrini, S., Privitera, A., Marega, C., Franco, L., et al., 2015. Synthesis and photochemical applications of processable polymers enclosing photoluminescent carbon quantum dots. ACS Nano 9, 4156–4164.

Nguyen-Tri, P., Nguyen, T.A., Carriere, P., Xuan, C.N., 2018. Nanocomposite coatings: preparation, characterization, properties, and applications. Int. J. Corros. 1–19.

Norouzian, R.S., Teija, A., Wilen, T.C.E., 2012. Flame retardant polyurethane nanocomposite: study of clay dispersion and its synergistic effect with dolomite. J. Appl. Polym. Sci. 129, 1678–1685.

Pramanik, S., Hazarika, J., Kumar, A., Karak, N., 2013. Castor oil based hyperbranched poly(esteramide)/polyaniline nanofibre nanocomposite as antistatic materials. Ind. Eng. Chem. Res. 16, 5700–5707.

Qiu, F., Xu, H., Wang, Y., Xu, W.J., Yang, D., 2012. Preparation, characterization and properties of UV-curable waterborne polyurethane acrylate/SiO_2 coating. J. Coat. Technol. Research. 9, 503–514.

Rahmatpour, A., Kaffashi, B., Maghami, S., 2011. Preparation and rheological properties of functionalized multiwalled carbon nanotube/waterborne polyurethane nanocomposites. J. Macromol. Sci. Part B 9, 1834–1846.

Rajabi, M., Rashed, G.R., Zaarei, D., 2015. Assessment of graphene oxide/epoxy nanocomposite as corrosion resistance coating on carbon steel. Corros. Eng. Sci. Technol. 50, 509–516.

Rajabia, M., Mahanpoora, K., Moradib, O., 2019. Prepararion of PMMA/GO and PMMA/GO-Fe_3O_4 nanocomposites for malachite green dye adsorption. Compos. Part B 167, 544–555.

Rattanabut, C., Wongwiriyapani, W., Muangrat, W., Bunjonfpru, W., Phonyiem, M., Song, Y.J., 2018. Graphene and poly(methyl methacrylate) composite laminates on flexible substrates for volatile organic compound detection. Jpn. J. Appl. Phys. 57, 04FP10.

Ray, S.S., Okamoto, M., 2003. Polymer/layered silicate nanocomposites: a review from preparation to processing. Prog. Polym. Sci. 28, 1539–1641.

Razak, S.I.A., Wahab, I.F., Fadil, F., Nuruljannah, D., Khudzari, A.Z., Adeli, H., 2015. A review of electrospun conductive polyaniline based nanofibre composites and blends: processing features, applications and future scopes. Adv. Mater. Sci. Eng. 19, 356286.

Razaka, A., Muhamad, I.I., Sharif, N.F.A., Nayan, N.H.M., Rahma, A.R., Yahyac, M.Y., 2015. Mechanical and electrical properties of electrically conductive nanocomposites of epoxy/polyaniline coated halloysite nanotubes. Dig. J. Nanomater. Bio. 10, 377–384.

Sadjadi, M.S., Farhadyar, N., 2009. Preparation and characterization of the hydrophilic coating based on epoxy resins and titanate on the glass substrate. J. Nanosci. Nanotechnol. 9, 1172–1175.

Sharma, S., Hussain, S., Singh, S., Islam, S., 2014. MWCNT-conducting polymer composite based ammonia gas sensors: a new approach for complete recoveryMWCNT-conducting process. Sens. Acutators B 194, 213–219.

Shi, X., Nguyen, T.A., Suo, Z., Liu, Y., Avci, R., 2009. Effect of nanoparticles on the anti-corrosion and mechanical properties of epoxy coatings. Surf. Coat. Technol. 204, 237–245.

Solouki, K.V., Yuan, B.D., Zloczower, I., 2018. Piezoresistive thermoplastic polyurethane nanocomposites with carbon nanostructures. Carbon 139, 52–58.

Spitalsky, Z., Tasis, D., Papagelis, K., Galiotis, C., 2010. Carbon nanotubes-polymer composites: chemistry, processing, mechanical and electrical properties. Prog. Polym. Sci. 35, 357–401.

Sridhar, L.N., Gupta, R.K., Bhardwaj, M., 2006. Barrier properties of polymer nanocomposites. Ind. Eng. Chem. Res. 45, 8282–8289.

Stander, L., Theodore, L., 2011. Environmental implications of nanotechnology-An Update. Int. J. Environ. Res. Public. Health 8, 470–479.

Tang, L., Weder, C., 2010. Cellulose whisker/epoxy resin nanocomposites. ACS Appl. Mater. Interfaces 2, 1073–1080.

Thakur, S., Karak, N., 2013. Castor oil-based hyperbranched polyurethanes as advanced surface coating materials. Prog. Org. Coat. 76, 157–164.

Thakur, S., Karak, N., 2014. Multi-stiluli responsive smart elastomeric hyperbranched polyurethane/reduced graphene oxide nanocomposites. J. Mater. Chem. A 2, 14867–14875.

Thakur, S., Karak, N., 2015. Tuning of sunlight-induced self-cleaning and self-healing attributes of an elastomeric nanocomposite by judicious compositional variation of the TiO_2-reduced graphene oxide. J. Mater. Chem. A 3, 12334–12342.

Theng, B.K.G., Walker, G.F., 1970. Interactions of clay minerals with organic monomers. Isr. J. Chem. 8, 417–424.

Tiwari, J.N., Tiwari, R.N., Kim, K.S., 2012. Zero-dimensional, one-dimensional, two-dimensional and three-dimensional nanostructured materials for advanced electrochemical energy devices. Prog. Mater. Sci. 57, 724–803.

Tomic, M., Dunjik, B., Bajat, J., Likic, V., Rogan, J., Donlajic, J., 2016. Anticorrosive epoxy/clay nanocomposite coatings: rheological and Protective properties. J. Coat. Technol. Res. 13, 439–456.

Triantafyllidis, K.S., LeBaron, P.C., Park, I., Pinnavaia, T.J., 2006. Epoxy-clay fabric film composites with unprecedented oxygen barrier properties. Chem. Mater. 18, 4393–4398.

Turri, S., Torlaj, L., Piccinini, F., Levi, M., 2010. Abrasion and nanoscratch in nanostructured coatings. J. Appl. Polym. Sci. 118, 1720–1727.

Vogel, V., Schubert, D., Kreuter, J., 2004. Comparison of scanning electron microscopy, dynamic light scattering and analytical ultracentrifugation for the sizing of poly(butyl cyanoacrylate) nanoparticles. Europ. J. Pharm. Biopharmaceutics 57, 369–375.

Wang, G., Wang, H., Ling, Y., Tang, Y., Yang, X., Fitzmorris, R.C., et al., 2011. Hydrogen-treated TiO_2 nanowire arrays for photoelectrochemical water splitting. Nano Lett. 11, 3026–3033.

Wang, L., Yin, Y., Jain, A., Zhou, H.S., 2014. Aqueous phase synthesis of highly luminescent, nitrogen-doped carbon dots and their application as bioimaging agents. Langmuir 30, 14270–14275.

Wang, Y., Cheng, Z., Liu, Z., Kang, H., Liu, Y., 2018. Cellulose nanofibre/polyurethane shape memory composites with fast water-responsivity. J. Mater. Chem. B. 6, 1668–1677.

Waseem, S., Khan, C.M., Asmatulu, R., 2012. Effects of Nanotechnology on global warming. ASEE Mdwest Section Conference, Rollo, MO, Septembeer 19–21, 13 pages.

Winnacker, M., Rieger, B., 2016. Poly(esteramide)s: recent insights into synthesis, stability and biomedical applications. Polym. Chem. 7, 7039–7046.

Yadav, S.K., Cho, J.W., 2012. Functionalized graphene nanoplatelets for enhanced mechanical and thermal properties of polyurethane nanocomposite. Appl. Surf. Sci. 266, 1–7.

Yu, H., Shi, R., Zhao, Y., Waterhouse, G.I.N., Wu, L.Z., Tung, C.H., et al., 2016. Smart utilization of carbon dots in semiconductor photocatalysis. Adv. Mater. 28, 9454–9477.

Zafar, F., Shaemin, E., Zafar, H., Shah, M.Y., Nishat, N., Ahmad, S., 2015. Facile microwave assisted preparation of waterborne polyesteramide/OMMT clay bionanocomposites for protective coating. Ind. Crop. Products 67, 484–491.

Zhang, S., Yang, Y., Gao, B., Li, Y.C., Liu, Z., 2017. Superhydrophobic controlled release fertilizers coated with bio-based polymers with organosilicon and nanosilica modification. J. Mater. Chem. A 5, 19943–19953.

Zhao, Y., Wang, F., Fu, Q., Shi, W., 2007. Synthesis and characterization of ZnS/hyperbranched polyester nanocomposite and its optical properties. Polymer 48, 2853–2859.

Zhu, H., Wang, X., Li, Y., Wang, Z., Yang, F., Yang, X., 2009a. Microwave synthesis of fluorescent carbon nanoparticles with electro chemiluminescence properties. Chem. Commun. 0, 5118–5120.

Zhu, H., Jiang, R., Xiao, L., Chang, Y., Guang, Y., Li, X., et al., 2009b. Photocatalytic decolorization and degration of congo red on innovative chitosan/nano-CdS composite catalyst under visible light irradiation. J. Hazard. Mater. 169, 933–940.

Zhu, X., Zhang, Z., Ge, B., Men, X., Zhou, X., 2014. Fabrication of a superhydrophobic carbon nanotubes coating with good reusuability and repairability. Colloids Surf. 444, 252–256.

Zou, W., Du, Z., Li, H., Zhang, C., 2011. Fabrication of carboxyl functionalized CdSe quantum dots via ligand self-assembly and CdSe/epoxy fluorescence nanocomposites. Polymer 52, 1938–1943.

CHAPTER

Synthesis of polymer nanomaterials, mechanisms, and their structural control

2

Rashmi Choubey[1], Neha Sonker[1], Jaya Bajpai[1], Preeti Jain[2] and Anamika Singh[2]

[1]*Bose Memorial Research Laboratory, Department of Chemistry, Government Autonomous Science College, Jabalpur, India*

[2]*Department of Chemistry, Medi-Caps University, Indore, India*

2.1 Polymer nanomaterials

Nanomaterials are the keystone of nanotechnology and nanoscience. They are synthetic materials or substances that are produced and utilized at a very small scale. The developed nanomaterials exhibit unique characteristics in comparison to the similar kind of bulk materials that do not exhibit nanoscale features, such as chemical reactivity, increased strength, or conductivity. Generally, nanomaterials are considered as materials at least having one external dimension that estimates 100 nm (or nanoscale, 1–100 nm) or lesser or having internal structures estimating 100 nm or lesser (i.e., 1–100 nm). The nanoscale-structured materials often acquire unique mechanical, optical, and electronic properties (Hubler and Osuagwu, 2010). The nanomaterials have been slowly expanding into commercialized materials and have started emerging as commodities (McGovern, 2010). In the formation of new materials the nanomaterials play a significant role as they can be utilized to impact and regulate physical properties and specific characteristics of other materials. These nanostructure materials include polymer multilayers, nanoporous materials, nanocapsules, nanoparticles (NPs), etc. The surface-areas-to-volume ratio of nanomaterials is much greater than their bulk counterparts, which leads to enhancement in their chemical reactivity and strength also. Likewise, at nanorange, quantum effects can turn out to be substantially more significant in determining the characteristics and materials properties, prompting novel electrical, optical, and magnetic behaviors.

Polymer nanomaterials are meant to be the largest and much versatile class of biomaterials, which have been studied extensively and applied progressively in drug-delivery fields (Elsabahy and Wooley, 2012; Gomes et al., 2012), tissue engineering and regenerative medicine (Kohane and Langer, 2008), and imaging (Achachelouei et al., 2019; Lu, 2010; Anderson et al., 2011). The incorporation of nanomaterials

Advances in Polymeric Nanomaterials for Biomedical Applications. DOI: https://doi.org/10.1016/B978-0-12-814657-6.00004-5

into polymer packaging in polymer nanomaterials tends to improve durability, barrier properties, physical performance, and biodegradation. Significant advancements in the polymer chemistry and the development of complex synthetic techniques have enabled the engineering of polymer nanomaterials with a high uniformity rate and precise control of its physicochemical properties (Elsabahy and Wooley, 2012). The most widely used polymer biomaterials include tissue-engineering scaffolds, drug delivery, diagnostics, and fabrication of medical devices. Polymer nanomaterials are developing progressively as more relevant materials in the medical field since they provide various advantages unlike other materials, such as high surface-to-volume ratio, large synthetic flexibility, pore size is small having a high porosity, biocompatibility, appropriate mechanical properties, and biodegradation. Various types of polymer are available, which are utilized for designing nanomaterials that are dependent on the advantages and the requirements they provide; these polymers are found as natural and synthetic polymers and may be degradable or nondegradable. Polymeric nanomaterials are available in single, agglomerated, aggregated, or fused forms with irregular, tubular, and spherical shapes. The most familiar category of polymeric nanomaterials involves dendrimers, quantum dots, nanotubes, and fullerenes. The polymer nanomaterials have applications in the nanotechnology field and show different physical and chemical attributes from normally available chemicals (e.g., silver nano, nanotubes of carbon, photocatalysts, silica, fullerene, and nanocarbon). Nanomaterials based on polymers have good biodegradability and biological safety, which can prevent the degradation of drugs or antigens (Burchiel et al., 2007). The most commonly used polymer nanomaterials involve polylactic acid (PLA), chitosan, poly(lactic-glycolic acid) (PLGA), polyglutamic acid, etc. Table 2.1 summarizes various polymer-based nanomaterials, their advantages, and disadvantages.

2.2 Types of polymer nanomaterials

Polymers utilized as biomaterials or nanomaterials can be obtained naturally, synthetically, or by combination of both. On the basis of their types, the polymers form nanomaterials: natural polymeric materials, biosynthesis materials, and chemosynthesis (copolymer) materials. There are different types of nanomaterials that depend on their dimensions and are classified into three categories, namely, zero dimensional, one dimensional, and two dimensional (Gusev and Rempel, 2004).

2.2.1 Based on types of polymer

2.2.1.1 Natural polymer–based nanomaterials

Natural polymers are one of the renewable resources acquired from different sources. They are easily degraded into small inorganic molecules, carbon dioxide, and water; also known as environment-friendly materials. Natural polymer–based

Table 2.1 Types of polymer-based nanomaterials and their application areas, advantages, and disadvantages (Dan et al., 2018).

Classification	Materials	Application areas	Advantages	Disadvantages
Natural polymeric material	Chitosan	Medical dressing, hemostasis material, gene transfer, carrier for drug delivery, hydrogel (Ravi Kumar, 2000)	Antimicrobial, biocompatibility, easily degradable, innocuous, film formation, absorbability (Badawy et al., 2004; Chou et al., 2005; Jayakumar et al., 2007)	Poor strength, poor spin ability, low solubility in water (Jayakumar et al., 2007)
	Starch	Tissue-engineered scaffold, hemostasis material, bone repair material, drug-delivery carrier (Cyras et al., 2013)	Safe degradation products and no toxicity, extensive sources, nonantigenic, low price (Sirivongpaisal et al., 2014)	Water resistant, poor mechanical properties, blocking performance are poor (Sirivongpaisal et al., 2014)
	Alginate	Medical dressing, complete pepcid, pharmaceutical excipient (Lee and Mooney, 2012; Rebecca, 2016; Amp et al., 2014)	Biocompatibility, hypotoxicity, enhances immunity, suppresses tumor growth (Lee and Mooney, 2012; Rebecca, 2016; Amp et al., 2014)	Poor cell attachment and biodegradability (Lee and Mooney, 2012; Rebecca, 2016; Amp et al., 2014)
	Cellulose	Pharmaceutical supplementary (Cyras et al., 2013)	Low price, large sources (Cyras et al., 2013)	Adverse reactions are rare (Cyras et al., 2013)
Biosynthesis material	PHB	Tissue-engineering material, carrier for drug delivery (Cazeneuve et al., 2016)	Nontoxic, biodegradable, safe, good chemical and physical properties (Cazeneuve et al., 2016; Aminabhavi et al., 2015)	Poor thermal stability, high crystallinity (Cazeneuve et al., 2016; Aminabhavi et al., 2015)

(Continued)

Table 2.1 Types of polymer-based nanomaterials and their application areas, advantages, and disadvantages (Dan et al., 2018). *Continued*

Classification	Materials	Application areas	Advantages	Disadvantages
Chemosynthesis material (copolymer)	PLA	Drug-delivery carrier, materials for antiadhesion, bone-fixing device, patch, suture, tissue-engineered scaffold (Cao et al., 2012; Chen et al., 2016)	Good mechanical properties, biocompatibility, nontoxic, safe (Cao et al., 2012; Chen et al., 2016)	Slow degradation speed, poor toughness, hydrophobicity, lack of reactive side chain groups (Cao et al., 2012; Chen et al., 2016)
	PLGA	Bone screw fixation, absorbable suture, tissue repair, drug delivery (Danhier et al., 2012)	Biocompatibility, controllable biodegradability (Danhier et al., 2012)	Stability and drug-loading capacity can be improved, higher cost (Danhier et al., 2012)
	PMMA	Dental materials, bone-fixation materials, artificial crystal (Ho et al., 2013)	Good biocompatibility, easy operation	Easy oxidation, monomer has cytotoxicity

PHB, *Poly-β-hydroxybutyrate;* PLA, *polylactic acid;* PLGA, *poly(lactic-glycolic acid);* PMMA, *polymethyl methacrylate resin.*

nanomaterials that are most commonly utilized are chitosan, cellulose, alginate, starch, chondroitin sulfate, hyaluronic acid, etc. Chitosan is a biodegradable material and has good biocompatibility; it can bind with protein having negative-charge or with plasmid DNA by means of electrostatic interaction for the formation of composites of polymer that prevent degradation of DNA and protein and therefore is suitable as drug-delivery carrier or an adjuvant. Also, chitosan comprises great absorbability, moisture retention, and permeability. Because of its significant intrinsic biological properties, including their nontoxicity and antimicrobial activity, the derivatives of chitosan have enormous potential in the medical fields.

A polysaccharide like alginate is found naturally and acquired mostly from the aquatic plants, specifically *Cyanophyceae*, *Chlorophyceae*, *Rhodophyceae*, and *Phaeophyceae*. Presently, the products of alginate that are widely utilized commercially are ammonium alginate, calcium alginate, and sodium alginate. Alginates have some beneficial functional properties such as high permeability of oxygen, great moisture absorption, simple evacuation, biodegradability, biocompatible, obstructive gelation, and adsorption of metal ions, which make them valuable in the biomedical field (Rebecca, 2016; Amp et al., 2014).

2.2.1.2 Biosynthesized polymer materials

The polymers acquired by the hydrolysis of enzyme (by using microbial enzymes) are coined as biosynthesized polymers. The microbial polysaccharides and microbial polyesters are present in these compounds. The type of biosynthesized polymers includes poly(3-hydroxybutyrate-*co*-3-hydroxyvalerate), poly-β-hydroxybutyrate (PHB), polyamino acid, bio fiber bundle, etc. PHB is a polymer of high molecular weight formed under ominous growth conditions by microorganisms (when limited nutrients are available). The properties of PHB are as good as synthetic polymers, such as biological degradability, biocompatibility, optical activity, piezoelectricity, and likewise extraordinary properties. Utility of this polymer cannot be limited to just as a carrier for drug delivery, but it can also be utilized as a scaffolding material for tissue engineering and as a material for bone fixing in surgical treatment. It is also utilized for repairing soft tissue (such as repairing of palatal tissue and skin), as well as in vascular substitutes, blood bags, and supportive material for wound due to the ability of desorption of PHB on fiber protein and serum protein (He et al., 2014).

2.2.1.3 Chemically synthesized polymer materials

The materials of polymer are chemically synthesized, including PLA, polyurethane (PU), PLGA, poly(methyl methacrylate), silicone rubber, polyester, polyvinyl alcohol, polyvinyl pyrrolidone, and so on, which are utilized as materials in the biomedical field, and have been developed via chemical techniques.

PLA as well as their copolymers are biodegradable and biocompatible and can be acquired from a broad range of raw material sources. They are nontoxic, renewable, and completely biodegradable. They comprise good thermal formability, mechanical strength, elastic modulus and are utilized in cartilage regeneration, repairing of cartilage, bone tissue engineering and in the controlled drug release formulation functioning as carrier. For a continuous drug-releasing system, it is utilized as a carrier; PLA supports in gradual drug release through its moderate degradation rate in vivo. The PU material comprises excellent fatigue resistance, good compatibility (blood, biological, and tissue compatibility), high elasticity, high strength, and wear resistance as compared to other polymeric materials. Therefore, in the biomedical field, materials such as PU are widely utilized in the polymeric capsules of drug, development of artificial organs, and catheter interventions (Noreen et al., 2016). The important properties of PU are low toxicity, excellent clotting, nonallergic, noncarcinogenic, and nonteratogenic. Being a biodegradable polymer, PLGA has good degradability and biocompatibility and is used broadly in the preparation of NPs, microspheres, pellets, microcapsules, film preparation, and implants. As another kind of controlled drug release material, copolymers of PLGA have been broadly utilized in the controlled release of antibiotic drugs, chemotherapeutic agents, peptides, proteins, polysaccharides, and different drugs.

2.2.2 Based on dimensions

2.2.2.1 *Zero-dimensional nanomaterials*

Nanodimensional materials (within 100 nm) of different thickness, length, and width are divided into nanomaterials of zero dimension, hydroxides, metals and metal oxides, sulfides, silica, carbonates; carbon quantum dots (CD), polyhedral-oligomeric silsesquioxanes; inorganic semiconductor quantum dots, NPs, etc. Various types of NPs are spherical in shape for example silver (Ag), gold (Au), iron (Fe), copper (Cu), etc. and some metal oxides like, oxides of copper (CuO or Cu_2O), oxides of iron (Fe_2O_3 or Fe_3O_4), titanium dioxide (TiO_2), oxides of zinc (ZnO), silica (SiO_2) or silicon dioxide, etc.; like quantum dots, inorganic semiconductor dots, for example, CdS, ZnS, SnTe, CdSe, so forth; and organic quantum dots such as CD, etc. There exist different shapes of zero-dimensional nanomaterials, though the most widely recognized one is spherical and thus might be nanocluster or spherical particles or likewise nanocrystals. They are utilized mainly in polymeric nanocomposites for the development or advancement of some specific properties such as sensor, antimicrobial, optical, catalytic, electronic, and so forth to intact matrix of polymer. For instance, remarkable properties of silver NPs such as antimicrobial, optical, catalytic, etc. The extraordinary catalytic action of NPs of zero dimension in the polymer nanocomposite is credited to their organization having very active features.

2.2.2.2 *One-dimensional nanomaterials*

If the thickness and width of materials are under nanometer range, but the length is in micrometer (μm) scale or more, in that case the nanomaterials are referred to as nanomaterials of one dimension. Nanorods, nanotubes, nanofibers, and nanowires are significant examples of nanomaterials of one-dimensional type, which are commonly utilized to form polymer nanocomposites having different types of polymers, therefore producing elongated structures. Hence, single-walled carbon nanotubes (SWCNTs), multiwalled CNTs (MWCNTs), cellulose nanofibers, carbon nanofibers, polyaniline nanofibers (PANi), nanorods, metal nanotubes, etc. are generally utilized as one-dimensional nanomaterial in various polymer nanocomposites. CNTs are mostly utilized among these, which comprise rolled layers of graphene having each carbon atom sp^2 hybridized and form covalent bonds with the three neighboring atoms of carbon. Among CNT, the SWCNT and MWCNT are commonly used for fabricating nanocomposites of polymers. They consist of unique electrical, mechanical, thermal, and optical properties. However, strong van der Waals forces and presence of layers in between the $\pi-\pi$ stacking make it hard to absorb them within the matrix of polymer without appropriate behavior. Likewise, polymer nanocomposites based on cellulose nanofibers are also known. They are linear polymers, comprising high strength and stiffness because of the large interhydrogen and intramolecular hydrogen bonding among molecules. Also, one-dimensional nanostructures of PANi (nanotube, nanorods, or nanofibers) recently achieve more attention in nanocomposites of polymer due to its remarkably increased dispersibility, processibility, and fundamentally advanced execution when compared with their mass analogs (colloidal and granular PANi) (Sapurina et al., 2010).

2.2.2.3 Two-dimensional nanomaterials

In two-dimensional nanomaterials, two of the parameters, width and length, are in micrometer (μm) range, while its diameter is in nanometer (nm) range; thus nanomaterials of such types are the flattened materials. Oxides of graphene (GO), graphene, reduced graphene oxide (RGO), double-layer hydroxide, nanoclays, and so forth are examples of such type of nanomaterials. Generally, they have exceptionally large surface areas, sufficient quantity of surface functionality, and high-aspect ratios; hence, these types of nanomaterials are best for the polymeric matrices reinforcement. Among a wide range of nanomaterials, nanomaterials of two-dimensional type are mostly applicable to polymer nanocomposites, in which layered silicates or nanoclays have been broadly inserted in polymer nanocomposites. The significant physicochemical properties of montmorillonite nanoclays that are modified organically include high modulus, strength, thermostability, barrier properties, and flame retardancy, which make them able nanomaterials into the domain of polymer nanocomposites. Therefore two-dimensional nanomaterials are present as films, layers, or sheets. Recently, nanomaterials having a combination of more than one nanomaterial have also been utilized in nanocomposites of polymer. In this framework the most usually studied nanomaterials are Fe_3O_4-embedded MWCNT, silver-embedded MWCNT, silver-embedded RGO, sulfur-embedded RGO, TiO_2-embedded RGO, TiO_2-embedded CD, silver-embedded Fe_3O_4, Ag-decorated CD, carbon dot–impregnated Cu_2O, etc. (Karak, 2017). All such nanomaterial mixtures are integrated into different polymer matrices to accomplish numerous wonderful properties for the polymer nanocomposites–end applications.

2.2.2.4 Three-dimensional nanomaterials

The three-dimensional nanomaterials are dimensionless on the nanoscale. These comprise multinanolayers, nanowires bundles, bulk powders, dispersions of nanotubes and NPs, etc. (Fig. 2.1).

2.3 Synthesis of polymer nanomaterials

The technique by which polymer structures can be altered has been made possible by the development of polymeric nanomaterials that have the ability to assimilate targeting moiety and develop multicomponent systems that can encapsulate multiple drugs with different chemical and physical properties. Polymers nanomaterial can be synthesized by many techniques, which are discussed in the following subsections.

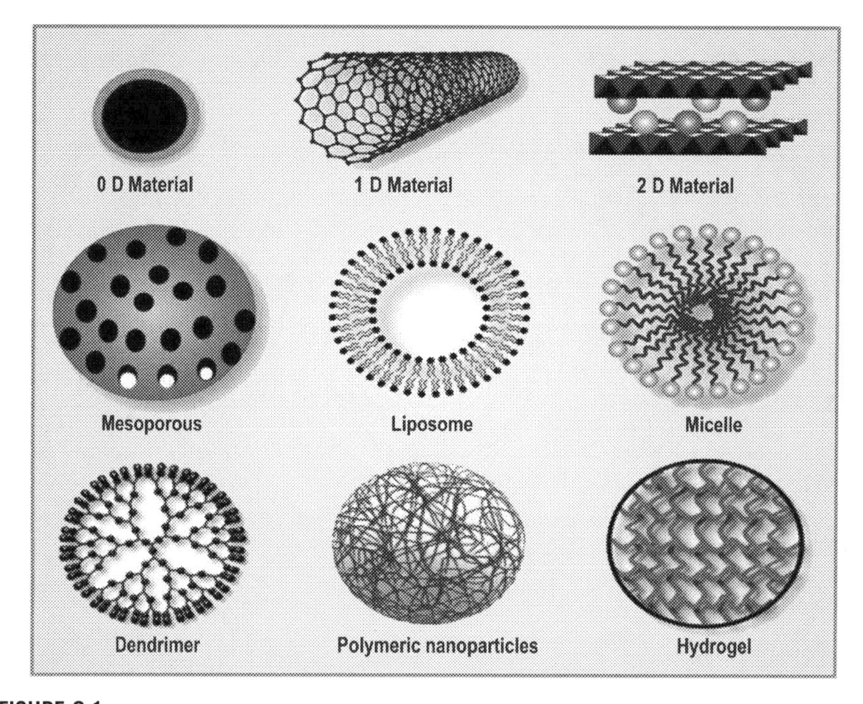

FIGURE 2.1

Different types of polymer nanomaterials.

2.3.1 Nanotubes

Nanotubes can be synthesized by the following techniques (Fig. 2.2):

1. *Chemical vapor deposition:* This method was discovered by Roy Gordon in 1970 at Harvard University (Bierman et al., 2010). This is the most commonly used method for CNTs, in which one or more volatile precursors are transported via the vapor phase to the reaction chamber where they decompose on a heated substrate (Rakszawski et al., 2009) (Fig. 2.3).
2. *Arc discharge:* By this method, one can synthesize CNTs. In this method a direct current arc voltage is applied across two graphite electrodes immersed in an inert gas such as He. This method was used in 1991 in carbon shoot of graphite electrodes and the principle of this technique is to vaporize carbon in the presence of catalyst (boron, yttrium, iron, nickel, cobalt, gadolinium, etc.) under reduced atmosphere of inert gas (argon and helium) (Coulombe et al., 2008) (Fig. 2.4).
3. *Laser ablation:* This technique was developed by Dr. Richard Smalley and coworker at Rice University and is more expensive than arc discharge and chemical vapor decomposition methods (Beecher et al., 2016) (Fig. 2.5).

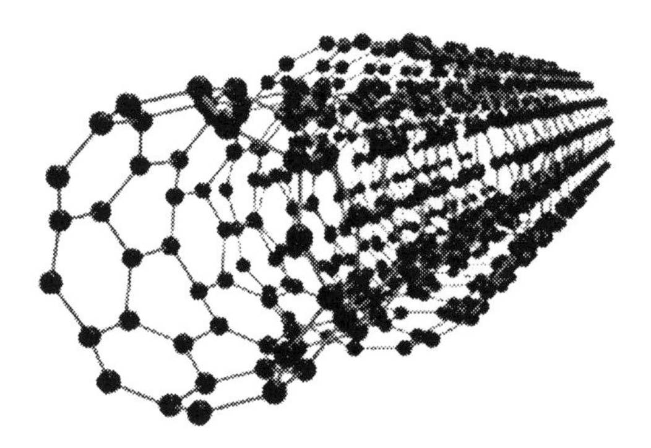

FIGURE 2.2

Schematic image of carbon nanotubes.

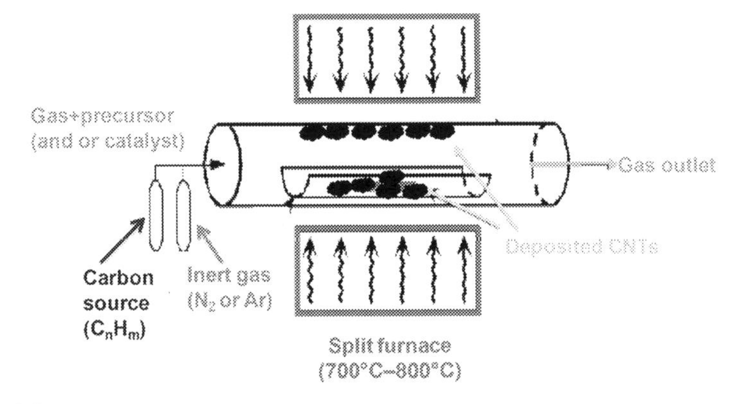

FIGURE 2.3

Schematic presentation of chemical vapor deposition method.

2.3.2 Nanowires

Nanowires are nanostructures with diameter of order of nanometer. There are different types of nanowires such as superconducting, metallic, semiconducting, and insulating (Jung and Yong, 2011). The technique for preparation of nanowires includes (Fig. 2.6):

1. *Vapor–liquid–solid method*: In 1964 this method was first reported by Wagner and Ellis for silicon whiskers. This is a common method for preparing nanowires having diameter ranging from hundred of nm to hundreds of μm (Christesen et al., 2013).
2. *Solution phase synthesis:* In this method, nanowires are grown in solution, and in comparison to other methods the solution phase synthesis can produce large number of nanowires; this is very a versatile technique for producing nanowires of gold, silver, platinum, and lead (DeBoef et al., 2013).

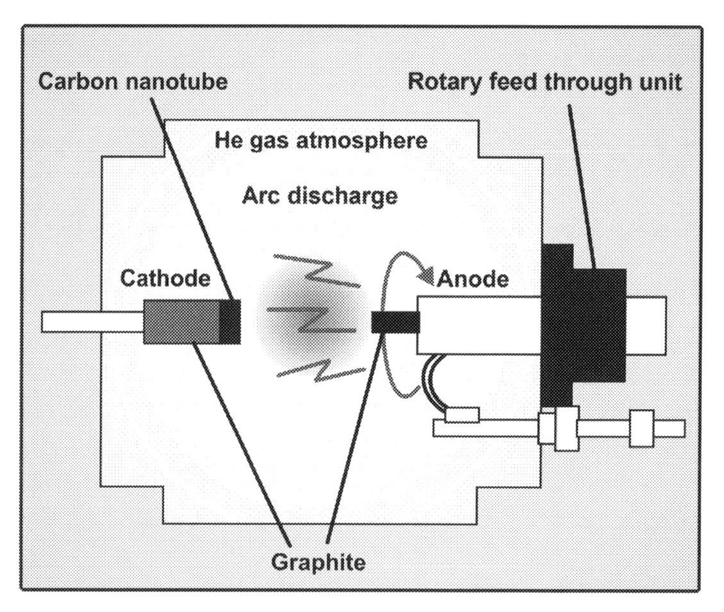

FIGURE 2.4

The image depicting arc discharge method.

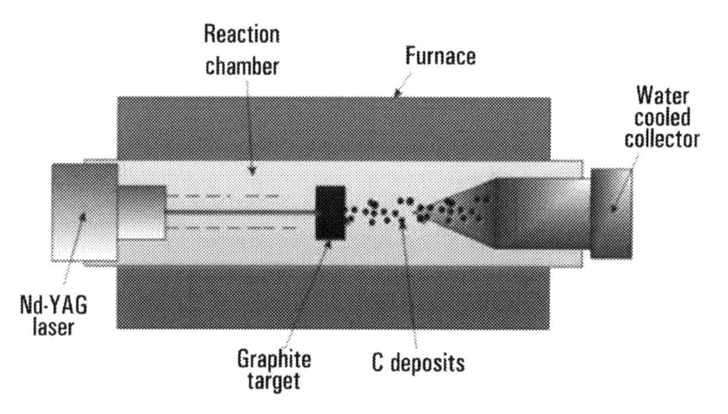

FIGURE 2.5

Pictorial presentation of laser ablation method.

3. *Noncatalytic growth:* Nanowires can also be produced with the help of catalyst, by which we get pure nanowires and the number of technological step is minimized. The simplest method to obtain nanowires is by heating of metals, that is, metal wires are heated with battery by joule heating in air (Jain and Rivest, 2013).

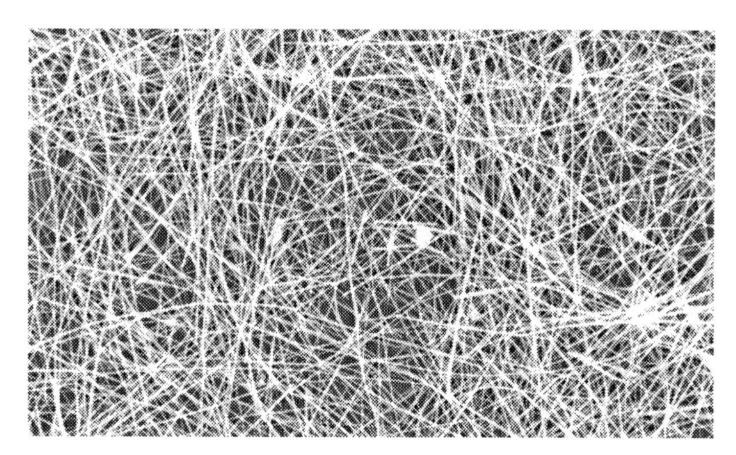

FIGURE 2.6

A typical SEM image of nanowires.

4. *DNA-template metallic nanowire synthesis:* For metallic nanowire synthesis an emerging field is to make use of DNA strand as scaffolds. This method was used for the synthesis of metallic nanowires in electronic components and for bio-sensing applications. This method allows transduction of DNA strand into metallic nanowires which can be detected electrically (Park et al., 2002).

2.3.3 Nanorods

In nanotechnology, nanorods are one of the morphologies of the nanoscale objects. Their dimensions range from 1 to 100 nm and they can be synthesized from metals or semiconducting materials. Synthesis of nanorods includes (Fig. 2.7):

1. *ZnO nanorods:* They are also known as nanowires; the optical band gap of ZnO nanorods can be regulated by changing the morphology, composition, size, etc. In comparison to this method the growth of nanorods from the vapor phase is a more developed method. By thermal oxidation processes, many metal oxide nanorods (ZnO, CuO, V_2O_5, Fe_2O_3) can be made simply by heating the starting metal in air (Guo et al., 2018) (Fig. 2.8).
2. *Gold nanorods:* One of the most common methods for synthesizing gold nanorods is the seed-mediated growth method. The growth solution is prepared by reduction of $HAuCL_4$ with ascorbic acid in the presence of cetyltrimethyl ammonium bromide surfactant and silver ions (Nazir et al., 2016) (Fig. 2.9).
3. *Cation exchange:* For the synthesis of new nanorods the cation exchange is a conventional technique. Cation exchanges in nanorods are kinetically favorable and often shape conversing also. In comparison to the bulk crystal systems, the cation exchange of nanorods is million times faster due to high surface area (Müller et al., 2017).

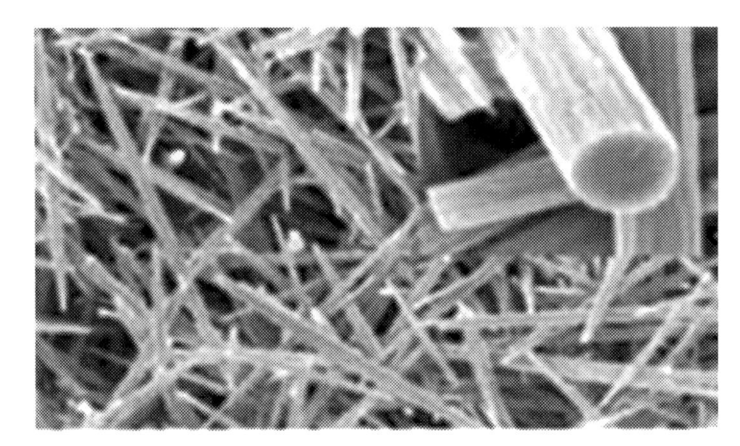

FIGURE 2.7

A typical SEM image of nanorods.

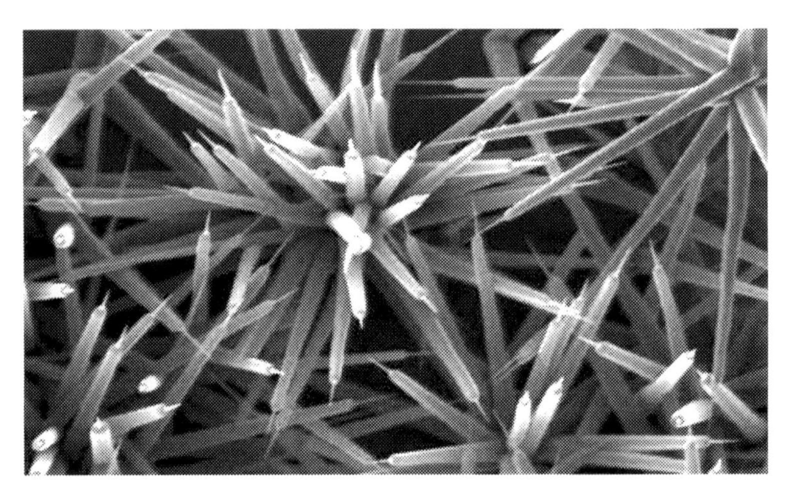

FIGURE 2.8

A SEM image of ZnO nanorods.

2.3.4 Nanocomposites

There are various widely used synthesis methods that are suitable for preparing nanocomposites, which are described as follows:

1. *Solution blending:* For fabrication of a nanocomposite the solution blending is the most commonly used method. The process involves mixing of polymer solutions and dispersed fillers in a suitable solvent. The most commonly used solvents are chloroform, water, and toluene (Dalod et al., 2017). By precipitation and simple filtration, nanocomposite can be obtained (Fig. 2.10).

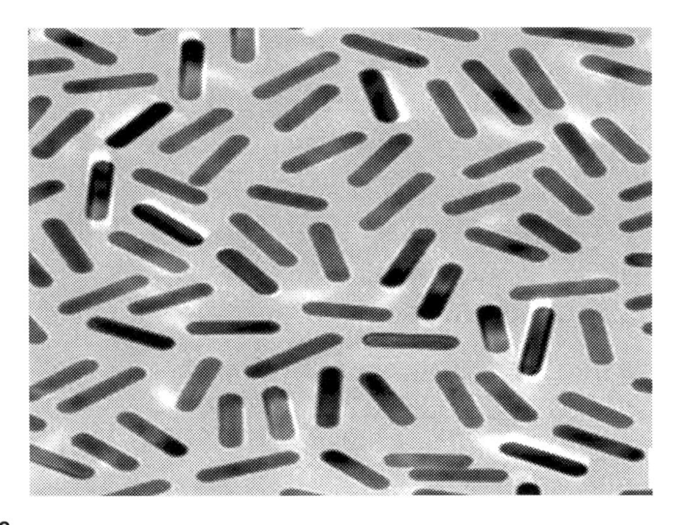

FIGURE 2.9

Image of gold nanorods.

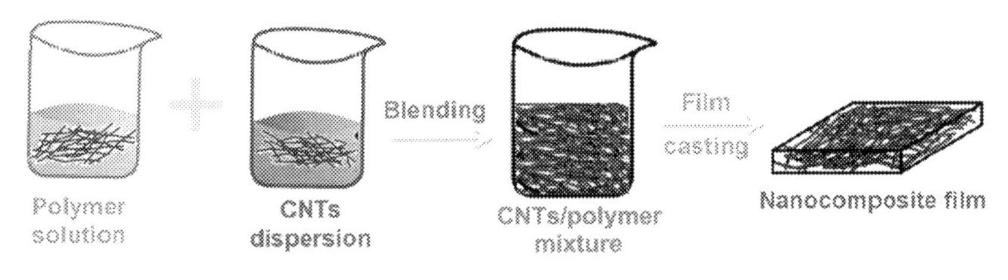

FIGURE 2.10

Images of solution blending method.

2. *Melt processing:* This process is also known as melt blending or melt compounding and is a cost-effective and simple technique that removes the use of toxic solvents. Blending can be done by injection molding or extrusion, due to high viscosity of thermoplastic polymers controlling the filler distribution in the matrix (Styskalik et al., 2017). High temperature is normally required in this process for the melting of polymer and mechanical or shear forces for uniform dispersion of the filler (Fig. 2.11).
3. *In situ polymerization*: This method yields a uniform distribution of fillers in polymer matrix and avoids the use of solvents. It involves preparation of a mixture of monomer and filler particles, which is further polymerized by some standard polymerization methods such as stirring, ultrasonication, and UV curing. Polymers that cannot be prepared by solution blending and melt processing can be dealt by this method. This method was reported to produce

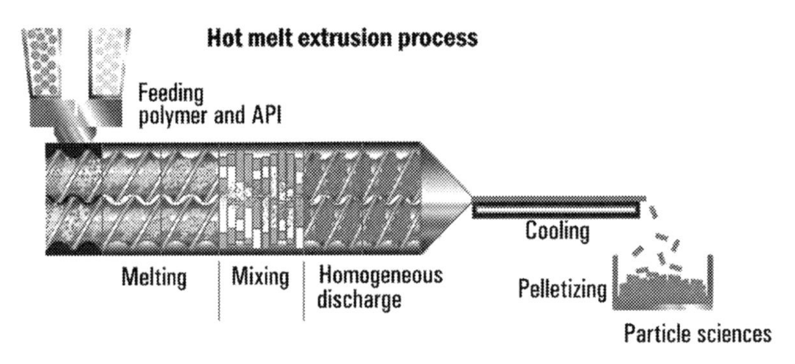

FIGURE 2.11

Image showing the melt processing method.

nanocomposites with noncovalent and covalent bonding between the constituent components (Cheng et al., 2015). Thermally unstable and insoluble polymers can also be prepared by this technique.

2.4 Mechanism of formation of nanoparticles

2.4.1 Sol–gel method

This process is a wet chemical technique, which is known as chemical solution deposition, and involves several steps in chronological order: hydrolysis and polycondensation, gelation, aging, drying, densification, and crystallization (Buchkremer et al., 2011). This process is used for the fabrication of both ceramic and glassy materials. In sol–gel method the solution involves gradual formation of gel-like network that contains both solid and liquid phases. By this method, one can produce solid materials from small molecules. This method is also used for fabrication of metal oxides, mainly the oxides of silicon and titanium (Fig. 2.12).

2.4.2 Hydrothermal

This method can be defined as a method of synthesis of single crystal that depends on the solubility of minerals in hot water at high pressure. The crystal growth is carried out in an apparatus that consists of a steel pressure vessel called autoclave, in which nutrients are supplied while maintaining water temperature between the opposite ends of the growth chamber. The nutrient solutes dissolve at the hotter end, and at the cooler end a seed crystal is deposited, thus achieving the growth of the desired crystal (Aldrich-Wright et al., 2016) (Fig. 2.13).

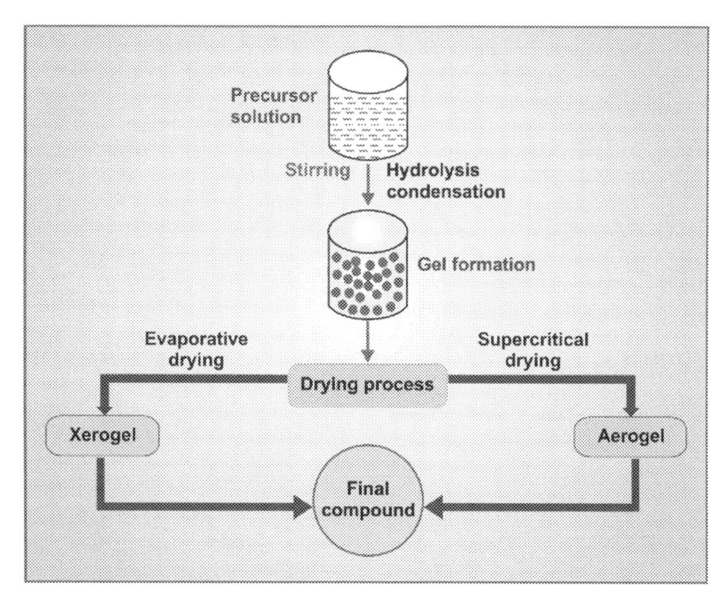

FIGURE 2.12

Schematic presentation of a sol–gel method.

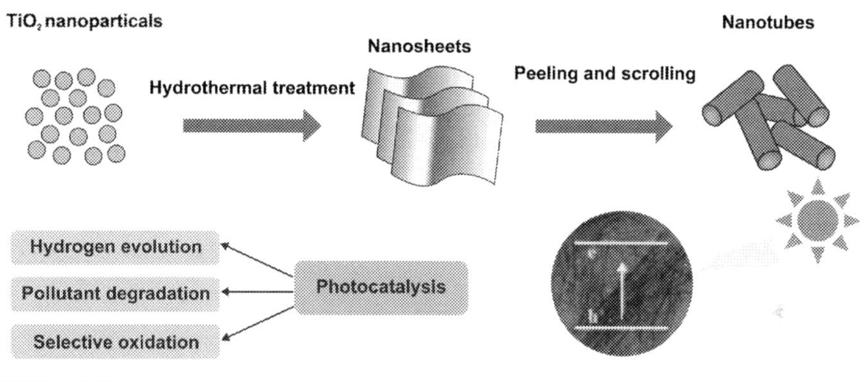

FIGURE 2.13

Image showing the presentation of a hydrothermal method.

2.4.3 Physical vapor deposition

This process is often known as the atomistic deposition process, and in this process the materials are vaporized from solid or liquid sources in the form of atoms or molecules and transported in the form of vapors through vacuum or low pressure gas (Haputhanthri et al., 2017). This process in some respect is similar to chemical vapor deposition method except that in this physical vapor deposition

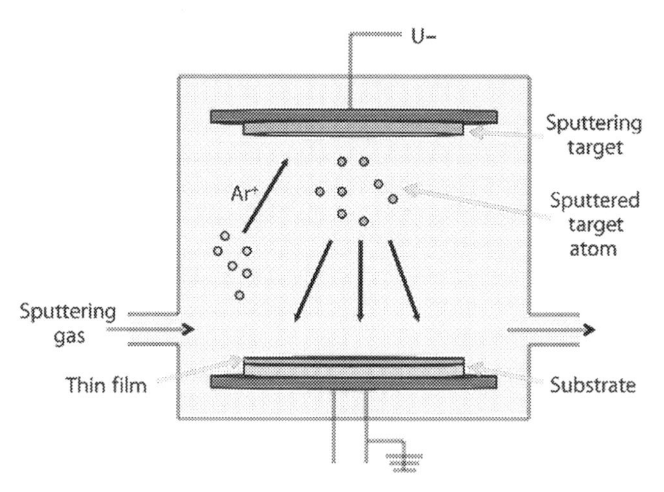

FIGURE 2.14

Schematic presentation of a PVD method. *PVD*, physical vapor deposition.

the precursors, that is, the materials, are deposited started out in solid form, while in chemical vapor deposition the precursors are introduced in reaction chamber in gas form (Fig. 2.14).

2.4.4 Hydrolysis

This is reverse of condensation reaction, and in this process, two molecules join together to form a large molecule and eject out water molecules. In this process, water is added to cause hydrolysis that breaks down the bonds; while in condensation process the molecule is build up by removing water and solvents. Some hydration reactions lead to hydrolyzes (Sá et al., 2017). In simple words, the hydrolysis is a chemical reaction in which water is used to break the bonds in particular molecules. Reactants other than water and products may be neutral molecules; in most hydrolysis processes, it involves organic compounds or ionic molecules such as hydrolysis of acids, bases, and salts.

2.5 Control of morphological parameters (factors controlling the shape and size of nanoparticles)

2.5.1 Concentration of monomer/polymer

In liquid-phase method to control the size and shape of NPs, it is essential to consider the balance between the available amount and the consumption rates of monomer and polymer, while in the case of open systems such as a semibatch reactor a monomer is continuously fed from outside the system using a constant rate pump etc.

The particle formation process involved various stages such as the prenucleation, nucleation, and growth stages. In prenucleation stage the concentration of monomer and polymer increases with time, and when the precursor monomer concentration reaches a critical value, generation of nucleus begins. The smallest diameter of stable nucleus is determined by the free energy of the aggregation of nuclei and the surface area. Then, in the growth stage, monomers/polymers supplied are consumed for the growth of the stable nuclei. To synthesize a monodisperse particle, it is desirable to separate the nucleation and the growth stages. However, in general, it is difficult to separate these stages. Consequently, the supplied monomers are consumed competitively by the nucleation and the growth of the generated nuclei. Thus to synthesize monodispersed particles, we can increase the nucleation rate or decrease the growth rate as much as possible.

In the case of polymeric NPs the control of size is not easy. On the basis of material the preparation method of polymeric NPs is classified into two types: monomers or polymers. Polyalkylcyanoacrylate NP is one of the typical polymeric NPs prepared from monomers with simultaneous polymerization. Bauduin et al. (1979) first reported this method in which alkylcyanoacrylate monomers are added into hydrochloric acid solution containing a surface-active agent (surfactant) at constant stirring. On the other hand, Al Khouri Falloug et al. (1986) described that nanocapsules were produced from monomers (isobutylcyanoacrylate) impregnated with drug by applying the interfacial polymerization technique.

2.5.2 By different methodologies

Different methodologies for the synthesis of NPs can play a major role to decide the crystalline behavior of the material. Several methods have been proposed for controlling the shape and size of NPs generated by the liquid-phase method: template synthesis using a surfactant (Gu et al., 2000), the solvothermal method (Yoshimura and Yu, 2002), the hot soap method (Peng et al., 2000), the solvothermal method, and the microemulsion method (Li et al., 1999).

The process for controlling the shape and size of particles is as follows: controlling the nucleation rate to increase the growth rate of nuclei or suppression of the aggregation of generated nuclei. If two-dimensional nucleation does not occur on the particle surface, the obtained particles are amorphous in nature. It is due to uncontrolled growth in any direction at the same growth rate in the generated nuclei. The typical example of this type of particle synthesis is the sol–gel method, for example, the surfactant or polymer in the solvent forms a hexagonal structure and a lamellar structure, etc., depending on the concentration. Using these structures as templates, rod-like particles, plate particles, etc. can be synthesized.

In the case of crystalline particles, it is necessary to keep a balance between the nucleation and the growth rates of nuclei. If the nucleation rate is faster than the growth rate, the generated particles are polycrystalline spherical particles. For example, for sulfide and oxide particles, the critical concentration is low and the growth rate of nuclei is fast so that the polycrystalline particles are formed.

2.5.3 By mechanical temperature

The effect of processing temperature on the composing process is a very important tool to discuss because the mechanical processing generates heat in the equipment. Therefore, to control the deformation of NPs, it is necessary to control the processing temperature. For example, when resin is used as the feed material, the processing temperature needs to be kept below its glass-transition temperature. On the other hand, it is reported that the higher the temperature is, the denser becomes the NP layer on the core particles when composing metal and ceramic particles (Abe et al., 2008). To investigate the processing temperature effect on the properties of particle composites, it is necessary to know the actual temperature at the particle surface during the composing process (Nogi et al., 1996). The particle-surface temperature was estimated thermodynamically from the reaction of oxide layer on the surface of metal particle and the added carbon. It is believed that the temperature at the particle surface reaches about 10 times higher than that of the composing vessel. This temperature effect can initiate highly specific phenomena at the particle surface and enhance the bonding strength between the particles to a great extent during the particle-composing process.

2.5.4 By revolution intensity of machine

The operating parameters of the machine can also affect the size and shape of particles including temperature, mechanical intensity, pressure, the type of the machine, etc. For example, in the case of the mechanical effect, it is considered that the higher the revolution of the machine is, the stronger is the force on the powder and on the particles between the interfaces so that on increasing the revolution, the frequency of the mechanical force on the particles also increases, which reduces the specific surface area of the NPs (Asahi et al., 1998).

In composite particles the mechanical force is responsible for the shape and size. The NPs are composed on the surface of core particle depending on the contact number between the particles and various effects, including the mechanical and thermal. The formation of nanocomposites generally involves two steps. In the first step, the surfaces of the core particles are activated and different kinds of NPs adhere to it. As a result, the adhesion ratio R of the NPs to the core particles increases, so that the specific surface area of the nanocomposites mixture decreases. In the second step, the NP layer itself bonded onto the surface of core particle (Kondo et al., 1993).

2.6 Characteristics of polymeric nanoparticles

2.6.1 Size

For achieving therapeutic efficacy the NPs size is a key factor in the biodistribution of long-circulating NPs in various physiological parameters such as hepatic filtration, tissue extravasation, tissue diffusion, and kidney excretion. In a study, in vivo biodistribution and varying particle sizes of 50 and 500 nm showed higher levels of agglomeration of the larger NPs in the liver. For example, for the passive drug delivery through the epidermis the prominent size limit is below 500 Da. The mesh spacing between mucin fibers of mucus ranges from 100 to 1000 nm, while the blood capillaries are in the range of $\sim 5-40\ \mu m$ in diameter. The mammalian vasculature has an average pore size of ~ 5 nm. NPs below this size range can easily transverse the endothelium and equilibrate with the extracellular space. The size of the NP was also observed to have a substantial effect on the protein absorption. Small (<100 nm), medium (100–200 nm), and large (>200 nm) pegylated poly(hexadecyl cyanoacrylate) NPs incubated with serum protein for 2 h showed a significant correlation between particle size and protein absorption (Fang et al., 2006). Protein absorption on small NPs (80 nm) was quantified (6%) and compared to the same NP formulation with a larger size (171 and 243 nm, 23% and 34%, respectively). In blood clearance kinetics and murine macrophages the effect of protein absorption on different sized NPs was confirmed by the analysis of NP. Blood clearance of the smaller NPs was twice as slow as with the larger NP formulations. Furthermore, the amount of drug encapsulated in NPs that accumulated in the tumor within 24 h was observed twice in comparison of the larger NP formulation. The size of NPs and its polydispersity can also significantly affect the biodistribution of NPs. Hennink et al. (2007) carried out crosslinking of micelles incubated in phosphate buffer saline (pH 7.4) at 37°C for more than 3 days and observed that they did not show substantial increases in size and polydispersity in contrast to noncross-linked micelles (PD ~ 0.5 after 10 h). Stable micelles showed a long circulation half-life of ~ 8 h due to a low rate of hepatic uptake (liver $\sim 10\%$ of the injected dose; spleen $\sim 2\%$ of the injected dose).

2.6.2 Shape

The physiochemical properties of NPs effectively depend on their morphology. Various research works have been focused on synthesizing nanomaterials with different shapes, such as nanooctahedrons, nanorods, nanocubes, nanohexagons, nanowires, nanotubes, nanoplates, nanoflowers, nanorings, and nanocapsules. Some authors performed an in vitro biocompatibility study on NPs with different morphologies including nanooctahedrons, nanorods, and nanocubes in human A549 lung tumor cells (Bao et al., 2012). These experiments were evaluated at different concentrations in the range of $10-1000\ \mu g/mL$ and the CCK-8 assay results revealed that after 24 h of incubation, more than 90% of cells survived which clearly indicated that these NPs were quite safe to the cells within the tested concentration range. Carboxyl-terminated poly(ethylene glycol)-phospholipids (DSPE-PEG)-coated iron oxide NPs with spherical, hexagonal, and wire-like shape for enhanced dispersion in water were tested in ECA-109 cells, and the results showed that such NPs were uptaken by cancer cells, and the particles induced negligible toxicity to the cells without laser irradiation (Chu et al., 2013; Xie et al., 2018).

2.7 Conclusion

In this chapter, we presented a detailed overview of NPs, their types, synthesis, and their structural control by different methodologies. Due to their nanosize, NPs have a large surface area that makes them a suitable candidate for various applications such as drug delivery, magnetic drug targeting, etc. Besides this, the physicochemical properties are also dominant at that size, which further increase the importance of these materials in applications. Synthetic techniques can be useful to control the specific morphology, size, and magnetic properties of NPs. Though NPs are useful for many applications, still there are some health hazard concerns due to their uncontrollable use and discharge to natural environment, which should be considered for making the use of NPs more convenient and ecofriendly.

References

Abe, I., Sato, K., Abe, H., Naito, M., 2008. Formation of porous fumed silica coating on the surface of glass fibers by a dry mechanical processing technique. Adv. Powder Technol. 19, 311–320.

Aldrich-Wright, J.R., Harper, B.W.J., Morris, T.T., Gailer, J.J., 2016. Inorg. Biochem. 163, 95–102.

Achachelouei, M.F., Knopf-Marques, H., Ribeiro da Silva, C.E., Barthès, J., Bat, E., Tezcaner, A., et al., 2019. Use of nanoparticles in tissue engineering and regenerative medicine. Front. Bioeng. Biotechnol. 7, 113.

Al Khouri Falloug, N., Fessi, H., Ph Devissaguet, J., Puisieux, F., Roblot-Treupel, L., 1986. Rapid communication: Nanocapsule formation by interfacial polymer deposition following solvent displacement. Int. J. Pharm. 28, 125–132.

Aminabhavi, T.M., Chaturvedi, K., Ganguly, K., Krauss, L., Kulkarni, A.R., Nadagouda, M.N., et al., 2015. Oral insulin delivery using deoxycholic acid conjugated PEGylated polyhydroxybutyrate co-polymeric nanoparticles. Nanomedicine 10, 1569–1583.

Amp, A.F., Dong, C.H., Guo, D., Gou, S., Liu, J., Zhu, P., 2014. Selective oxidized modification of alginate fiber. Dyeing Finish. 8, 482–490.

Anderson, C.J., Fiamengo, A.L., Hagooly, A., Hawker, C.J., Pressly, E.D., Ramos, N., et al., 2011. Evaluation of multivalent, functional polymeric nanoparticles for imaging applications. ACS Nano 5, 738–747.

Asahi, A., Endo, S., Hatta, T., Naito, M., Tanimoto, T., 1998. Kagaku Kogaku Ronbunshu 24, 99–103.

Badawy, M.E.I., Hofte, M., Rabea, E.I., Rogge, T., Stevens, C.V., Smagghe, G., et al., 2004. Synthesis and fungicidal activity of new *N,O*-acyl chitosan derivatives. Biomacromolecules 5, 589–595.

Bao, S., Han, Y., Ren, L., Shi, Y., Wu, S., Zhou, X., 2012. Controllable synthesis, magnetic and biocompatible properties of Fe_3O_4 and α-Fe_2O_3 nanocrystals. J. Solid. State Chem. 196, 138–144.

Bauduin, P., Couvreur, P., Guiot, P., Kante, B., Roland, M., Speiser, P., 1979. Polycyanoacrylate nanocapsules as potential lysosomotropic carriers: preparation, morphological and sorptive properties. J. Pharm. Pharmacol. 31, 331–332.

Beecher, S.J., Eason, R.W., Grant-Jacob, Hua, P., James, A., Parsonage, T.L., et al., 2016. An 11.5 W Yb:YAG planar waveguide laser fabricated via pulsed laser deposition. Opt. Mater. Express 6.

Bierman, M.J., Jin, S., Morin, S.A., Tong, J., 2010. Mechanism and kinetics of spontaneous nanotube growth driven by screw dislocations. Science 328 (5977), 476–480.

Buchkremer, H.P., Nedelec, R., Sebold, D., Stoever, D., Uhlenbruck, S., 2011. ECS Trans. 35, 2275.

Burchiel, S., Gao, J., Gigliotti, A., Mcdonald, J., Mitchell, L., Wal, R.V., 2007. Pulmonary and systemic immune response to inhaled multiwalled carbon nanotubes. Toxicol. Sci. 100, 203–214.

Cao, H.L., Peng, W., Yuan, L.I., Zhao, S.S., 2012. Preparation and characterization of PLA/MMT nanocomposites with microwave irradiation. J. Mater. Eng. 2, 4.

Cazeneuve, S., Tao, F., Wang, T., Wen, Z., Wu, L., 2016. Effective recovery of poly-β-hydroxybutyrate (PHB) biopolymer from Cupriavidus necator using a novel and environmentally friendly solvent system. Biotechnol. Prog. 32, 678–685.

Chen, Z., Sha, L., Yang, Z., Zhang, A., 2016. Polylactic acid based nanocomposites: promising safe and biodegradable materials in biomedical field. Int. J. Polym. Sci. 2016, 1–11.

Cheng, D., Jin, A., Hu, L., Yang, H., Yu, D., Zhang, Q., 2015. Scandium and gadolinium codoped $BaTiO_3$ nanoparticles and ceramics prepared by sol-gel-hydrothermal method: facile synthesis, structural characterization and enhancement of electrical properties. Powder Technol. 283, 433–439.

Chou, C., Li, C., Yang, T., 2005. Antibacterial activity of *N*-alkylated disaccharide chitosan derivatives. Int. J. Food Microbiol. 97, 237–245.

Christesen, J.D., Cahoon, J.F., Grumstrup, E.M., Papanikolas, J.M., Pinion, C.W., 2013. Nano Lett. 13, 6281–6286.

Chu, M., Dai, X., Peng, J., Li, H., Shao, Y., Wu, Q., 2013. Near-infrared laser light mediated cancer therapy by photothermal effect of Fe_3O_4 magnetic nanoparticles. Biomaterials 34, 4078–4088.

Coulombe, S., Swanson, E.J., Tavares, Jason, 2008. Plasma synthesis of coated metal nanoparticles with surface properties tailored for dispersion. Plasma Process. Polym. 5 (8), 759.

Cyras, V.P., Moran, J.I., Vazquez, A., 2013. Bio-nanocomposites based on derivatized potato starch and cellulose, preparation and characterization. J. Mater. Sci. 48, 7196–7203.

Dalod, A.R.M., Grendal, O.G., Skjærvø, S.L., Inzani, K., Selbach, S.M., Henriksen, L., et al., 2017. Controlling oriented attachment and in situ functionalization of TiO_2 nanoparticles during hydrothermal synthesis with APTES. J. Phys. Chem. C 121, 11897–11906.

Dan, L., Dandan, Z., Jinyu, H., Kai, Z., Xiaohua, W., Zheng, J., 2018. Polymer-based nanomaterials and applications for vaccines and drugs. Polymers 10, 31.

Danhier, F., Ansorena, E., Silva, J.M., Coco, R., Breton, A.L., Preat, V., 2012. PLGA-based nanoparticles: an overview of biomedical applications. J. Controlled Release 161, 505–522.

DeBoef, B.A., Del Padre, N.A., Hooper, M.M., Naumiec, R.G., St. Germaine, A., 2013. Modern apparatus for performing flash chromatography: an experiment for the organic laboratory. J. Chem. Educ. 90, 376–378.

Elsabahy, M., Wooley, K.L., 2012. Design of polymeric nanoparticles for biomedical delivery applications. Chem. Soc. Rev. 41, 2545–2561.

Fang, C., et al., 2006. In vivo tumor targeting of tumor necrosis factor-alpha-loaded stealth nanoparticles: effect of MePEG molecular weight and particle size. Eur. J. Pharm. Sci. 27, 27–36.

Gomes, M.E., Mano, J.F., Santo, V.E., Reis, R.L., 2012. From nano- to macro-scale: nanotechnology approaches for spatially controlled delivery of bioactive factors for bone and cartilage engineering. Nanomedicine (Lond.) 7, 1045–1066.

Gu, Z., Li, Y., Wan, J., 2000. The formation of cadmium sulfide nanowires in different liquid crystal systems. Mat. Sci. Eng. A 286, 106.

Guo, et al., 2018. Efficient DNA-assisted synthesis of trans-membrane gold nanowires. Microsyst. Nanoeng. 4, 17084.

Gusev, A.I., Rempel, A.A., 2004. Nanocrystalline Materials. Cambridge International Science Publishing, Cambridge, p. 354.

Haputhanthri, R., Ojha, R., Izgorodina, E.I., Guo, S.X., Deacon, G.B., McNaughton, D., et al., 2017. Vib. Spectrosc. 92, 82–95.

He, H., Lin, X., Lu, W., Tang, X., Tian, B., Yang, H., et al., 2014. PEG-PLGA copolymers: their structure and structure-influenced drug delivery applications. J. Controlled Release 183, 77–86.

Hennink, W.E., Nostrum, C.F., Rijcken, C.J., Schiffelers, R.M., Snel, C.J., 2007. Hydrolysable core-crosslinked thermosensitive polymeric micelles: synthesis, characterisation and in vivo studies. Biomaterials 28, 5581–5593.

Ho, H.K., Pastorin, G., Tan, A., Zhao, C., 2013. Nanomaterial scaffolds for stem cell proliferation and differentiation in tissue engineering. Biotechnol. Adv. 31, 654–668.

Hubler, A., Osuagwu, O., 2010. Digital quantum batteries: energy and information storage in nanovacuum tube arrays. Complexity 15, 5.

Jain, P.K., Rivest, J.B., 2013. Cation exchange on the nanoscale: an emerging technique for new material synthesis, device fabrication, and chemical sensing. Chem. Soc. Rev. 42, 89–96.

Jayakumar, R., Nwe, N., Tokura, S., Tamura, H., 2007. Sulfated chitin and chitosan as novel biomaterials. Int. J. Biol. Macromol. 40, 175–181.

Jung, S., Yong, K., 2011. Fabrication of CuO-ZnO nanowires on a stainless steel mesh for highly efficient photocatalytic applications. Chem. Commun. 47 (9), 2643–2645.

Karak, N., 2017. Biobased Smart Polyurethane Nanocomposites: From Synthesis to Applications. The Royal Society of Chemistry, Cambridge, p. 26.

Kohane, D.S., Langer, R., 2008. Polymeric biomaterials in tissue engineering. Pediatr. Res. 63, 487–491.

Kondo, A., Naito, M., Yokoyama, T., 1993. Application of comminution techniques for the surface modification of powder materials. ISIJ Int. 33, 915–924.

Lee, K.Y., Mooney, D.J., 2012. Alginate: properties and biomedical applications. Prog. Polym. Sci. 37, 106–126.

Li, M., Mann, S., Schnablegger, H., 1999. Coupled synthesis and self-assembly of nanoparticles to give structures with controlled organization. Nature 402, 393.

Lu, Z.R., 2010. Molecular imaging of HPMA copolymers: visualizing drug delivery in cell, mouse and man. Adv. Drug. Deliv. Rev. 62, 246–257.

McGovern, C., 2010. Commoditization of nanomaterials. Nanotechnol. Percept. 6 (3), 155–178.

Müller, K., Bugnicourt, E., Latorre, M., Jorda, M., Echegoyen Sanz, Y., Lagaron, J.M., et al., 2017. Review on the processing and properties of polymer nanocomposites and nanocoatings and their applications in the packaging, automotive and solar energy fields. Nanomaterials 7, 74.

Nazir, M.S., Kassim, M.H.M., Mohapatra, L., Gilani, M.A., Raza, M.R., Majeed, K., 2016. Characteristic properties of nanoclays and characterization of nanoparticulate and nanocomposites. Nanoclay Reinforced Polymer Composites. Springer, Singapore, pp. 35–55.

Nogi, K., Naito, M., Kondo, A., Nakamura, A., Niihara, K., Yokoyama, T., 1996. New method for elucidation of temperature at the interface between particles under mechanical stirring. Powder Metall. 43, 396–401.

Noreen, A., Tabasum, S., Zia, K.M., Zahoor, A.F., Zuber, M., 2016. Bio-based polyurethane: an efficient and environment friendly coating systems: a review. Prog. Org. Coat. 91, 25–32.

Park, W.I., Kim, M., Pennycook, S.J., Yi, G.C., 2002. ZnO nanoneedles grown vertically on Si substrates by non-catalytic vapor-phase epitaxy. Adv. Mater. 14, 1841–1843.

Peng, X., Manna, L., Yang, W., 2000. Shape control of CdSe nanocrystals. Nature 404 (6773), 59–61.

Rakszawski, J.F., Walker Jr., P.L., Imperial, G.R., 2009. Carbon formation from carbon monoxide-hydrogen mixtures over iron catalyst. I. Properties of carbon formed. J. Phys. Chem. 63 (2), 133–140.

Ravi Kumar, M.N.V., 2000. A review of chitin and chitosan applications. React. Funct. Polym. 46, 1–27.

Rebecca, J., 2016. Alginate fiber from brown algae. Der Pharm. Lett. 8, 68–71.

Sá, J., Fernandes, D.L.A., Pavliuk, M.V., Szlachetko, J., 2017. Catal. Sci. Technol. 7, 1050–1054.

Sapurina, I., Stejskal, J., Trchová, M., 2010. Polyaniline nanostructures and the role of aniline oligomers in their formation. Prog. Polym. Sci. 35, 1420–1481.

Sirivongpaisal, P., Wittaya, T., Woggum, T., 2014. Properties and characteristics of dual-modified rice starch based biodegradable films. Int. J. Biol. Macromol. 67, 490–502.

Styskalik, A., Skoda, D., Barnes, C., Pinkas, J., 2017. The power of non-hydrolytic sol-gel chemistry: a review. Catalysts 7, 168.

Xie, W., Guo, Z., Gao, F., Gao, Q., Wang, D., Bor-shuang, L., et al., 2018. Shape-,size- and structure-controlled synthesis and biocompatibility of iron oxide nanoparticles for magnetic theranostics. Theranostics 8, 12.

Yoshimura, M., Yu, S., 2002. Shape and phase control of ZnS nanocrystals: template fabrication of wurtzite ZnS single-crystal nanosheets and ZnO flake-like dendrites from a lamellar molecular precursor $ZnS{\cdot}(NH_2CH_2CH_2NH_2)_{0.5}$. Adv. Mater. 14, 296.

CHAPTER

Polymeric nanomaterials in drug delivery

3

Anil Kumar Bajpai[1] and Rajesh Kumar Saini[2]

[1]*Government Model Science College, Jabalpur, India*

[2]*Government Post Graduate College, Tikamgarh, India*

3.1 Introduction

Drugs are low-molecular-weight chemical compounds given for a short duration or on the regular basis and that are not endogenous biochemical, show therapeutic response, and prescribed for prevention or diagnosis of diseases ("Drug", 2007; Drug Definition, 2014). The treatments of acute disease or chronic illnesses have been achieved by delivering drugs in various dosage forms or by various routes of administration at predetermined and controlled rate required to the body during treatment of disease because the rate of the drug uptake not only depends on the drug properties such as solubility, charge, molecular size, and so on but also on site of administration as well as the external stimuli such as pH, temperature, presence of enzyme, active transport mechanisms, and so on.

Since ancient times, plant-originated compounds have been used as drugs for the treatment of various diseases including cancer, skin disease originated by microbes, cough and cold, diabetes, cardiovascular, inflammatory by human due to their unique properties such as less toxicity, extraordinary chemical diversity, low price, good therapeutic potential, and macromolecular specificity. Despite several advantages, there are many challenges in the clinic trails of natural products such as large size, low biocompatibility, in vivo instability, poor absorption, less effectiveness, poor bioavailability and solubility, and problems in delivering to target-specific sites. Therefore there is a need of developing new controlled, targeted drug delivery systems that may be able to deliver drugs to specific body effectively and efficiently without any adverse side effects (Martinho et al., 2011; Jahangirian et al., 2017).

Drug delivery is an advanced technology that is applied in biomedical fields for cure and diagnosis of various types of diseases (Cregg and Mardinoglu, 2012). Ideally, drug delivery systems that are used to deliver drug molecules at site of action under controlled rate for either short time or longer duration as per needs of the body over the period of treatment are coined as controlled drug delivery systems that transport active agent solely to the site of action (Kaur et al., 2019). In practice, this means that controlled delivery systems attempt to control the

Advances in Polymeric Nanomaterials for Biomedical Applications. DOI: https://doi.org/10.1016/B978-0-12-814657-6.00010-0

amount of drug molecules delivered in the target tissue or cells. This can partly be achieved by sustainable control release systems that prolong the concentration of drug in the blood plasma or tissue levels for desired period of time. On the other hand, drug targeting is a form of controlled release, which exercises spatial control of the drug released in the body. With the idea of controlled drug delivery in minds, the researchers are still on their way to reach this ultimate goal (Wang and Von Recum, 2011).

All those techniques and approaches such as tablets, injections, suspensions, creams, ointments, liquids, and aerosols, which can be used to deliver drug molecules safely at target site in the body, are referred to as drug delivery technologies. Drug delivery technologies involve the multidisciplinary areas for development and advancement in fabricating novel drug delivery carriers to achieve the desirable therapeutic effects of drug and protect the drug molecules from hydrolysis, chemical and enzymatic degradation, reduce its toxicity, achieve the release under controlled rate, as well as improve its bioavailability (Lee, 2000). All those systems that are used to deliver drug molecules or therapeutic agents inside the human body are termed as drug delivery systems (Bayer and Peppas, 2008). These systems possess many advantages such as biocompatibility, biodegradability, protection of drug molecules, or active therapeutic agents from hydrolysis, enzyme and other chemicals, nontoxic nature, release of drug molecules in controlled rate at the site of action, and improved bioavailability (Sykes, 2000).

Nanotechnology plays an important role to develop nanocontrolled drug delivery carriers (1–100 nm) to overcome the biological and physical barriers, increase safety and patent adherence by implementing the use of knowledge and benefits of nanoscience. These advanced controlled nano-drug delivery carriers can easily and freely migrate in the human body compared to macromolecular materials with immense success. Such nano-drug delivery carriers improve the efficacy of the drugs, and can also be used for diagnosis and cure of chronic diseases and ultimately reduce health care costs because of their unique structural, chemical, mechanical, magnetic, electrical, and biological properties (Safari and Zarnegar, 2014; Orive et al., 2004; Razzacki et al., 2004; Arayne et al., 2007). Nanotechnology term was first used by Taniguchi in Japan who was dealing with manufacturing and studying nanosized materials for various applications. Nanotechnology may play an important role in the improvement of bioactivity of those drugs that are unable to pass clinical trial phases due to their low uptake ability, high toxicity and short half-life because nano-drug delivery carriers easily cross the physiological barriers and provide improved drug targeting and enhanced cellular uptake, as well as reduce the toxicity of free drug molecules, transported via the circulation to desired site and help in systemic treatments (Sundar et al., 2010; Narayani and Rao, 1993; Berthold et al., 1996).

Since early 1970, the concept of controlled and targeted drug delivery systems has gained much attention, which aims at delivering the therapeutic agents at controlled rates at a definite time interval, and at the target site (Jeong et al., 2002). The micelles- and liposomes-based drug delivery systems are first-generation nanomaterials that have been approved by the FDA as drug delivery systems for delivery of active therapeutic molecules and imaging because they show higher oral bioavailability, protect sparingly water-soluble drugs from degradation in gastrointestinal region, prolong stability in blood circulation, facilitate easy uptake of the drug by cells, deliver drug in controlled and specific dose to target sites, and reduce side effects.

In several last decades, the field of nanotechnology has gained much attention for the development of novel nanoformulation systems as effective controlled targeted drug delivery systems to deliver drug under controlled rate at the target site in limited dosage frequency to achieve a precise targeting, reduce side effects, prevent degradation, and improve bioactivity. These nanoformulation systems possess various unique properties such as response to a stimulus (pH, temperature, etc.), large surface area, biocompatibility, biodegradability, ease of surfaces functionalization, high drug-loading capacity, controlled and sustainable release rate to mitigate the side effects, site-specific action of the drug for precise targeting (Fig. 3.1).

In all the stages of clinic trials, nano-drug delivery systems have demonstrated potentially successful drug-delivery carriers to deliver drugs with poor solubility and absorption for the treatment and diagnosis of diseases because of their size-dependent efficiency, shape, improved biocompatibility, reduction in fed/fasted variability, smaller dosage forms, and biodegradable nature. Stimuli-responsive polymers can be used in developing advanced drug delivery systems, because they offer a large change in their structure in response to small alternation in external stimuli (Sagadevan and Periasamy, 2014; Hruby et al., 2015; Rossi et al., 2016).

In this chapter, the authors are providing details of various types of smart nanomaterials for developing intelligent drug delivery systems, their properties, challenges, and prospects in clinical trials of nano-drug delivery systems in medicine and pharmacy.

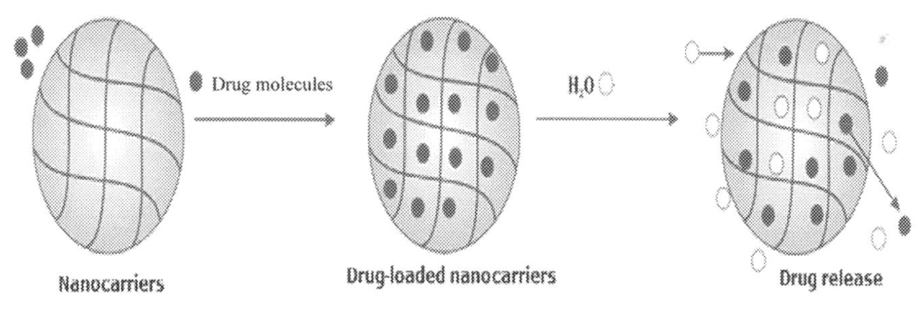

FIGURE 3.1

Schematic presentation of drug release mechanism.

3.2 Conventional delivery systems

In the previous years, drug molecules have been used as conventional dosage forms such as orally administered pills, tablets, suspensions, creams, ointments, liquids and aerosols, subcutaneous or intravenous injections for cure and treatment, and management of acute or chronic disease (Lee, 2000). These conventional routes of administration of drug molecules follow first-order kinetics. Therefore conventional route of drug delivery suffers many problems such as not maintaining the drug level concentrations in blood plasma for required time period for effective treatment of disease, not providing ideal pharmacokinetic profiles, requirements of extra dosages, and high toxicity due to free drug that may damage normal cells and tissues (Fig. 3.2) (Li et al., 2001; Kiesel et al., 2002). In conventional methods of drug administration, the concentration of drug is very high at the time of administration and slowly decreases with time. For the effectiveness of traditional method, however, the concentration should be between the maximum and the minimum levels because if concentration is higher than the maximum level, it may create high toxicity and if lower than the minimum level, it no longer remains effective.

The effectiveness of the traditional conventional routes of drug delivery is low as rate of delivery and uptake of drug molecules in body at cellular level depend upon various parameters such as type of drug (hydrophilic/hydrophobic), charge, composition of drug, size, pH, temperature, enzyme and transport mechanisms at the site of administration (Fig. 3.3). The major disadvantages of traditional methods are:

1. Non-uniform distribution of therapeutic agents throughout the body
2. Drug is not delivered at the active site
3. Wasteful, potential toxic responses at other sites

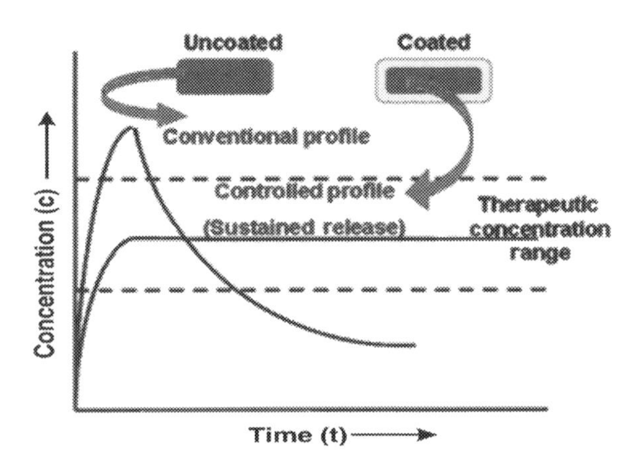

FIGURE 3.2

Concentration profiles for drug delivered by tablet, sustained release device, or controlled release device.

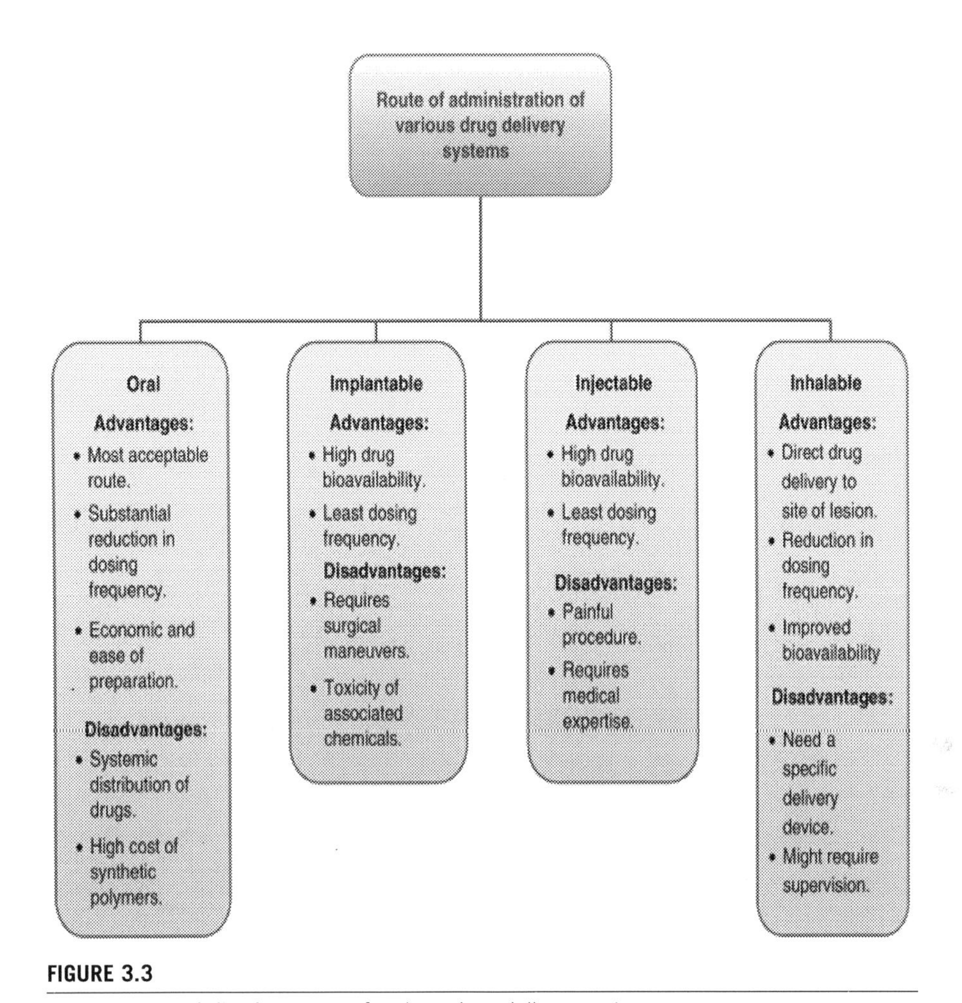

FIGURE 3.3

Advantages and disadvantages of various drug delivery systems.

4. Lack of drug-specific affinity toward a philological site
5. Regular and extra dosage to achieve high plasma concentration
6. The drug does not reach the active sites in the desired concentration
7. Expensive and ineffective at applied dose (Orive et al., 2003; Shen et al., 2008)

3.3 Controlled drug delivery

The concept of drug delivery has been developed from the need to deliver direct therapeutic agents to specific biological targets at optimum doses for a prolonged time for the effective and sustainable release of drugs in the body. The technology that delivers the therapeutic agents from a reservoir to specific target sites at action at the required rate and maintains its concentration level for a predetermined time period, and provides an intended effect are called controlled release systems (Friedman et al., 2013; Saltzman, 2001; Sershen and West, 2002). Controlled-release systems show many advantages over the conventional route of drug administration such as maintaining an optimum level of drug concentration in blood plasma for specific long time periods, improved drug efficiency and bioactivity, need for fewer administrations, reduced toxicity, delivery of difficult drugs such as hydrophobic and short half-life drug effectively, and providing higher patient compliance (Fleming and Salzman, 2002). Thus controlled drug delivery has been used to achieve:

- Sustainable controlled release of drug for a specific time period at optimum dosage (Tiwari et al., 2012)
- Reduced toxicity of drug (Tao and Desai, 2003)
- Targeted delivery of drug
- Minimized dosages of drug
- Ease of drug administration
- Higher patient compliance (Smith et al., 1990)

3.4 Types of controlled drug delivery

The mechanism of release of entrapped drug molecules from nanomaterials-based drug delivery carriers depends on various factors such as nature of the drug, nature of materials, and mode of fabrication because the main problems associated with drug delivery carriers are prevention of drug molecules from biodegradation, easy passage to target site, and lower toxicity. There are three main mechanisms of drug release from the nanocarriers. These can be categorized as (Fig. 3.4) (Leong and Langer, 1988),

1. Diffusion-controlled system
2. Swelling-controlled system
3. Erosion-controlled system

3.4.1 Diffusion-controlled systems

Diffusion-controlled drug-delivery devices have been the subject of numerous studies (Sobol et al., 1998). The release characteristics can be applied to such systems as long as the matrix remains intact and its permeability remains unchanged until the drug it contains is released (Fig. 3.4A).

Release of dispersed drug from a polymer matrix by diffusion occurs in four steps:

1. Dissolution of drug into the surrounding polymer or pores
2. Molecular diffusion of the drug across or through the polymer barrier along its concentration gradient

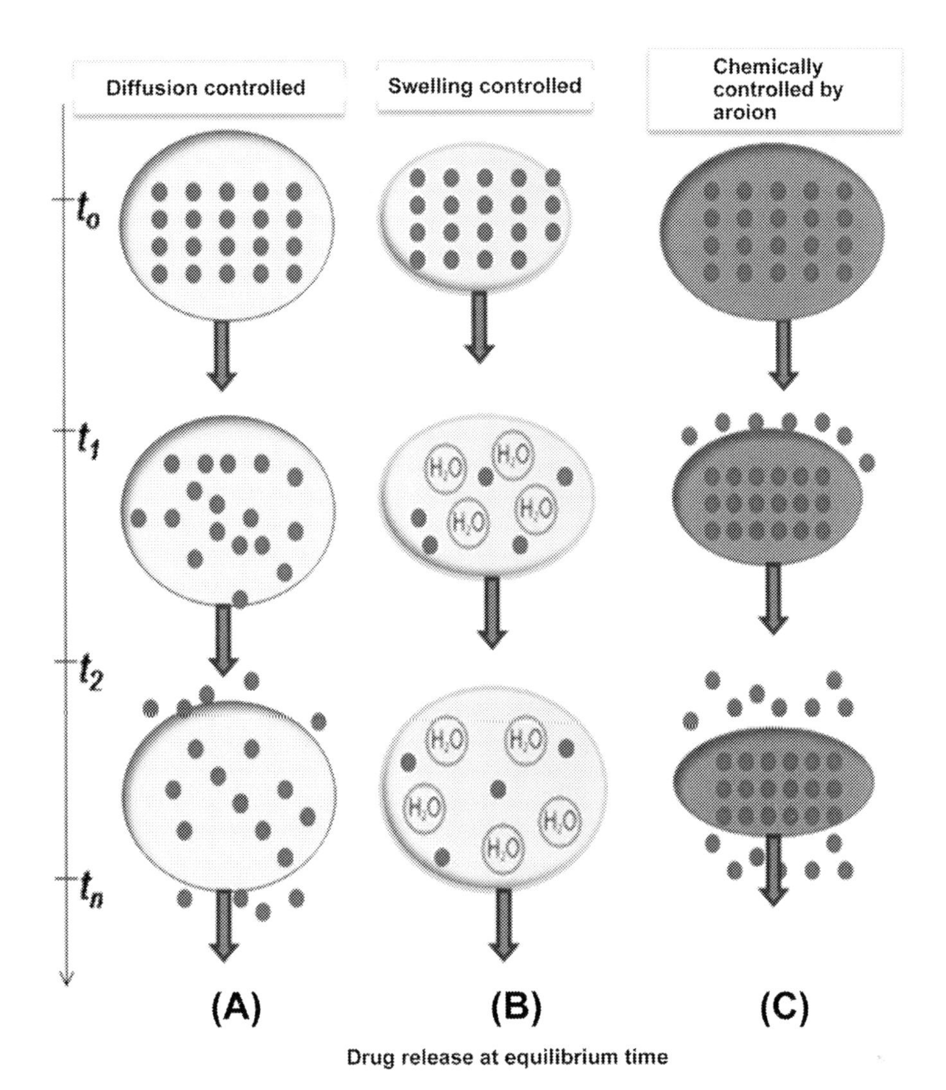

FIGURE 3.4

Schematic diagram illustrating the three mechanisms of controlled drug release from a polymer matrix.

3. Drug desorption from the polymer
4. Diffusion into the external medium or tissue

When a drug is dissolved in the delivery matrix and the mechanism for delivery is diffusional, then the thermodynamic driving force is the concentration gradient (Mourgues et al., 2004; Chow et al., 2007). There are two types of diffusion-controlled device (matrix devises, reservoir devises) that have been used in drug delivery as shown in Fig. 3.5.

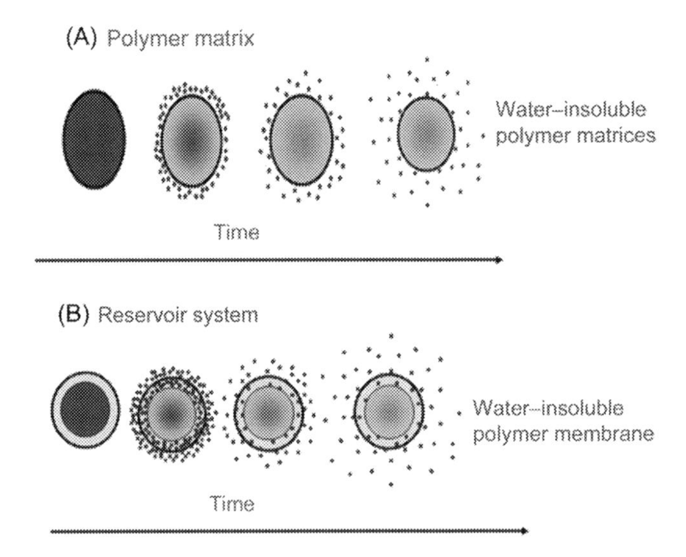

FIGURE 3.5

Schematic representations of matrix and reservoir devices.

3.4.1.1 Reservoir devices

Reservoir devices contain drug molecules in central compartment surrounded by polymer membrane in the form of either hollow fibers or microcapsule and release entrapped central compartment drug at constant rate as per Fick's first law of diffusion (Mourgues et al., 2004). The diffusion of drug molecules takes place through the surrounding polymeric membrane. The rate of release of drug molecules through the surrounded polymeric membrane depends on the nature of polymers, its surface functional groups, nature of sink solution, pH, method of fabrication, and presence of size of pores (Fig. 3.5A) (Mathowitz and Jacob, 1999; Muller and Keck, 2004).

3.4.1.2 Matrix devices

Matrix devices are easily fabricated devices for controlled drug delivery of drug that follow Fick's second law of diffusion. They contain dispersed drug molecules throughout the polymer matrix by functional groups present on the polymeric chains (Fig. 3.5B). They do not show burst release of drug from matrix because in matrix devices the drug is not present in the central compartment in higher concentration as in the case of reservoirs devices. If accidentally polymer membrane ruptures, no extra dosage of drug releases in the matrix devices but reservoir devices immediately release high dosage that may cause high toxicity. This property makes matrix devices superior to the reservoirs devices; they cannot undergo sudden dose-dumping to achieve zero-order release.

3.4.2 Swelling-controlled systems

Swelling-controlled systems show release of entrapped drug molecules through the interface of glassy and rubbery states of polymeric nanoparticle matrix. In this type of system, when polymer chains of matrix swell in a suitable medium, the glassy state of matrix is slowly changed into rubbery state and the molecules present at the rubbery state show fast and rapid diffusion while the molecules of drug present in glassy state remain immobile. The rate of diffusion of drug depends on the swelling rate of polymeric nanomaterial matrix (Figs. 3.4B and 3.6).

3.4.3 Chemically controlled systems

In chemically controlled release systems, the entrapped drug molecules are released through the polymeric nanomaterials matrix due to chemical reactions such as degradation occurring at the surface or bulk of matrix. It can be classified as surface or bulk erosion and entrapped drug molecules start rapid diffusion through the degradation of pendant chains of the polymer backbone (Fig. 3.4C). It can be further classified as:

3.4.3.1 Kinetically controlled systems

In these systems, the diffusion of drug molecules from polymeric matrix depends on the rate of degradation and not on the diffusional rate of drug. It is further classified into two types:

Pendant chain systems

In these systems, the drug molecules are bonded covalently with cleavable spacers in polymeric chains and show pendant chain system type chemical controlled release. The rate of release of drug molecules depends on the degradation or breaking of cleavable spacers during chemical reaction.

Surface eroding systems

In this type of system, rate of drug release depends on the rate of surface erosion.

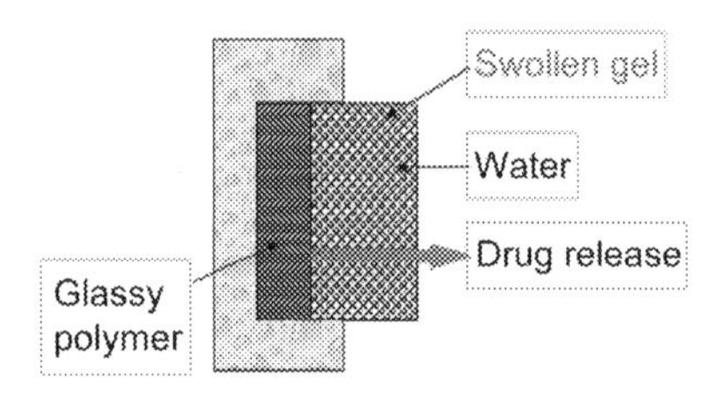

FIGURE 3.6

Swelling-controlled drug delivery system.

3.4.3.2 Reaction diffusion–controlled systems

This system involves both polymer degradation and diffusion combined to predict drug release. It is further classified into (1) bulk degrading systems and (2) affinity hydrogel systems.

3.4.4 Targeted drug delivery systems

Targeted drug delivery systems are the smart drug delivery systems. have been developed for prolonged, localized, and targeted delivery of drug molecules to specific targeted diseased area without any side effects to body with maintaining the required level of drug levels in the body (Fig. 3.7) (Saltzman et al., 2008; Stolnik et al., 1995). It may use various external stimuli such as pH, temperature, external magnetic field, electric field, light, and so on to control the rate of release of entrapped drug molecules through the drug carriers. However, the effect of such external stimuli is less on the rate of release of drug molecules to target a specific site such as cells or tissues if applied from outside the body. This type of system can be further classified as:

3.4.4.1 Passive targeting

The passive targeting (Fig. 3.7A) delivers the active therapeutic agents at desired site following the physio-anatomic conditions of the body and its effectiveness depends on the nature of the drug and carrier. Only those drug carriers, which are smaller in size and have enhanced penetration and retention (EPR) effect, crossed barriers such as disrupted endothelial lining of tumor tissues and reached its destination allowing release of drug at the targeted site for a long period of time in controlled rate. The physicochemical factors such as size of nanocarriers, its zeta

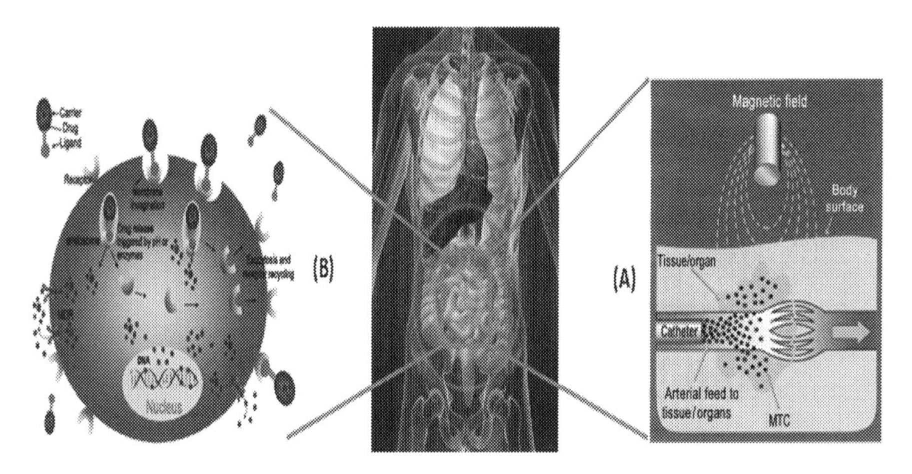

FIGURE 3.7

Targeted drug delivery systems (A) passive, and (B) active targeting.

potential, nature (hydrophilicity/hydrophobicity), and so on affect the clearance kinetics and in vivo biodistribution of carriers (Jin et al., 2006). Generally, when carriers are injected intravenously they are taken up by the reticular-endothelial system (RES) which are mainly fixed macrophages in the liver and spleen after opsonization by proteins present in the bloodstream (Davis, 1997).

3.4.4.2 Active targeting

For active targeting (Fig. 3.7B) it is required that the surface is fabricated with specific antibodies, functional groups for direct delivery of drug molecules at specific site of action through specific recognition mechanisms to improve the efficiency and uptake of drug by specific cells, tissues, or organ systems (Illum et al., 2002; Zhang and Chu, 2002).

The targeting drug delivery has the following advantages:

1. Medical: Optimum dose without toxic side effects, at the right time, and in the specific location.
2. Industrial: Efficient use of inexpensive ingredients, low-cost material production.
3. Societal: Enhanced patient's compliances, better effective low-cost therapy, improve the standard of living.

3.4.5 Stimuli-responsive drug delivery

3.4.5.1 pH-sensitive release systems

All the pH-sensitive nanoparticles contain pendant acidic (COOH) or basic groups (NH_2) that are able to ionize in response to change of pH of external medium by either accepting or releasing protons (Fig. 3.8). The polymers with a large number of ionizable groups are known as polyelectrolyte and nanomaterials based on such polyelectrolyte can swell or deswell with changing pH of the external

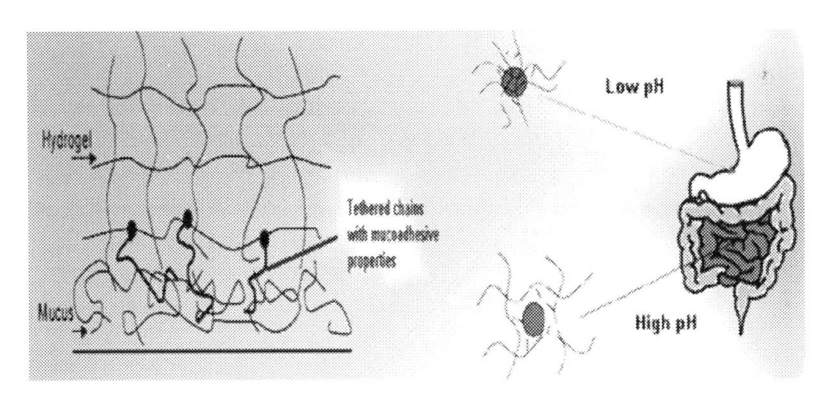

FIGURE 3.8

The swelling phenomena of a hydrogel in a buffered pH solution.

medium. Mostly, nanoparticles with weak acidic groups show higher swelling in basic medium due to an increase in ionization of weak acidic groups present on chains, and swelling of nanomaterials is increased due to repelling action of electrostatic forces. However, weak basic groups containing nanoparticles show just the opposite nature in basic medium and, consequently, show less swelling. pH-sensitive nanoparticles are produced on the basis of polymers which have free ionic groups and play an important role in developing advanced controlled targeted drug delivery systems for tumor, ulcerative colitis, colorectal cancer, Cohn's disease, and cellular compartments (e.g., endosomers) (Lai and Shum, 2016; Tannock and Rotin, 1989; Litzinger and Huang, 1992). pH-responsive nanoparticles can be utilized to deliver antitumor drugs at specific site of tumor without side effect because these sites have low pH than other sites as well as deliver those drugs which are destroyed in the stomach by acid metabolized by pancreatic enzymes as GIT- and colon-specific drug-delivery systems in the treatment of colonic diseases (Fig. 3.8) (Kshirsagar, 2000; Onuki, 1993).

3.4.5.2 Temperature-sensitive release systems

Temperature-sensitive nanocarriers have ability to release drug molecules to desired site in definite amount for prolonged time period because their sensitivity depends on hydrogen bonding and hydrophobic interactions (Baltes et al., 1999). When temperature-sensitive nano-drug delivery systems are put at higher temperature, polymeric chains get collapsed due to an increase in hydrophobic interaction arising due to breaking of hydrogen bonds and result in lower swelling of carriers, but at lower temperature, water molecules are highly hydrogen-bonded in the vicinity of hydrophobic polymer chains and lower the free energy of mixing thus resulting in greater swelling (Jeong et al., 2002). The rapid sigmoidal swelling response with temperature of polymeric carriers makes such materials an ideal system for pulsatile release applications of drug molecules at a specific site in a controlled manner. Under certain conditions, this effect can also be reversed, as illustrated in Fig. 3.9 (Shibayama and Tanaka, 1993; McBain et al., 2008).

3.4.5.3 Magnetic-sensitive drug delivery systems

Magnetic nanoparticles are nanosize carriers (1–100 nm) that show response in respect to change in alternating magnetic field and open new horizons for immobilization and transport of biologically active agents in many applications such as cancer treatments and magnetic resonance imaging (MRI) due to their typical unique properties, such as superparamagnetic behavior at room temperature, high stability physiological environment, small dimension, surface charge, show both steric and Coulombic repulsions subject to Coulomb's law (Laurent et al., 2008; Ma and Liu, 2007; Pankhurst et al., 2003). Presently many superparamagnetic nanomaterials-based drug delivery carriers are being used as vectors and substance carriers for release of antitumor drugs at specific tumor sites (Ruiz-Hernandez et al., 2008; Levy et al., 2008). Superparamagnetic nanoparticles become heated up when they come in contact with the alternating magnetic field due to transfer of energy from field to

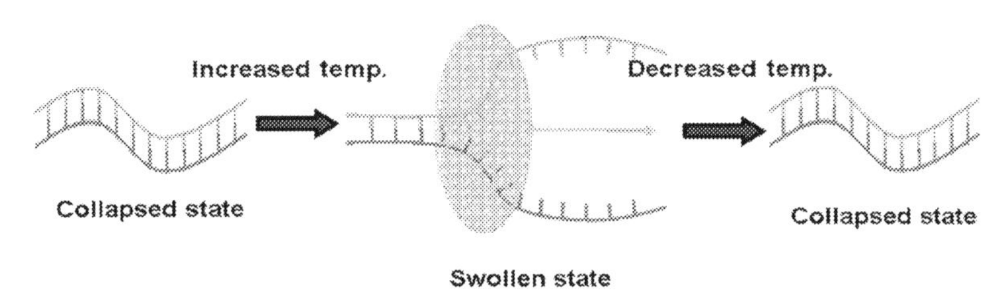

FIGURE 3.9

An illustration of the hydrogen bonding mechanism that controls swelling and deswelling with temperature in certain interpenetrating polymers networks referred to as the "Zipper Effect."

nanoparticles. This property of superparamagnetic nanomaterials can be used to develop advanced nanocarriers for cure and treatment of hyperthermia or release of therapeutic active agents at site of action with reduced toxicity. The hyperthermia effect of superparamagnetic nanomaterials under changing alternating magnetic fields leads to an increased temperature at the tumor sites and kills or destructs the cancerous cells efficiently (Goya et al., 2008; Shersen and West, 2002). Superparamagnetic nanoparticles encapsulated in biocompatible polymers have been developed and gained much attention as ideal carriers for in vivo applications due to their lower toxicity and biocompatible nature that prevent degradation and changes in the original structure and formation of large aggregates.

3.4.5.4 Light-sensitive drug delivery systems

Light-sensitive drug delivery systems show responsive changes in their properties by absorbing energy from innocuous electromagnetic radiation and such responses can be used to develop modulating drug delivery systems to deliver drug at the specific site in controlled rate on demand as well as delimited sites of the body with optimized manner preventing toxicity as well as improving patient comfort (Wang et al., 2007). Light-sensitive drug delivery systems can be categorized into two types: single-switchable carriers which show an irreversible change in structure when exposed to specific radiation and release drug at a time while others are multiswitchable carriers that show reversible change in structure in response to on/off of incident radiation and release drug in the pulsatile manner (Sershen et al., 2000). At present, many nanomaterials which belong to self-assembled colloids such as liposomes, micelles have gained much attention as novel carriers for modulated drug delivery in response to light because the rate of release of drug can be controlled by many factors such as control of the wavelength of the light, nature of materials, exposure time, and intensity of the incident beam. Fig. 3.10 shows a light-sensitive drug delivery system.

Gold nanoparticles incorporated poly(NIPAAM-co-AAm) nanocomposite materials have been developed to deliver proteins in response to exposure of near infrared light. Gold nanoparticles contain a thin layer of dielectric core that enables it to show optical activity because they absorb the near infrared light and heat up which

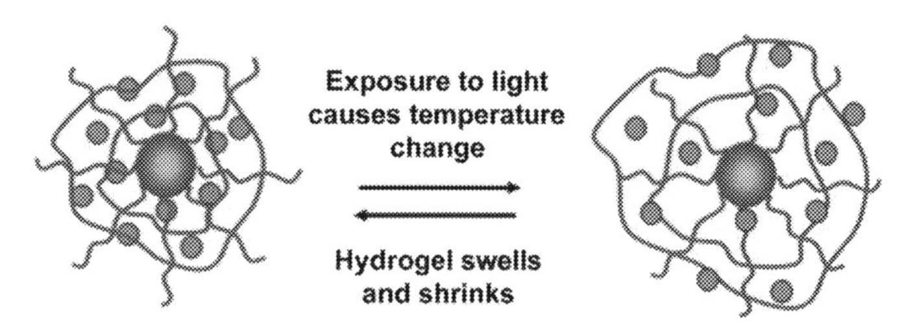

FIGURE 3.10

Light-sensitive drug delivery system.

increased the temperature of poly(NIPAAM-co-AAm) above its lower critical solution temperature (40°C) and phase transition occurs and polymer chains get collapsed that triggered the release of soluble drug embedded in the matrix. Therefore these materials can be used to modulate the release of various proteins from a composite material (Avenitt et al., 1999; Jong and Borm, 2008).

3.5 Significance of nanomaterials in drug delivery

Nanotechnology is a revolutionary field that involves the concept of multidisciplinary sciences for the development, creation, synthesis, manipulation of nanosized materials for targeting and delivering drugs at a controlled rate for prolong time, tissue regeneration, cell culture, biosensors, and other biomedical areas because of large surface area and quantum effects. Nanotechnology provides a variety of drug delivery carriers that have unique properties such as easily transportable along with bloodstream, high uptake by cells, ability to penetrate tissues, targeted delivery of drugs and imaging agents, reduced toxicity and low drug wastage, improved loading efficiency, easily circulate in the body, high biodegradability, and stability and long shelf life. The nanocarriers are very small in size compared to eukaryotic or prokaryotic cells and, therefore, easily reach inaccessible areas in significant amount via intravenous injections or other administration routes due to their EPR effect, and capacity to deliver drug at a controlled rate, quicker and much cheaper, increased comfort, safety, and patent compliance, and ultimately reduce health care costs (Cole et al., 2011).

3.6 Nanocarriers for drug delivery: basic properties

According to National Nanotechnology Initiative (NNI), nanoparticles are submicron moieties (1–100 nm) made of inorganic, organic, or hybrid materials having many novel properties compared with the bulk materials (Fig. 3.11). Nanocarriers such as liposomes, solid lipids nanoparticles, dendrimers, polymers, silicon or carbon materials, and magnetic nanoparticles with optimized physicochemical and

Just how small is nano ?

Name	Abbrev.	Sci. Unit	Representative objects with this size scale
metre	m	100	Height of a 7-year-old child.
deci-	dm	10^{-1}	Size of our palm.
centi-	cm	10^{-2}	Length of a bee.
milli-	mm	10^{-3}	Thickness of ordinary paperclip.
micro-	μm	10^{-6}	Size of typical dust particles.
nano-	nm	10^{-9}	The diametre of a C60 molecule is about 1 nm.
pico-	pm	10^{-12}	Radius of a Hydrogen Atom is about 23 pm.
femto-	fm	10^{-15}	Size of a typical nucleus of an atom is 10 fm.
atto-	am	10^{-18}	Estimated size of an electron.

Scale of things

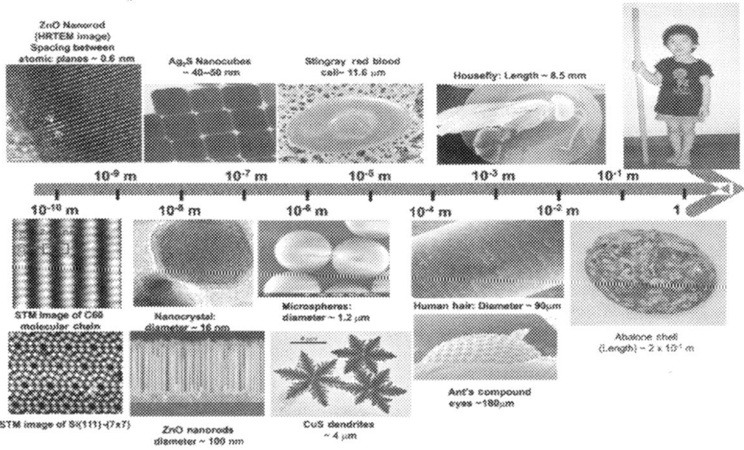

Scaling down to nanometer

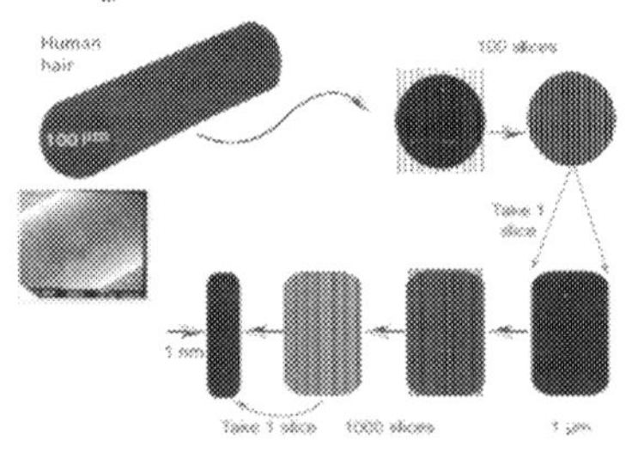

Micrograph of a looped nanowire against a human hair

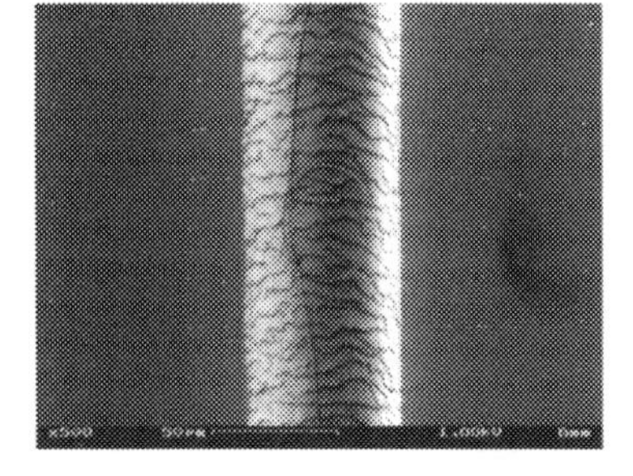

FIGURE 3.11

Size scale of nanotechnology.

biological properties can be fabricated for developing an ideal drug delivery system to deliver a variety of therapeutic agents because they show high cellular uptake in comparison to bulk molecules. The drug molecules can be conjugated with nanocarriers either by covalently or physically linking for achieving the targeted therapy. The way of covalent linking of drug is more precise than physical encapsulation for controlling the amount of drug within the nanocarriers. The delivery of drug molecules from nanocarriers can be accomplished by using active (EPR), or passive targeting (using external stimuli, e.g., temperature, pH, alternate magnetic field, light, enzymatic activity). The nanocarriers that are used as drug delivery systems must have optimal pharmacokinetic properties, size in the range of 10–100 nm, nontoxicity, biocompatibility, and biodegradability, because their undesired effects strongly depend on their surface chemistry (greater surface area make more reactive), size and shape, concentration, and route of administration, stay time in bloodstream, and reaction with immune system. Therefore toxicological studies of nanocarriers-based drug delivery systems are needed before clinical trials for in vivo applications (Nevozhay et al., 2007; Arsawang et al., 2011; Ai et al., 2011; Couvreur et al., 2006).

Nanoparticles can be classified as natural (made by natural polymers like chitosan, pectin, casein, alginate, and silk protein) and synthetic nanoparticles [made by synthetic polymers like polycyanoacrylate or poly(D-L-lactite) and poly(lactate-co-glycolide) (PLGA)] on the basis of sources from which nanoparticles are obtained. Natural nanoparticles have many advantages over synthetic nanoparticles such as good biodegradability, biocompatibility, nontoxicity, and noncarcinogenic nature (Kwon, 2003; Mesiha et al., 2005; Whatmore, 2006). Nanocarriers can be further classified on the basis of dimensions of the dispersed particles such as isodimensional nanoparticles (have all three dimensions in nanosize, e.g., spherical silica nanoparticles), elongated structures like nanotubes or whiskers (have two dimensions are in the nanometer scale and the third is larger), and filler in the form of nanometer-thick sheets (have only one dimension in nanosize) (Fig. 3.12).

The terminologies very often applied in nanoscience and nanotechnologies are listed as follows:

- Nanoparticles: particles that have size in the range of 1–100 nm are called "nanoparticles" (ISO, 2004; Klaine et al., 2008).
- Nanocomposites: the composite materials in which nanosize materials are dispersed in polymeric matrix of macrodimension.
- Nanomaterials: nanoscale materials have size in the range of 1–100 nm and either internal or surface structure such as nanoparticles, nanocomposites, nanopowder, nanocrystals, and so on.

Nanoparticles can be further classified as incidental and engineered nanoparticles on the basis of their source of generation. Those nanoparticles, which are produced in an uncontrolled manner as byproducts of various reactions or processes such as combustion of fuel, vaporization, weathering, or agricultural practices and release into the environment, can be termed as incidental nanoparticles (DHHS, 2009; NNI, 2009). However, those nanoparticles which are synthesized and fabricated with specific design and properties for various biomedical and

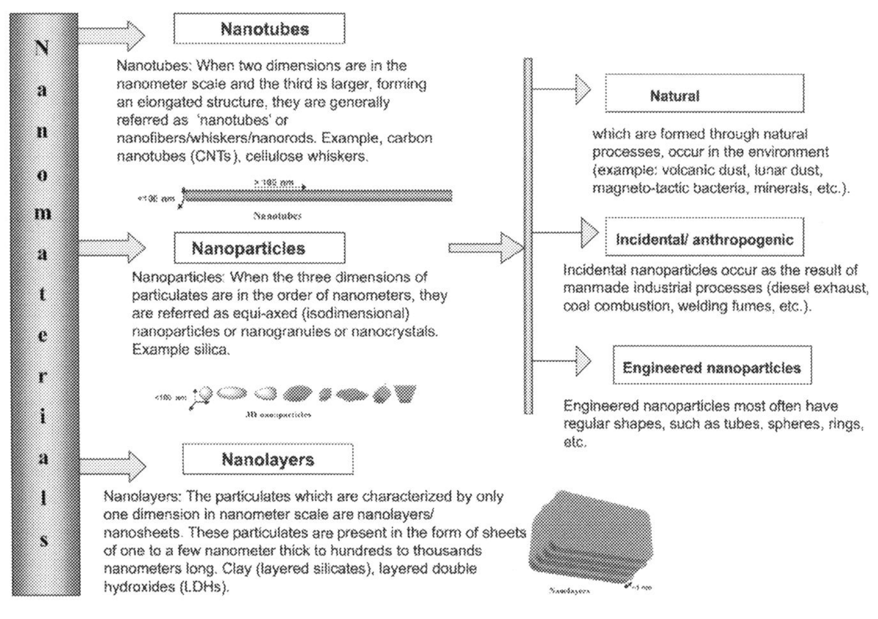

FIGURE 3.12

Schematic classifications of nanobiomaterials.

industrial applications belong to engineered nanoparticles (NNI, 2009; Kawasaki and Player, 2005).

3.7 Various nanoscale drug delivery systems

In the last decades, many advanced nanoscale smart systems have been designed for efficient transport of drug molecules to the target sites under a controlled manner with reduced dosage to minimize the side effects experienced by patients (Allen and Cullis, 2004; Yu et al., 2016). In particular, smart nanocarriers resolve the problems associated with traditional therapies such as nonspecific and non-uniform distribution of drug molecules, uncontrolled delivery at target sites, low bioavailability, rapid clearance, toxicity issues related to drugs, and degradation of drug molecules within the specific biological media (Yin et al., 2016; Liu et al., 2016; Werner et al., 2018; Marianecci et al., 2016).

3.7.1 Vesicular nanocarriers

In the present time, vesicular nanocarriers (liposomes and niosomes) have gained much attention as novel drug delivery systems for delivery of various bioactive agents in specific site because they have size below 100 nm, more surface to volume ratio, and have the ability to control the pharmacokinetic and pharmacodynamic profiles of incorporated therapeutic drugs (Moghassemi and Hadjizadeh, 2014). However, these vesicular nanocarriers have some disadvantages such as physical instability arising due to accumulation or aggregation, fusion, or hydrolysis of incorporated drugs and mechanisms of drug release are not clear at cellular level (Tavano and Muzzalupo, 2016).

3.7.1.1 Nanoliposomes

Liposomes are small spherical unilamellar nanosize vesicles composed of bilayered phospholipids (synthesized from cholesterol and nontoxic phospholipids containing one or more concentric bilayers of amphipathic phospholipids), with an aqueous interior that can incorporate imaging agents, peptides, proteins, nucleic acids, and low-molecular-weight anticancer and antiviral drugs for the sustained and targeted release to the site of action (Lombardo et al., 2018). They possess many unique properties such as small particle size, neutral in nature, bilayer charge, bilayer composition, a lipid membrane surrounding an aqueous cavity, incorporate water-soluble drugs in central aqueous core as well as lipophilic drugs in the outer phospholipid layer, easily functionalized with "stealth" materials, harmless carriers that can circulate in the bloodstream for a long time, and high encapsulation ability. Nanoliposomes have size from 25 nm to micrometer and are preferred as passive (transport the drug molecules for a definite time interval) and active targeting (incorporate antibody, ligands, etc.), and show many advantages over liposomes such as they neither degrade rapidly nor clearance by liver macrophages, as well as lead to the long eliminating half-life of drug molecules, ease of modification of size, hydrophobic/hydrophilic character, reduced toxicity, and high biocompatibility (Lombardo et al., 2016; Pogodin et al., 2012; Dan, 2018; Chang and Yeh, 2012). Natural and synthetic lipid-based drug delivery vesicles consist of hydrophilic head with one or more hydrophobic tails and are prevalent in the market and widely used in clinical trials because of ease of preparation by easily available phosphor lipid compounds, and prevent degradation of drug molecules in harsh bio-environment as well as controlled drug release kinetics. Liposome formulations are mostly administrated intravenously and currently under clinical trials as novel carriers for treating multidrug-resistant cancer and delivery of various anticancer drugs such as daunorubicin, cisplatin, doxorubicin, paclitaxel, and vincristine (Table 3.1).

The circulation times of nanoliposomes can be improved by conjugation with polymers because this process not only overcomes the problems such as the interception by the immune system, toxicity, biocompatibility issues but also improves the specificity during the drug release process. The PEGylated liposomes possess highly hydrophilic polymer brushes that hinder the protein adsorption, prevent the hydrophobic and electrostatic interactions with plasma proteins or cells and stop uptake in the RES, and show improved cellular uptake by cancer cells as well as good on/off switching behavior in the presence of external stimuli (Fan and Zhang, 2013; Bozzuto and Molinari, 2015; Coviello et al., 2015).

Table 3.1 Date showing the list of some marketed nanoformulations used in clinical trials that are approved by the FDA.

Trade name	Drug	Indication	Applied technology	Company	Status
RapamuneÂ	Rapamycin	Immunosuppressive	ElanNanocrystalÂ	Wyeth	Marketed
Emend Â	Aprepitant	Antiemetic	ElanNanocrystalÂ	Merck	Marketed
Tricor Â	Fenofibrate	Hypercholesterolemia	ElanNanocrystalÂ	Abbott	Marketed
Megace ESÂ	Megestrol	Antianorexic	ElanNanocrystalÂ	Par Pharmaceutical Companies	Marketed
AvinzaÂ	Morphine sulfate	Pain relief	ElanNanocrystalÂ	King Pharmaceutical	Marketed
Focalin ÂXR	Dexmethylphenidatehydrochloride	Immediate and a second delayed-release CNS stimulant	ElanNanocrystalÂ	Novartis	Marketed
Ritalin ÂLA	Methylphenidate hydrochloride	Extended-release CNS stimulant	Elan NanocrystalÂ	Novartis	Marketed
Zanaflex Capsules	Tizanidine hydrochloride	Centrally acting Î ± 2-adrenergic agonist	Elan NanocrystalÂ	Acorda	Marketed
Triglide Â	Fenofibrate	Hypercholesterolemia	IDD-PÂ Skyepharma	Sciele Pharma Inc.	Marketed
Semapimod Â	Guanylhydrazone	TNF-Î ± inhibitor	Own	Cytokine Pharmasciences	Phase II
Paxceed Â	Paclitaxel	Antiinflammatory	Unknown	Angiotech Pharmaceuticals Inc.	Phase III
Theralux Â	Thymectacin	Anticancer		Celmed BioSciences Inc.	Phase II
Nucryst Â	Silver	Antibacterial	Own	Nucryst Pharmaceuticals	Phase II
Genexol-PM	Paclitaxel	Nonsmall Cell lung cancer	Amphiphilic diblock copolymer forming micelle	Samyang Biopharmaceutical Corp.	Phase I

(Continued)

Table 3.1 Date showing the list of some marketed nanoformulations used in clinical trials that are approved by the FDA. *Continued*

Trade name	Drug	Indication	Applied technology	Company	Status
Docetaxel-PNP	Docetaxel	Advanced solid malignancies	Polymeric nanoparticles	Samyang Biopharmaceutical Corp.	Phase I
CYT-6091	TNF (Tumor necrosis factor)	Unspecified adult solid tumor	AuNP (Gold nanoparticles)	NCI (National Cancer Institute)	Phase I
Paclitaxel poliglumex	Paclitaxel	Prostate cancer	Drug polymer conjugate	OHSU Knight Cancer Institute	Phase III
Kogenate FS	Recombinant factor VIII	Hemophilia A	PEG (polyethylene glycol)-liposome	Bayer	Phase I
Long-circulating liposomal prednisolone disodium phosphate	Prednisolone	Rheumatoid arthritis	Liposome	Radboud University	Phase II
LE-DT	Docetaxel	Pancreatic cancer	Liposome	Insys Therapeutics Inc.	Phase II
Cisplatin and Liposomal Doxorubicin	Cisplatin and doxorubicin	Advanced cancer	Liposome	M.D. Anderson Cancer Center	Phase I
Liposomal doxorubicin and bevacizumab	Doxorubicin and bevacizumab	Kaposi's sarcoma	Liposome	NCI (National Cancer Institute)	Phase II
AP5346	AP5346 and oxaliplatin	Head and neck cancer	Drug polymer conjugate	AP5346 and oxaliplatin	Not stated
Renagel	Sevelamer	Chronic kidney disease	Poly(allylamine hydrochloride)	Sanofi	FDA approved
Eligard	Leuprolide	Prostate cancer	Leuprolide acetate and polymer PLGA (poly (DL-lactide-co-glycolide))	Tolmar	FDA approved

Estrasorb	Estradiol	Menopausal therapy Crohn's disease	Micellar estradiol	Novavax	FDA approved
CIMZIA	Cimzia/certolizumab pegol	Rheumatoid/psoriatic arthritisAnkylosing spondylitis	PEGylated antibody fragment (certolizumab)	UCB	FDA approved
Marqibo	Vincristine sulfate	Acute lymphoblastic leukemia	Liposomal vincristine	Talon Therapeutics Inc.	FDA approved
Onivyde	Irinotecan	Pancreatic cancer	Liposomal irinotecan	Merrimac	FDA approved
GastroMARK; umirem	Iron	Imaging agent	SPION coated with silicone	AMAG Pharmaceuticals	FDA approved
NanoTherm	Iron oxide	Glioblastoma	Iron oxide	MagForce	FDA approved

3.7.1.2 Niosomes

Niosomes are multilamellar or unilamellar structures vesicles containing both hydrophilic (head) and hydrophobic (tail) groups, and created mainly by combing cholesterol or its derivatives and alkyl or dialkyl polyglycerol ether, alkyl esters alkyl ethers, alkyl amides, fatty acids (act as nonionic surfactants), and amino acids. The amino acids, which are used in fabrication of niosomes, possess good biocompatibility, biodegradability, nontoxicity, and nonimmunogenic nature. Niosomes contain bilayer structure originated due to self-spontaneous arrangement of surfactant monomer. During self-spontaneous fabrication process, hydrophilic heads, that is, polar groups attached to aqueous solvents while the nonpolar groups of hydrophobic tails arrange away from aqueous solvents. They are capable to transport both water-soluble and lipid-soluble drug molecules at target sites at a controlled rate in response to the external stimuli, as well as the ability to prolong blood circulation, and can easily penetrate across peptide channels inside the cell. The stability of niosomes is higher than that of the liposomes due to presence of surfactants (Carafa et al., 2010; Malhotra and Jain, 1994; Udupa, 2002; Amoabediny et al., 2018).

3.7.2 Particulate carriers

3.7.2.1 Polymeric nanoparticles

In the past decades, many biodegradable and biostable polymer-based nanoparticles have been extensively investigated as one of the most promising novel nanomaterials for drug delivery applications because of special characteristics such as striking physicochemical properties, core—shell structure, controllable size, surface charge, hydrophilicity and hydrophobicity, low cost, easy modification of surface by incorporation of specific functional groups, good pharmacokinetic control, physically or chemically entrapment or encapsulation of drug molecules to the surface, diffusion-controlled release of drug molecules, excellent optimum drug loading and bioavailability, minimum drug leakage, sustainable targeted release at specific pathological site and/or target cells, biocompatible and fair biodegradable nature, nontoxic byproducts, high stability, good mechanical properties, excellent versatile behaviors and easily conjugated with peptides, aptamers, or antibodies (Couvreur, 2013; Ernsting et al., 2012; Ganta et al., 2008).

Stimulus-responsive polymers-based nanoparticles have been actively pursued as "intelligent," "smart," or "environmentally sensitive" nanoparticles because they release incorporated drug molecules to specific sites in response to a spontaneous change in structural properties of carrier under on/off switching of either internal or external stimulus (temperature, solvents, light, reactants, pH, ions in solution, redox, magnetic, and chemical recognition), and offer many advantages such precise control on concentration of released drug through a remote apparatus on/off switching. The in vitro and/or in vivo drug release performance of stimuli-responsive nanocarriers can be further improved by introducing two or more signals in a single polymer nanoparticle. When stimuli-responsive nanocarriers show rapid physiocochemical transition with respect to response of two or more external or internal stimuli called dual- or multi-stimuli responsive nanocarriers that have high precise control over the rate of release of drug molecules and show site-specific target delivery with minimum toxicity, as well as possess programmed drug release features due to combined sequential response take place at the pathological site (Meng et al., 2009; Rapoport, 2007; Chan et al., 2013; Pardeike et al., 2009).

3.7.2.2 Solid lipid nanoparticles

Solid lipid nanoparticles (SLNs) (nanostructure lipid carriers and the lipid drug conjugate nanoparticles) also referred to as lipospheres are composed of solid lipids, for example, highly purified mono-, di-, and tri-glycerides, fatty acids, complex glyceride mixtures or waxes stabilized by various surfactants prepared by spray drying, ultrasonication processes, and have been exploited as most promising approaches for transport of anticancer drugs to colon or breast. SLNs form a physically stable strongly lipophilic matrix (avoidance of organic solvents in the preparation process) and exist as solid particles at body temperature 37°C. They can entrap the drug molecules in its lipophilic matrix, prevent its degradation, as well as show controlled drug release and good tolerability. Mostly they follow diffusion-controlled mechanism for drug release with simultaneous degradation of lipid. However, they suffer from many disadvantages such as poor drug encapsulation capacity, burst drug release after crystallization (unordered matrix), and relatively high water content of the dispersions (Ogawara et al., 2009).

3.7.2.3 Dendrimers

In 1985 the term dendrimer was proposed by Tomalia. Dendrimers are three-dimensional highly branched architectures having low polydispersity and high functionality with an inner core (diameter size 2.5–10 nm). The structure of dendrimer resembles the structure of a tree. The main three parts of dendrimers are focal core, building blocks (interior layers of repeated monomers), and multiple peripheral functional groups. They can be prepared either by divergent approach or convergent approach and are able to encapsulate drug molecules either by dendritic structure (at inside core by physical bonds with nonpolar cavities) or drug conjugation (at surface by covalent bonds with large numbers of positively or negatively charged functional groups). Dendrimers-based drug delivery systems show many advantages over other delivery systems such as enhanced water solubility, prevent drug molecules from degradation, specific and sustained release of drug to the target sites, carry many drug molecules (targeting moieties, imaging chemicals) using a variety of functional groups, and improved pharmacodynamic and pharmacokinetic behaviors (Duncanand and Izzo, 2005; Yang and Kao, 2006; Kannan et al., 2014; Astruc et al., 2010; Ballauff and Likos, 2004).

3.7.3 Inorganic nanocarriers

In the past decade, many inorganic nanoparticles of metal oxide or metallic composition such as superparamagnetic iron oxide nanoparticles, gold nanoparticles, and so on have gained much attention as an ideal carrier for transportation of drug molecules at a specific site in the biomedical field. These inorganic nanoparticles show many distinct and special properties, nanoscale size, fair biocompatibility and stability, reduced toxicity, easy synthesis (sol-gel process, spray drying, or microemulsion process), good hydrophilicity, and antimicrobial nature over other nanomaterials.

3.7.3.1 Superparamagnetic iron oxide nanoparticles

In recent years, magnetic nanoparticles (metals, alloys, metal oxides) have gained much considerable attention for applications such as designing carrier for MRI, treatment of in-stent thrombosis, pigments, catalysis, photocatalysis, delivery of antitumor or anticancer drugs, due to their unique properties such as superparamagnetic nature, susceptibility to the external magnetic field, good biocompatibility, better uptake and function at cellular and molecular levels. Superparamagnetic iron oxide nanoparticles [maghemite (γ-Fe_2O_3) and magnetite (Fe_3O_4)] have been approved by food and drug administration for clinical use because of their favorable and unique chemical and biological properties such as easy synthesis (alkaline coprecipitation of Fe^{2+} and Fe^{3+}), good biocompatibility and nontoxicity (present in human heart, spleen, and liver), easily tailoring to properties by inorganic, organic, or polymer coating, tendency to promote activation of phagocytotic and cytokine-release functions of macrophages, fair stability in physiological conditions, and excellent superparamagnetic property. These special properties depend on the crystallinity, route of administration, hydrodynamic sizes, and shape of iron oxide nanoparticles. Drug molecules can be easily loaded in superparamagnetic iron oxide nanoparticles by various methods such as physical or chemical bonding, adsorption due to charge on surface, or by encapsulation process and used as carriers for passive (good EPR effect) and active targeting (attached antibodies like recognized ligands) of drug at desire site with the help of external alternating magnetic field as stimuli. Superparamagnetic iron oxide nanoparticles encapsulation with drug molecules can be guided and heated by the use of external alternating magnetic field and triggered to release drug at defined sites at a controlled rate. Therefore these materials are widely used as contrasting agents, separating agents, carriers for antitumor or anticancer drug, magnetic guided delivery of cells, and hyperthermia for tumor therapy (Chen et al., 2008; Pankhurst et al., 2003; Xie et al., 2007; Cao et al., 2004) as depicted in Fig. 3.13.

3.7.3.2 Metallic nanoparticles

Metallic nanoparticles of gold, silver, copper, and so on possess distinct and unique optoelectrical properties, easy tailoring of properties to binding with recognized ligands, and broad adsorption range in visible region. Therefore they have been developed for various biomedical applications such as nanoprobes for bioimaging, nanobiosensors for biosensing more specific and highly sensitive biomolecular diagnostics, sustainable transport of therapeutic agents, and photoguided delivery of antitumor drug or hyperthermia as shown in Fig. 3.14 (White et al., 2009; Juan, 2013; Blackman, 2009; Snyder et al., 2007). Gold nanoparticles

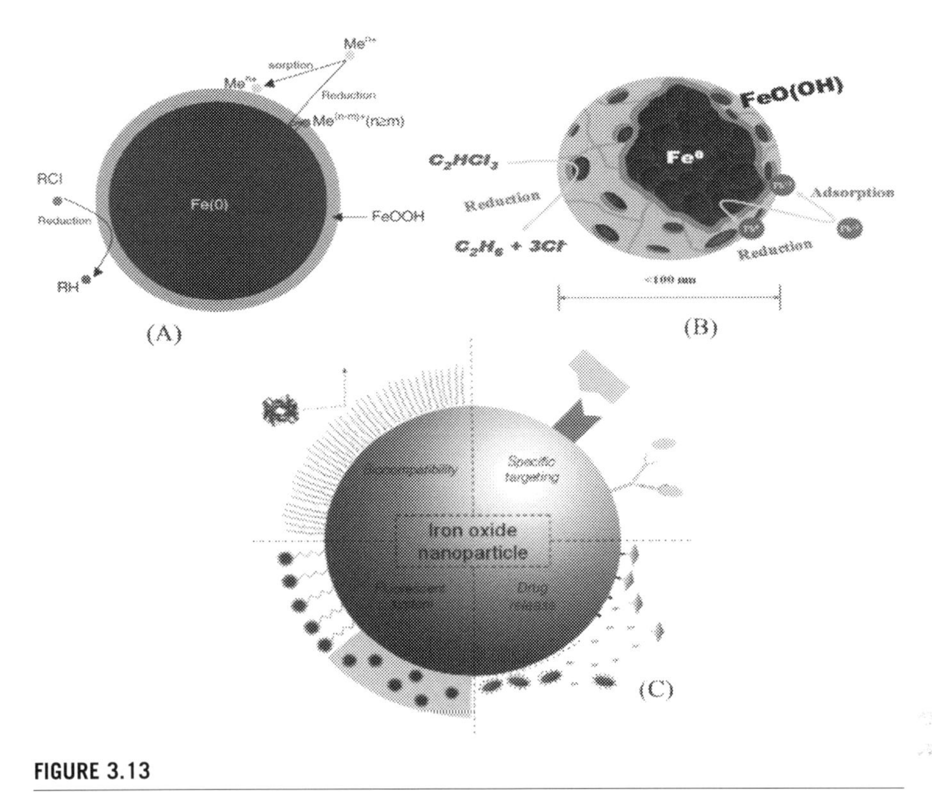

FIGURE 3.13

(A) The core–shell model of zero-valent iron nanoparticles. (B) A three-dimensional view of zero-valent iron nanoparticles. (C) Overview of possible modifications on iron oxide nanoparticle surface.

have gained much importance in the biomedical filed as promising materials for drug delivery, biosensors because of their special properties such as nanosize (5–100 nm), good biocompatibility, easy synthesis by the reduction of chloroauric acid, and tailoring of surface by Ovalbmin peptide antigen and CpG adjuvant, good immune responses, low toxicity, excellent optical and electrical properties which lead to heat and ablate the tumor by absorbing light. Gold nanoparticles can be functionalized with recognized ligands probes such as antibodies, nucleotides, and so on to fulfill the demand of biomedical applications in bioimaging or biosensing (Mirsadeghi et al., 2016; Colvin, 2007; Baszkin and Norde, 1999). Recently, gold nanoparticles with oligonucleotide have been developed to detect DNA strands because of their special optical properties. Gold nanoparticles are widely applied as carriers for transport of peptides, proteins, or nucleic acid GNPs have shown the success in delivery of peptides, proteins, or nucleic acid (Hamley et al., 2012; Guo et al., 2005; Laurent et al., 2012; Mahmoudi et al., 2013). Silver nanoparticles show fair biocompatibility and antibacterial nature for broad-spectrum microorganisms, and low toxicity to human mammal cells.

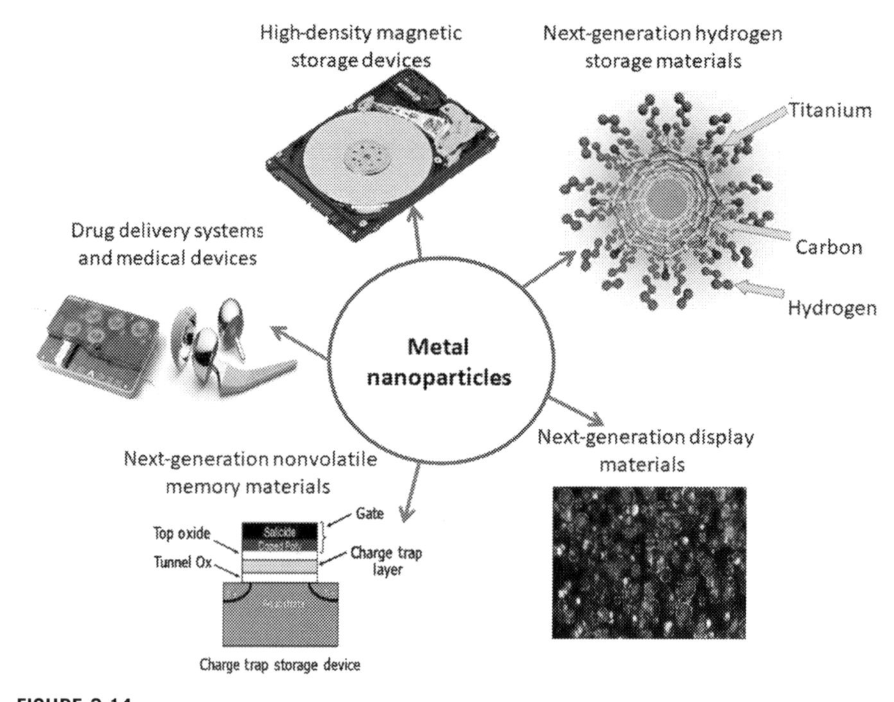

FIGURE 3.14

Applications of metal nanoparticles in various fields.

3.7.3.3 Carbon nanotubes

Since 1991, carbon nanotubes (1–2 nm elongated and tabular shaped nanomaterials named as single, double, or multiwalled nanotubes) have been developed as promising materials for biomedical applications such as biosensor, drug delivery carriers, and biomedical devices due to their excellent structural, mechanical, and electrical properties such as high electrical conductivity, high strength, easy preparation by deposition of carbon precursor or by vaporization of graphite (Beg et al., 2011; Arsawang et al., 2011) (Fig. 3.15). However, carbon nanotubes are insoluble in many solvents and show cytotoxicity. Therefore functionalized carbon nanotubes have been developed to improve their biocompatibility and solubility for various biomedical applications (Di Crescenzo et al., 2011). Carbon nanotubes can be functionalized by oxidation followed by carboxyl coupling or addition reaction (attachment of organic functional group at sidewall or tip) (Foldvari and Bagonluri, 2008). The oxidation followed by carboxyl coupling method shows many advantages over addition approach because therapeutic agents or bioactive materials (proteins, peptides, nucleic acids) can be easily bonded with carboxyl groups through amide or ester linkage, show high loading capacity and solubility, easily cross through cell membranes (hydrophilic and

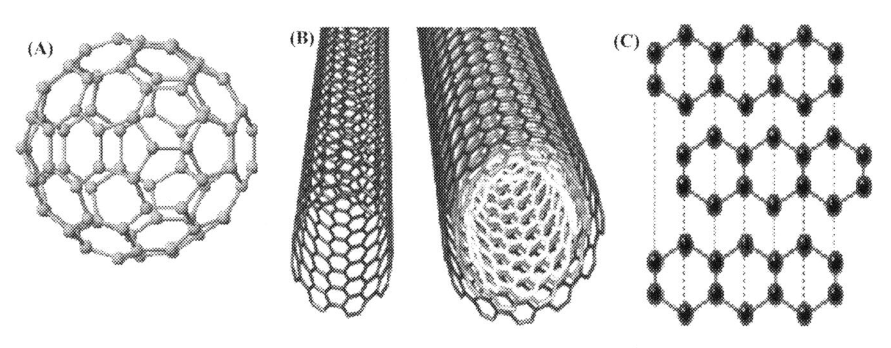

FIGURE 3.15

The chemical structure of carbon allotropes. (A) 0D fullerene, (B) 1D carbon nanotubes, (C) 3D graphite.

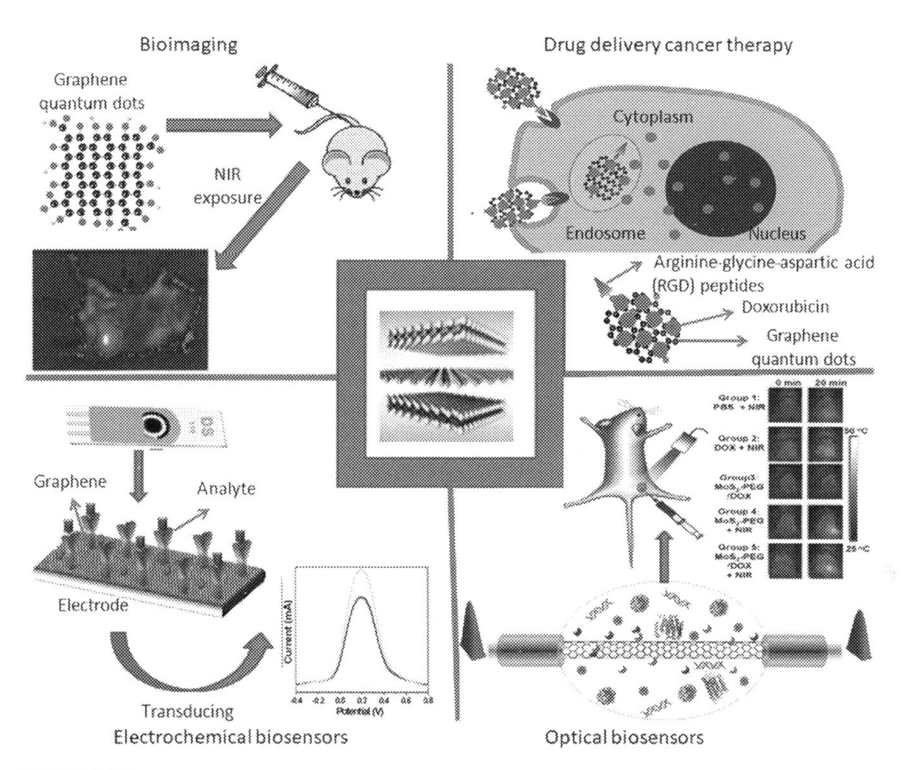

FIGURE 3.16

Image showing biomedical, biosensor, and drug delivery application of graphene.

hydrophobic nature and small size), which are essential requirements for biological uses basically for drug delivery strategy and delivery covalently or electrostatic bonded drugs to target cells (Dhar et al., 2008) (Fig. 3.16). Functionalized carbon nanotubes–based drug delivery carriers can release drugs either in an electrically or chemically controlled manner and burst release can be stopped or prevented by using polypyrrole films that act as seal at open ends.

3.8 Nanomedicine formulations: clinical development and approved materials

In the past three decades, scientists have been attempting to develop various types of advanced pharmaceutical nanocarriers such as nanoparticles, nanospheres, nanocapsules, nanoemulsion, and nanosized vesicular carriers (liposomes and niosomes) for the site-specific targeted delivery of therapeutic agents (small or large size) in human body (Fig. 3.17). Table 3.1 shows a list of some marketed nanoformulations used in clinical trials that are approved by the FDA (Lombardo et al., 2019; Jain and Thareja, 2019; Chakroborty et al., 2013; Couvreur, 2013; Sahoo et al., 2007).

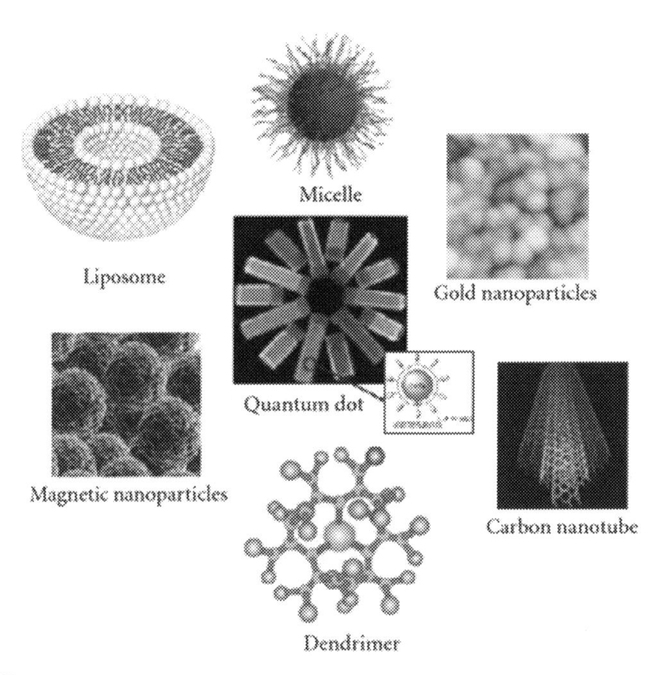

FIGURE 3.17

Different types of nanocarriers.

3.9 Conclusions and future perspectives

Nanoparticles-based drug delivery systems show many advantages over the conventional route of administration of drug such as ease of modification of surface functionality, control over the size of particles, controlled release, biodegradability, greater drug encapsulation, late clearance of the drug, diminished undesired effects, easy penetration intravenously; hence, allowing optimum drug concentration at the target site. Despite a large number of advantages, nanoparticles possess certain drawbacks also which mainly include particle aggregation as well as difficulty in handling nanoparticles in liquid and dry states, toxicity issues, and so on, which restrict the successful clinical and commercial use of nanoparticles. The key aspects of using nanotechnology in drug delivery technology have to fulfill the following specific objectives:

- Development of improved carriers for poorly water-soluble drugs
- Prolong sustainable drug release system for site-specific targeting
- To decrease toxicity issues related with materials
- To improve the bioactivity of drug by protecting it from biological barriers
- Retention of drug in the body for a longer period of time for effective treatment
- Cost-effective and biodegradability
- Easy transport of drug across epithelial and endothelial barriers
- Combined therapeutic and diagnostic modalities into one agent

Nanotechnology in drug delivery strategy is just an emerging field and requires more time and effort and provides opportunities to scientists to overcome the challenges in the clinical trials and make it a promising approach in reality.

References

Ai, J., Biazar, E., Montazeri, M., Majdi, A., Aminifard, S., Safari, M., Akbari, H.R., 2011. Nanotoxicology and nanoparticle safety in biomedical designs. Int. J. Nanomed. 6, 1117–1127.

Allen, T.M., Cullis, P.R., 2004. Drug delivery systems: entering the mainstream. Science 303 (5665), 1818–1822.

Amoabediny, G., Haghiralsadat, F., Naderinezhad, S., et al., 2018. Overview of preparation methods of polymeric and lipid-based (niosome, solid lipid, liposome) nanoparticles: a comprehensive review. Int. J. Polym. Mater. Polym Biomater. 67, 383–400.

Arayne, M.S., Sultana, N., Qureshi, F., 2007. Nanoparticles in delivery of cardiovascular drugs. Pak. J. Pharm. Sci. 20, 340–348.

Arsawang, U., Saengsawang, O., Rungrotmongkol, T., Sornmee, P., Wittayanarakul, K., Remsungnen, T., Hannongbua, S., 2011. How do carbon nanotubes serve as carriers for gemcitabine transport in a drug delivery system? J. Mol. Graph. Model. 29, 591–596.

Astruc, D., Boisselier, E., Ornelas, C., 2010. Dendrimers designed for functions: from physical, photophysical, and supramolecular properties to applications in sensing, catalysis, molecular electronics, photonics, and nanomedicine. Chem. Rev. 110 (4), 1857–1959.

Avenitt, R.D., Wescott, S.L., Halas, N.J., 1999. Linear optical properties of gold nanoshells. J. Opt. Soc. Am. B 16, 1814–1823.
Ballauff, M., Likos, C.N., 2004. Dendrimers in solution: insight from theory and simulation. Angew. Chem. 43 (23), 2998–3020.
Baltes, T., Garret-Flaudy, F., Freitag, R., 1999. Investigation of the LCST of polyacrylamides as a function of molecular parameters and the solvent composition. J. Polym. Sci., Part A: Polym. Chem. 37, 2977–2989.
Baszkin, A., Norde, W., 1999. Physical Chemistry of Biological Interfaces. CRC Press.
Bayer, C.L., Peppas, N.A., 2008. Advances in recognitive, conductive and responsive delivery systems. J. Control. Rel. 132, 216–221.
Beg, S., Rizwan, M., Sheikh, A.M., Hasnain, M.S., Anwer, K., Kohli, K., 2011. Advancement in carbon nanotubes: basics, biomedical applications and toxicity. J. Pharm. Pharmacol. 63, 141–163.
Berthold, A., Cremer, K., Kreuter, J., 1996. Preparation and characterization of chitosan microspheres as drug carrier for prednisolone sodium phosphate as model for anti-inflammatory drugs. J. Control. Rel. 39, 17–25.
Blackman, J., 2009. Metallic Nanoparticles, First ed. Elsevier.
Bozzuto, G., Molinari, A., 2015. Liposomes as nanomedical devices. Int. J. Nanomed. 10, 975–999.
Cao, J.Q., Wang, Y.X., Yu, J.F., Xia, J.Y., Zhang, C.F., Yin, D.Z., Hafeli, U.O., 2004. Synthesis of Fe_3O_4 nanoparticles and their magnetic properties. J. Magn. Magn. Mater. 277, 165–174.
Carafa, M., Marianecci, C., Di Marzio, L., De Caro, V., Giandalia, G., Giannola, L.I., Santucci, E., 2010. Potential dopamine prodrug-loaded liposomes: preparation, characterization, and in vitro stability studies. J. Liposome Res. 20, 250–257.
Chakroborty, G., Seth, N., Sharma, V., 2013. Nanoparticles and nanotechnology: clinical, toxicological, social, regulatory and other aspects of nanotechnology. J. Drug Deliv. Ther 3 (4), 138–141.
Chan, A., Orme, R.P., Fricker, R.A., Roach, P., 2013. Remote and local control of stimuli responsive materials for therapeutic applications. Adv. Drug. Deliv. Rev. 65 (4), 497–514.
Chang, H.I., Yeh, M.K., 2012. Clinical development of liposome-based drugs: formulation, characterization, and therapeutic efficacy. Int. J. Nanomed. 7, 49–60.
Chen, Z.P., Zhang, Y., Zhang, S., Xia, J.G., Liu, J.W., Xu, K., Gu, N., 2008. Preparation and characterization of water-soluble monodisperse magnetic iron oxide nanoparticles via surface double-exchange with DMSA. Colloids Surf. A: Physicochem. Eng. Asp. 316, 210–216.
Chow, A.H.L., Tong, H.H.Y., Chattopadhyay, P., Shekunov, B.Y., 2007. Particle engineering for pulmonary drug delivery. Pharm. Res. 24 (3), 411–437.
Cole, A.J., Yang, V.C., David, A.E., 2011. Cancer theranostics: the rise of targeted magnetic nanoparticles. Trends Biotechnol. 29, 323–332.
Colvin, V.L., 2007. Nanoparticles as catalysts for protein fibrillation. Proc. Natl. Acad. Sci. U. S. A. 104, 8679–8680.
Couvreur, P., Gref, R., Andrieux, K., Malvy, C., 2006. Nanotechnologies for drug delivery: application to cancer and autoimmune diseases. Prog. Solid State Chem. 34, 231.
Couvreur, P., 2013. Nanoparticles in drug delivery: past, present and future. Adv. Drug Deliv. Rev. 65 (1), 21–23.
Coviello, T., Trotta, A.M., Marianecci, C., Carafa, M., Di Marzio, L., Rinaldi, F., Di Meo, C., Alhaique, F., Matricardi, P., 2015. Gel-embedded niosomes: preparation, characterization

and release studies of a new system for topical drug delivery. Colloids Surf. B Biointerfaces 125, 291–299.

Cregg, P.J., Mardinoglu, K.M.A., 2012. Inclusion of interactions in mathematical modelling of implant assisted magnetic drug targeting. Appl. Math. Model. 36, 1–34.

Dan, N., 2018. Chapter 14: Structure and kinetics of synthetic, lipid-based nucleic acid carriers: Lipoplexes. Lipid Nanocarriers for Drug Targeting. Elsevier, pp. 529–562.

Davis, S.S., 1997. Biomedical applications of nanotechnology—implications for drug targeting and gene therapy. Trends Biotechnol. 15, 217–224.

Dhar, S., Liu, Z., Thomale, J., Dai, H., Lippard, S.J., 2008. Targeted single-wall carbon nanotube-mediated Pt(IV) prodrug delivery using folate as a homing device. J. Am. Chem. Soc. 27 (130), 11467–11476.

DHHS, 2009. Department of Health and Human Services, Centers for Disease Control and Prevention and National Institute for Occupational Safety and Health. Approaches to Safe Nanotechnology: Managing the Health and Safety Concerns Associated with Engineered Nanomaterials. Publication No. 2009-125.

Di Crescenzo, A., Velluto, D., Hubbell, J.A., Fontana, A., 2011. Biocompatible dispersions of carbon nanotubes: a potential tool for intracellular transport of anticancer drugs. Nanoscale 3, 925–928.

"Drug Definition", 2014. Stedman's Medical Dictionary. Archived from the original on 2014-05-02. via Drugs.com. (Accessed 01 May 2014).

"Drug". Dictionary.com Unabridged. v 1.1. Random House. 20 September 2007. Archived from the original on 14 September 2007. via Dictionary.com.

Duncanand, R., Izzo, L., 2005. Dendrimerbiocompatibilityandtoxicity. Adv. Drug Deliv. Rev. 57 (15), 2215–2237.

Ernsting, M.J., Foltz, W.D., Undzys, E., Tagami, T., Li, S.D., 2012. Tumor-targeted drug delivery using MR-contrasted docetaxel-carboxymethyl cellulose nanoparticles. Biomaterials 33, 3931–3941.

Fan, Y., Zhang, Q., 2013. Development of liposomal formulations: from concept to clinical investigations. Asian J. Pharm. Sci. 8 (2), 81–87.

Fleming, A.B., Salzman, W.M., 2002. Pharmacokinetics of the carmustine implant. Clin. Pharmacokine. 41, 403–419.

Foldvari, M., Bagonluri, M., 2008. Carbon nanotubes as functional excipients for nanomedicines: I. Pharmaceutical properties. Nanomedicine 4, 173–182.

Friedman, A.D., Claypool, S.E., Liu, R., 2013. The smart targeting of nanoparticles. Curr. Pharm. Des. 19, 6315–6329.

Ganta, S., Devalapally, H., Shahiwala, A., Amiji, M., 2008. A review of stimuliresponsive-nanocarriers for drug and gene delivery. J. Control. Rel. 126 (3), 187–204.

Goya, G.F., Grazú, V., Ibarra, M.R., 2008. Magnetic nanoparticles for cáncer therapy. Curr. Nanosci. 4, 1–16.

Guo, M., Gorman, P.M., Rico, M., Chakrabartty, A., Laurents, D.V., 2005. Charge substitution shows that repulsive electrostatic interactions impede the oligomerization of Alzheimer amyloid peptides. FEBS Lett. 579, 3574–3578.

Hamley, I.W., Callaway, D.J.E., Tjernberg, A., Hahne, S., Lilliehöök, C., Terenius, L., Thyberg, J., Nordstedt, C., 2012. The amyloid beta peptide: a chemist's perspective. Role in Alzheimer's and fibrillization. Chem. Rev. 112, 5147–5192.

Hruby, M., Filippov, S.K., Stepanek, P., 2015. Smart polymers in drug delivery systems on crossroads: which way deserves following? Eur. Polym. J. 65, 82–97.

Illum, L., Davis Brigger, I., Dubernet, C., Couvreur, P., 2002. Nanoparticles in cancer therapy and diagnosis. Adv. Drug Deliv. Rev. 54 (5), 631–651.

ISO, 2004. Occupational ultrafine aerosol exposure characterization, assessment. Draft technical report number 6. ISO/TC146/SC2WG1 Particle size selective sampling and analysis (workplace air quality).

Jahangirian, H., Lemraski, E.G., Webster, T.J., Rafiee-Moghaddam, R., Abdol-lahi, Y., 2017. A review of drug delivery systems based on nanotechnology and green chemistry: green nanomedicine. Int. J. Nanomed. 12, 2957.

Jain, A.K., Thareja, S., 2019. In vitro and in vivo characterization of pharmaceutical nanocarriers used for drug delivery. Artif. Cells Nanomed. Biotechnol. 47 (1), 524–539.

Jeong, B., Kim, S.W., Bae, Y.H., 2002. Thermosensitive sol-gel reversible hydrogels. Adv. Drug Deliv. Rev. 54, 37–51.

Jin, Y., Tong, L., Ai, P., Li, M., Hou, X., 2006. Self-assembled drug delivery systems. 1. Properties and in vitro/in vivo behavior of acyclovir self-assembled nanoparticles (SAN). Int. J. Pharm. 309, 199–207.

Jong, W.H.D., Borm, P.J.A., 2008. Drug delivery and nanoparticle applications and hazards. Int. J. Nanomed. 3 (2), 133–149.

Juan, M., 2013. Campelo Book Titled As Sustainable Preparation of Supported Metal Nanoparticles and Their Applications in Catalysis. RSC Green Chemistry, Thomas Graham House, Science Park, Cambridge, United Kingdom.

Kannan, R.M., Nance, E., Kannan, S., Tomalia, D.A., 2014. Emerging concepts in dendrimer-based nanomedicine: from design principles to clinical applications. J. Intern. Med. 276 (6), 579–617.

Kaur, G., Arora, M., Ganugula, R., Ravi Kumar, M.N.V., 2019. Double-headed nanosystems for oral drug delivery. Chem. Commun. 55, 4761–4764.

Kawasaki, E.S., Player, A., 2005. Nanotechnology, nanomedicine, and the development of new, effective therapies for cancer. Nanomedicine 1 (2), 101–109.

Kiesel, T., Li, Y., Unger, F., 2002. ABA-triblock copolymers from biodegradable polyester A-blocks and hydrophilic poly(ethylene oxide) B-blocks as a candidate for in situ forming hydrogel delivery systems for proteins. Adv. Drug Deliv. Rev. 54, 99–134.

Klaine, S.J., Alvarez, P.J., Batley, G.E., Fernandes, T.F., Hand, R.D., Lyon, D.Y., Mahendra, S., McLaughlin, M.J., Lead, J.R., 2008. Nanomaterials in the environment: behavior, fate, bioavailability, and effects. Environ. Toxicol. Chem. 27, 1825–1851.

Kshirsagar, N.A., 2000. Drug delivery systems. Indian J. Pharma 32, S54–S61.

Kwon, G.S., 2003. Polymeric micelles for delivery of poorly water-soluble compounds. Crit. Rev. Ther. Drug Carr. Syst. 20, 357–403.

Lai, W.F., Shum, H.C., 2016. A stimuli-responsive nanoparticulate system using poly(ethylenimine)-*graft*-polysorbate for controlled protein release. Nanoscale 8, 517–528.

Laurent, S., Ejtehadi, M.R., Rezaei, M., Kehoe, P.G., Mahmoudi, M., 2012. Interdisciplinary challenges and promising theranostic effects of nanoscience in Alzheimer's disease. RSC Adv. 2, 5008–5033.

Laurent, S., Forge, D., Port, M., Roch, A., Robic, C., Elst, L.V., Muller, R.N., 2008. Magnetic iron oxide nanoparticles: synthesis, stabilization, vectorization, physicochemical characterizations, and biological applications. Chem. Rev. 108, 2064–2110.

Lee, R.R., 2000. The Science and Practice of Pharmacy, 21st ed. Lippincott Williams & Wilkins, Philadelphia, PA, USA.

Leong, K.W., Langer, R., 1988. Polymeric controlled drug delivery. Adv. Drug Rev. 1, 199–233.
Levy, M., Wilhelm, C., Siaugue, J.M., Horner, O., Bacri, J.C., Gazeau, F., 2008. Magnetically induced hyperthermia: size-dependent heating power of γ-Fe_2O_3 nanoparticles. J. Phys. Condens. Matter. 20, 204133.
Li, S., Bueno, M.M., Vart, M., 2001. Protein release from physically crosslinked hydrogels of the PLA/PEO/PLA triblock copolymer-type. Biomaterials 22, 363–369.
Litzinger, D.C., Huang, L., 1992. Phosphatidylethanolamine liposomes: drug delivery, gene transfer and immunodiagnostic applications. Biochim. Biophys. Acta 1113, 201–227.
Liu, D., Yang, F., Xiong, F., Gu, N., 2016. The smart drug delivery system and its clinical potential. Theranostics 6 (9), 1306–1323.
Lombardo, D., Calandra, P., Barreca, D., Magazù, S., Kiselev, M., 2016. Soft interaction in liposome nanocarriers for therapeutic drug delivery. Nanomaterials 6 (7), 125.
Lombardo, D., Calandra, P., Magazù, S., Wanderlingh, U., Barrecad, D., Kiselev, M.A., 2018. Soft nanoparticles charge expression within lipid membranes: the case of amino terminated dendrimers in bilayers vesicles. Colloids Surf. B: Biointerfaces 170, 609–616.
Lombardo, D., Kiselev, M.A., Caccamo, M.T., 2019. Smart nanoparticles for drug delivery application: development of versatile nanocarrier platforms in biotechnology and nanomedicine. J. Nanomater. 2019, 3702518. Available from: https://doi.org/10.1155/2019/3702518.
Ma, Z., Liu, H., 2007. Synthesis and surface modification of magnetic particles for application in biotechnology and biomedicine. China Particuol 5, 1–10.
Mahmoudi, M., Quinlan-Pluck, F., Monopoli, M.P., Sheibani, S., Vali, H., Dawson, K.A., Lynch, I., 2013. Influence of the physiochemical properties of superparamagnetic iron oxide nanoparticles on amyloid β protein fibrillation in solution. ACS Chem. Neurosci. 4, 475–485.
Malhotra, M., Jain, N.K., 1994. Niosomes as drug carriers. Indian Drugs 31, 81–86.
Marianecci, C., Petralito, S., Rinaldi, F., Hanieh, P.N., Carafa, M., 2016. Some recentadvances on liposomal and niosomal vesicular carriers. J. Drug Deliv. Sci. Technol 32, 256–269.
Martinho, N., Damgé, C., Reis, C.P., 2011. Recent advances in drug delivery systems. J. Biomater. Nanobiotechnol 2, 510.
Mathowitz, E.C.D., Jacob, S.J., 1999. Encyclopedia of Controlled Drug Delivery. John Wiley& Son Inc., New York.
McBain, S.C., Yiu, H.P., Dobson, J., 2008. Magnetic nanoparticles for gene and drug delivery. Int. J. Nanomed. 3, 169–180.
Meng, F.H., Zhong, Z.Y., Feijen, J., 2009. Stimuli-responsive polymersomes for programmed drug delivery. Biomacromolecules 10 (2), 197–209.
Mesiha, M.S., Sidhom, M.B., Fasipe, B., 2005. Oral and subcutaneous absorption of insulin poly(isobutylcyanoacrylate) nanoparticles. Int. J. Pharm. 288, 289–293.
Mirsadeghi, S., Shanehsazzadehc, S., Atyabi, F., Rassoul, Dinarvand, R., 2016. Effect of PEGylated superparamagnetic iron oxide nanoparticles (SPIONs) under magnetic field on amyloid beta fibrillation process. Mater. Sci. Eng. C 59, 390–397.
Moghassemi, S., Hadjizadeh, A., 2014. Nano-niosomes as nanoscale drug deliverysystems: an illustrated review. J. Controlled Rel. 185, 22–36.

Mourgues, A., Charmette, C., Sanchez, J., Marti-Mestres, G., Gramain, P., 2004. EO/EP copolymer membranes as reservoir in a transdermal therapeutic system for caffeine delivery: modeling and simulation. J. Membr. Sci. 241, 297–304.

Muller, R., Keck, C., 2004. Challenges and solutions for the delivery of biotech drugs—a review of drug nanocrystal technology and lipid nanoparticles. J. Biotechnol. 113 (1–3), 151–170.

Narayani, R., Rao, K.P., 1993. Preparation, characterization and in vitro stability of hydrophilic gelatin microspheres using a gelatin-methotrexate conjugate. Int. J. Pharm. 95, 85–91.

Nevozhay, D., Kañska, U., Budzyñska, R., Boratyñski, J., 2007. Current status of research on conjugates and related drug delivery systems in the treatment of cancer and other diseases (Polish). Postepy Hig. Med. Dosw 61, 350–360.

NNI, 2009. National Nanotechnology Initiative. Leading to a Revolution in Technology and Industry.

Ogawara, K.I., Un, K., Tanaka, K., Higaki, K., Kimura, T., 2009. In vivo anti-tumor mal doxorubicin (DOX) in Dox-resistant tumor-bearing mice: involvement of cytotxic effect on vascular endothelial cells. J. Controlled Rel. 133 (1), 4–10.

Onuki, A., 1993. Theory of phase transition in polymer gels. Adv. Polym. Sci. 109, 63–121.

Orive, G., Hernández, R.M., Rodríguez Gascón, A., Domínguez-Gil, A., Pedraz, J.L., 2003. Drug delivery in biotechnology: present and future. Curr. Opin. Biotechnol. 14, 659–664.

Orive, G., Gascon, A.R., Hernández, R.M., Domínguez-Gil, A., Pedraz, J.L., 2004. Techniques: new approaches to the delivery of biopharmaceuticals. Trends Pharmacol. Sci. 25, 382–387.

Pankhurst, Q.A., Connolly, J., Jones, S.K., Dobson, J., 2003. Applications of magnetic nanoparticles in biomedicine. J. Phys. D: Appl. Phys. 36, 167–181.

Pardeike, J., Hommoss, A., Müller, R.H., 2009. Lipid nanoparticles (SLN, NLC) in cosmetic and pharmaceutical dermal products. Int. J. Pharm. 366 (1–2), 170–184.

Pogodin, S., Werner, M., Sommer, J.U., Baulin, V.A., 2012. Nanoparticle-induced permeability of lipid membranes. ACS Nano 6 (12), 10555–10561.

Rapoport, N., 2007. Physical stimuli-responsive polymeric micelles for anti-cancer drug delivery. Prog. Polym. Sci. 32 (8-9), 962–990.

Razzacki, S.Z., Thwar, P.K., Yang, M., Ugaz, V.M., Burns, M.A., 2004. Integrated microsystems for controlled drug delivery. Adv. Drug Deliv. Rev. 56, 185–198.

Rossi, S., Donadio, S., Fontana, L., Porcaro, F., Battocchio, C., Venditti, I., Bracci, L., Fratoddi, I., 2016. Negatively charged gold nanoparticles as dexamethasonecarrier: stability and citotoxic activity. RCS Adv. 6, 99016–99990.

Ruiz-Hernandez, E., Lopez-Noriega, A., Arcos, D., Vallet-Regı, M., 2008. Mesoporous magnetic microspheres for drug targeting. Solid State Sci. 10, 421–426.

Safari, J., Zarnegar, Z., 2014. Advanced drug delivery systems. Nanotechnology of health design A review. J. Saudi Chem. Soc. 18, 85–99.

Sagadevan, S., Periasamy, M., 2014. A review on role of nanostructures in drug delivery systems. Rev. Adv. Mater. Sci. 36, 112–117.

Sahoo, S.K., Parveen, S., Panda, J.J., 2007. The present and future of nanotechnology in human healthcare. Nanomed. Nanotech. Biol. Med. 3 (1), 20–31.

Saltzman, W., Torchilin, M., Vladimir, P., 2008. Drug Delivery Systems. Access Science, McGraw-Hill Companies.

Saltzman, W.M., 2001. Drug Delivery. Oxford University Press, New York.

Sershen, S., West, J., 2002. Implantable, polymeric systems for modulated drug delivery. Adv. Drug Deliv. Rev. 54, 1225–1235.
Sershen, S.R., Westcott, S.L., Halas, N.J., West, J.L., 2000. Temperature-sensitive polymer-nanoshell composites for photothermally modulated drug delivery. J. Biomed. Mater. Res. 51, 293–298.
Shen, Z.Y., Ma, G.H., Dobashi, T., Maki, Y., Su, Z.G., 2008. Preparation and characterization of thermo-responsive albumin nanospheres. Int. J. Pharm. 346, 133–142.
Shersen, S., West, J., 2002. Implantable, polymeric systems for modulated drug delivery. Adv. Drug Deliv. Rev. 54, 1225–1235.
Shibayama, M., Tanaka, T., 1993. Volume phase transition and related phenomena of polymer gels. Adv. Polym. Sci. 109, 1–62.
Smith, K.L., Schimpf, M.E., Thompson, K.E., 1990. Bioerodible polymers for delivery of macromolecules. Adv. Drug Deliev. Rev. 4, 343–357.
Snyder, M.A., Lee, J.A., Davis, T.M., Scriven, L.E., Tsapatsis, M., 2007. Silica nanoparticle crystals and ordered coatings using lys-sil and a novel coating device. Langmuir 23, 9924–9928.
Sobol, E.N., Bagratashvili, V.N., Popov, V.K., Sobol, A.E., Said-Galiev, E.E., Nikitin, L. N., 1998. Kinetics of diffusion of organometallic compounds into polymers from solutions in supercritical carbon dioxide. Russ. J. Phys. Chem. 72 (1), 17–20.
Stolnik, S., Illum, L., Davis, S.S., 1995. Polymers in drug delivery. Adv. Drug Deliv. Rev. 16, 195–214.
Sundar, S., Kundu, J., Kundu, S.C., 2010. Biopolymeric nanoparticles. Sci. Technol. Adv. Mater. 11 (1), 014104.
Sykes, R., 2000. Towards the magic bullet. Int. J. Antimicrob. Agent 14, 1–12.
Tannock, I.F., Rotin, D., 1989. Acid pH in tumors and its potential for therapeutic exploitation. Cancer Res. 49, 4373–4384.
Tao, S.L., Desai, T.A., 2003. Microfabricated drug delivery systems: from particles to pores. Adv. Drug Deliv. Rev. 55, 315–328.
Tavano, L., Muzzalupo, R., 2016. Multi-functional vesicles for cancer therapy: the ultimate magic bullet. Colloids Surf. B: Biointerfaces 147, 161–171.
Tiwari, G., Tiwari, R., Sriwastawa, B., Bhati, L., Pandey, S., Pandey, P., Bannerjee, S.K., 2012. Drug delivery systems: an updated review. Int. J. Pharm. Investig. 2 (1), 2–11.
Udupa, N., 2002. Niosomes as drug carriers. In: Jain, N.K. (Ed.), Controlled and Novel Drug Delivery, first ed. CBS Publishers and Distributors, New Delhi, India.
Wang, Y., Ma, N., Wang, Z., Zang, X., 2007. Photocontrolled reversible supramolecular assemblies of an azobenzene-containing surfactant with alpha-cyclodextrin. Angew. Chem. Int. Ed. 46, 2823–2826.
Wang, N.X., Von Recum, H.A., 2011. Affinity based drug delivery. Macromol. Biosci. 11, 321–332.
Werner, M., Auth, T., Beales, P.A., Fleury, J.B., Höök, F., Kress, H., Van Lehn, R.C., Müller, M., Petrov, E.P., Sarkisov, L., Sommer, J.U., Baulin, V.A., 2018. Nanomaterial interactions with biomembranes: bridging the gap between soft matter models and biological context. Biointerphases 13 (8), 028501.
Whatmore, R.W., 2006. Nanotechnolgy - what is it? Should we be worried? Occup. Med. 56, 295–299.
White, R.J., Luque, R., Budarin, V.L., Clark, J.H., Macquarrie, D.J., 2009. Supported metal nanoparticles on porous materials. Methods and applications. Chem. Soc. Rev. 38, 481–494.

Xie, J., Xu, C., Kohler, N., Hou, Y., Sun, S., 2007. Controlled PEgylation of monodisperse Fe_3O_4 nanoparticles for reduced non-specific uptake by cells.macrophage. Adv. Mater. 19, 3163–3166.

Yang, H., Kao, W.J., 2006. Dendrimers for pharmaceutical and biomedical applications. J. Biomater. Sci., Polym. Ed. 17 (1-2), 3–19.

Yin, J., Chen, Y., Zhang, Z.H., Han, X., 2016. Stimuli-responsive block copolymer-based assemblies for cargo delivery and theranostic applications. Polymers 8 (7), 268.

Yu, X., Trase, I., Ren, M., Duval, K., Guo, X., Chen, Z., 2016. Design of nanoparticle-based carriers for targeted drug delivery. J. Nanomater. 2016, 1087250.

Zhang, Y., Chu, C.C., 2002. Thermal and mechanical properties of biodegradable hydrophilic-hydrophobic hydrogels based on dextran and poly (lactic acid). J. Mater. Sci. Mater. Med. 13 (8), 773–781.

CHAPTER

Nanostructures in gene delivery

4

Sarthak Bhattacharya[1,2]

[1]*Department of Pharmaceutics and Pharmaceutical Technology, Shri R.D. Bhakt College of Pharmacy, Jalna, India*

[2]*Dr. Babasaheb Ambedkar Marathwada University (BAMU), Aurangabad, India*

4.1 Introduction

Since the inception of human civilization in this mortal world, disease or disorders or illness has become an integral part of our lives. Looking back to the past, we have witnessed the rational use of several chemicals and chemical compounds to treat these ailments. Some of them have shown some astonishing results to treat these but in some times we have faced challenges too to make them bio-friendly.

The chemical compounds in the early civilization dates were not known to us. The one and only option was to identify the herbs by the local people and based on the observations, those herbs were made palatable to fight the illness. Later on when scientific advancements have started to initiate its course of path, lots of discoveries leading to maintain normal healthy life have been surfaced out. These discoveries can be elaborated in multiple directions starting from identification of chemical compounds, their structures, and structure–activity relationships (SAR) to formulation developments of these compounds into various dosage forms, that is, tablets, capsules, ointment, suppositories, and so many which are endless in count.

The scientific discoveries in the later stage have targeted mainly two domains; one is the chemical compounds division. This chemical compound domain is more specifically related to isolation, nomenclature, structural identification and modification, SAR, in vitro and in vivo pharmacological activities, and quantitative SAR (QSAR). The domain is formulation strategies of chemical compounds with multiple biological activities. Formulation strategies conjugate formulation development, in vitro and in vivo testing, biocompatible materials development, and targeted delivery systems.

Formulation development often synonymously known as dosage form development, delivery systems, targeted delivery systems are very important and integral part of research related to some scintillating discoveries in the field of medicine, pharmaceutical, and biomedical field. Numerous materials are often tested under this domain for targeting a particular disease or group of ailments. Materials with good biocompatibility, less tissue toxicities, better absorption

Advances in Polymeric Nanomaterials for Biomedical Applications. DOI: https://doi.org/10.1016/B978-0-12-814657-6.00007-0

portfolios, solubility, and bioavailability are some of the main criteria for primary selection. Another aspect of these materials is that they should show targeting, especially organ > tissue > cells targeting should be achieved.

Targeted therapies which are now the latest boom in biomedical research are not the conventional approaches falling under formulation development. A conventional approach means old dosage form development which can be tablets, capsules, semisolids, parenteral preparations, suppositories, and pessaries. These conventional dosage form developments however lack so many disadvantages which are to be rectified to get maximum therapeutic efficacies. Bioavailability, clinical efficacy, drug biomaterials interactions, and targeting organs at molecular levels are of great concerns in today's biomedical research. Numerous ailments are now surfaced out which cannot be treated with these conventional formulations. For example, earlier we approached shops for purchasing our daily needs but with the progression of time, our definition of needs is being modified even changed. We approach now the online e-commerce sites for direct delivery of our daily needs at our doorstep, which reveals that our mind is constantly searching for new methodologies and new concepts to make our lives more generous, more healthy, and more beautiful.

To make our life healthier, one has to be ailment-free. The subject "ailments" is a big phrase in our life starting from simple cough and cold to cancer. Cough and cold may be overcome with conventional formulations but in case of cancer, can we fight with conventional approaches. The answer is a big NO. The obvious reason is that conventional formulations have so many limitations and using conventional formulations with limitations, cancer cannot be cured. Not only cancer, HIV-AIDS, cardiovascular disorders, diabetes, nephrological emergencies like kidney stones, blockage of urethra, some gynecological diseases such as polycystic ovary syndrome and so many are in the lists of biomedical research field for urgent attention. We have to act like e-commerce sites where delivery is fast, specific, and timely (FST). This FST concept we have to adopt in biomedical research field also.

FST concept first starts with "Fast." It means we have to think fast, act fast, and deliver fast. The next one comes specific which means we have to act precisely. Specific has a distinct meaning in biomedical research. It further elaborates that the site of action should be precisely been chosen, and site of action is directly linked to the site of application. The conventional formulations act on the site of application and from there to the site of action. This involves multiple steps [adsorption, distribution, metabolism, and excretion (ADME) phenomenon] which significantly reduce the therapeutic effectiveness of the bioactive moiety. Moreover, it also affects the bioavailability which is an effective index in therapeutic effectiveness. Other limitations are solubility, penetration through PLP membrane, distribution in biological fluid, metabolism pathway, and excretion pathway. Conventional formulations still have these limitations and site-specificity is a big challenge for such formulations. In the latest biomedical research, the aim is to deliver the bioactive molecules at its specific site where it will show its remedial effectiveness. To accomplish such goal, scientists are now working at ground 0 level, that is, molecular levels. So many pathways are hypothetically derived to address molecular microenvironment.

Addressing molecular microenvironment through pathways is a big challenge. Concept of DNA, RNA, amino acids and genes play a significant role in such pathways approach. Abnormalities found in cellular components significantly contribute to the progression of a disease or disorder. To address such abnormalities in cellular components, nanostructures loaded with biomolecules, probiomolecules, and other NCEs (novel chemical moieties) have been proved to be precious. Nano-sized structures have, in recent period, gained methodical research awareness owing to their only one of its kind and precious properties compared with conventional materials used for biomedical applications.

Nanomaterials can be used in diverse applications, including biomaterial development, drug delivery, tissue targeting, and so many noncountable applications in biomedical research fields. Numerous advantages attend biomaterials on the nanoscale, which typically ranges from tens to hundreds of nanometers. For example, some nanometer-sized materials show enhanced permeability and retention effect in vivo delivery, which may be helpful for the selective delivery of nanomaterials to a cancer or malignant tumor site. Coating nanomaterials with multiple bioactive ligands may be used to take multiple advantages of the multivalent effect, whereby the binding affinity and specificity of biomolecular interactions can be increased significantly.

Nanostructures or in simple "Nanomaterials" (backbones of nanostructures) are almost similar in size to cellular organelles, biomacromolecules, and microorganisms. These biological nanostructures can be referred to as "natural bionanostructures." On the other hand, specifically designed "man-made bionanostructures" can substitute the function of the natural bionanostructures and can even have improved properties or have functions that are unparalleled. One of the most fascinating aspects of the man-made bionanostructure development is that its numerous beneficial properties can be combined and incorporated into a single nanomaterial to create a multifunctional bionanomaterial.

Nanomaterials can be prepared in two different ways, namely, a top-down approach and a bottom-up approach. In the top-down approach, the final nanostructure is carved from a larger block of matter into the desired shape and order, consequently without atomic-level control. By contrast, in the bottom-up approach, the desired nanostructures can be built from molecular building blocks that self-assemble by means of principles of molecular recognition.

In the bottom-up approach, the structure of the molecular building blocks, atomic and molecular-level control may be manipulated which may ultimately turn into self-assembled nanostructures. The configuration of most natural bionanostructures is determined by bottom-up processes, which are quite often seen in protein folding, phospholipids into cellular membranes, DNA and RNA structures, and microorganisms coated proteins.

So many synthetic molecules are now being used as building blocks for self-assembly. Block copolymers are one of the most widely used for such applications. Self-assembled nanostructures made up of block copolymers have been used in diversified applications, including novel biomaterials developments, carrier molecules for targeted therapies, and so many. Other commonly used building blocks include peptides, DNA and RNA, dendrimers, and other types of amphiphilic molecules. In addition, hybrid nanostructures composed of organic soft materials and inorganic hard materials and vice versa have been manufactured with improved properties compared with their pure forms. Nanostructures, depending on their physical parameters such as shape and size, show improved therapeutic activities. Gold nanoparticles of different sizes show therapeutic responses based on their different sizes. On the other hand, functionalized nanoparticles with different shapes have been shown improved therapeutic goals. Carbon nanotubes (CNTs) have size-dependent cellular uptake efficiency, in which shorter CNTs more readily penetrate through an energy-independent pathway. It has also been reported that ligand-coated nanostructures have size and shape-dependent binding modes when they interact with their binding partner in a multivalent manner (Kono et al., 1999; Raffa et al., 2008).

Apart from their biological activity, nanostructures can display size- and shape-dependent cytotoxicity and other therapeutic profiles. Recent toxicological studies have shown that the degree of accumulation of rigid multi-walled CNTs (MWCNT) longer than 20 μm is significantly higher compared with low aspect ratio (ratio of length to width) CNTs and tangled nanotube aggregates (Kostarelos, 2008; Poland et al., 2008). Gold nanoparticles are acknowledged to be almost nontoxic. It is evident that gold nanoparticles of very small size show relatively high toxicity (Connor et al., 2005; Goodman et al., 2004; Pernodet et al., 2006; Pan et al., 2007), thus cellular responses to gold nanoparticles appear to be size-dependent. Hence, the control of physical properties of nanostructures is highly important for their successful utilization in biological systems to address therapeutic effectiveness and thus nanostructures manufactured to have specific shapes and sizes contribute to advanced biomedical research.

4.2 Management of physical properties in self-assembled nanostructures

4.2.1 Driving forces for self-assembly: noncovalent interactions

Self-assembly is an autonomous formation of well-defined nanostructures from building blocks. Self-assembly is a force balance process between three classes of force: a driving force that brings self-assembly units together, an opposing force that balances with the driving force, and a functional force that determines the directionality and functionality of self-assembled aggregates (Lee, 2008). The most important driving force underlying self-assembly is noncovalent interactions or weak covalent bonds, such as Van der Waals interactions, the hydrophobic effect, electrostatic interactions, hydrogen bonding, and coordination bonding. Noncovalent interactions are weaker and longer than covalent bonds but collectively have a very significant influence on the detailed structures of self-assembled nanostructures.

4.2.1.1 Van der Waals interaction

Van der Waals interactions are the attractive or repulsive forces between molecules other than those due to covalent bonds or to the electrostatic interaction of ions. The Van der Waals interaction is a dispersion force, of which there are three different types, namely, dipole–dipole, dipole–induced dipole, and induced dipole–induced dipole interactions (London dispersion force). Depending on conditions, Van der Waals interactions can be either attractive or repulsive. Hence, it is important to understand the nature of Van der Waals interactions both at the molecular level and in relation to nano-objects ranging from supramolecular to macroscopic in size.

4.2.1.2 Hydrophobic effect

Many of the synthetic building blocks for self-assembly are amphiphiles. For the aggregation of amphiphiles in an aqueous medium, hydrophobic interactions are one of the most significant factors. Many cellular molecules (e.g., cell membrane consisting of P–L–P; Protein–Lipid–Protein), for example, proteins and lipids are also amphiphilic due to their both polar and nonpolar regions. The self-assembly of amphiphiles is directed by microphase separation of two dissimilar blocks. During usage of the polar solvent as selective solvent in the self-assembly, the nonpolar regions of the amphiphile cluster together to expose the minimum possible hydrophobic area to the polar solvent, whereas the polar-regions arrange to maximize their interaction with such solvent. The forces that hold the nonpolar regions of the molecules together are called hydrophobic interactions. Hydrophobic interactions are not due to any intrinsic attraction between nonpolar-regions but rather are the result of the system's tendency to achieve the greatest thermodynamic stability by minimizing the number of ordered polar solvents molecules required to surround hydrophobic portions of the amphiphilic molecules.

4.2.1.3 Electrostatic interaction

Forces that originate from electrostatic interactions have high impact on many self-assembled nanostructures. The electrostatic interaction, which can be either an attractive or a repulsive force, occurs between two charged atoms, ions, or molecules, leading to Coulomb interaction. Electrostatic interactions play a significant role in synthetic nanostructures linked with biomolecules, cationic molecule–DNA complex system (Pack et al., 2005; Mastrobattista et al., 2006; Han et al., 2007; Xu et al., 2008). Specifically, when cationic molecules such as cationic polymers or lipids are mixed with negatively charged DNA (or RNA), they form multiple intermolecular electrostatic interactions, resulting in the formation of condensed nanostructures. From this, it is understood that the interactions between charged particles in a liquid medium, the total force acting on colloidal objects, are to be taken into consideration.

Moreover, in addition to the noncovalent forces, other types of noncovalent interactions, such as hydrogen bonding, p–p stacking interactions, steric and depletion forces, and solvation and hydration forces and energies, should also be taken into consideration to control the preparation of self-assembled nanostructures for obtaining optimum therapeutic effectiveness.

4.2.1.4 Hydrogen bond

Hydrogen bond is the electrostatic attraction between H atom and a highly electronegative atom nearby, for example, O, F, Cl, or others. Hydrogen bond attractions can occur both between molecules (intermolecular) and within different parts of a single molecule (intramolecular). It is very common both in inorganic molecules (e.g., water) and in organic molecules (e.g., DNA and proteins). For instance, hydrogen bond exists between the amides and carbonyls in the backbone of β-sheets formed by the self-assembly of peptides and enhances the stability of the self-assembled nanostructures.

4.2.1.5 $\pi-\pi$ Stacking

$\pi-\pi$ Stacking also plays a significant role in the stability of the nanostructures from self-assembly. In the multiscale self-assembly of diphenylalanine (FF), the backbone hydrogen bonds and $\pi-\pi$ interactions from the aromatic peptide side chains hold the self-assembled FF structures together (Pan et al., 2007). In alkaline solution, folic acid can self-assemble via the formation of Hoogsteen-bonded nanoscale tetrameric discs, which then stack through $\pi-\pi$ interactions and inter-disc hydrogen bonding to form chiral columns (Gottarelli et al., 1996; Kamikawa et al., 2004). However, due to the lack of hydrogen bond, methotrexate was unable to form any well-defined nanostructures with similar treatment (Lock et al., 2013).

At the end, it is crystal clear evident that noncovalent interactions play an important role in the formation and stability of nanostructures. The controlling factors in terms of physical properties of nanostructures are very important consideration in their successful preparation and delivery at the targeting site.

4.3 Strategies of drug delivery by nanostructures

4.3.1 Passive delivery

In drug and/or gene delivery by nanostructures, biomolecules are often associated with nanocarriers by physical encapsulation or chemical conjugation (Choi et al., 2012) and therefore passively delivered by nanocarriers on to the site of action. In the former method, biomolecules are physically incorporated into the internal cavity of the nanocarriers and stabilized by noncovalent interactions between biomolecules and nanocarriers, particularly hydrophobic effect (Keith and Cui, 2014; Liu and Fréchet, 1999). Many nanostructures, for example, nanomicelles, nanocapsules, and porous nanoparticles, have hydrophobicity to stabilize the entrapped drug molecules (Chung et al., 2014). When the nanostructures release drug or other biomolecules at target sites of action, the release rate plays a pivotal role. However, physical encapsulation into hydrophobic compartments often results in very low drug loading (DL), typically on the order of 2%–5% by weight (Lin et al., 2013). It is one of the vital challenges posed by nanostructures on delivery of therapeuticals. The second method is to attach biomolecules or NCEs, biomolecules such as peptides, DNA/RNA, and gene to the nanocarriers by direct chemical conjugation. To get good control over the release of biomolecules or NCEs, biomolecules such as peptides, DNA/RNA, and gene, the conjugation between nanocarriers and biomolecules or NCEs, biomolecules such as peptides, DNA/RNA, and gene should be easily delinked at target sites. If biomolecules cannot be delinked from their nanocarriers in time, their bioactivity and efficacy will be reduced at significant level. On the other hand, if biomolecules or NCEs, biomolecules such as peptides, DNA/RNA, and gene tend to be dissociated or portioned from their nanocarriers too quickly, they will fail to reach the target sites of action in a considerable dose. The ADME profile of these biomolecules will also be speeded up and elimination of such biomolecules will take place at faster rate than expected. Therefore realistic design of the chemical conjugation between biomolecules and its nanocarriers is of great importance and should be studied thoroughly.

4.3.2 Self-delivery

It seems that the common strategies discussed earlier simply consider biomolecules as active therapeuticals, which need to be delivered at the site of action at a predetermined rate for obtaining better therapeutic response. However, their physiochemical properties, such as self-assembly ability and solubility, are uncared for on numerous occasions. In recent years, there is a growing trend to build well-defined nanostructures with biomolecules as building units. Through this approach, the volume of distribution and content of biomolecules in the nanostructures can be precisely controlled. Rational analysis, design, and fabrication, lots of self-delivering nanostructures with high and fixed drug contents have been created for thorough understanding of such processes.

4.4 Various nanostructures for gene delivery and gene therapies

In recent advancements, nanostructures with various shapes and sizes have been manufactured and applied for many biomolecules. Various nanostructures manufactured by different materials and their applications in gene delivery are discussed in detail. RNAi (RNA interface), miRNA (MicroRNA), and siRNA (Small interfering RNA) play an important role in gene delivery. RNAi is considered as effective therapeutic agent for different types of virus-mediated and neoplastic disorders. miRNA and siRNA are also used as additional therapeutic agents as they regulate gene expression with high selectivity. RNAi noncoding can develop so many therapeutic agents due to their noncoding capabilities.

4.4.1 Liposomes nanostructures

In the past five decades, many important scientific breakthrough, such as remote DL, extrusion for homogeneous size, long-circulating (PEGylated) liposomes (stealth liposomes), triggered release liposome, liposomes containing nucleic acid polymers, ligand-targeted liposome, and liposome containing combinations of biomolecules, have led to plentiful clinical trials in the delivery of multiple therapeutic agents, such as anticancer, antifungal, and antibiotic biomolecules, gene medicines, anesthetics, and anti-inflammatory biomolecules (Allen and Cullis, 2013).

Liposomes are very attractive choice among nanoscientists as drug delivery vehicles. Particularly, hydrophobic biomolecules can place themselves inside the bilayer of liposome and hydrophilic biomolecules are entrapped within the aqueous core or at the bilayer interface (Çağdaş et al., 2014). Liposome has the multiple benefits in the nanodesign of biomolecules starting from preventing drug degradation, reducing side effects, and targeting biomolecules to the site of action with better therapeutic index (Ochekpe et al., 2009; Mishra et al., 2011; Soppimath et al., 2001). Hydrophobic biomolecules are usually formulated in surfactants and organic co-solvents to increase their solubility in polar solvents. However, these solubilizers themselves may cause tissue and cell toxicity at the doses needed to deliver the drug. In contrast, liposome, which are nontoxic, biocompatible, and biodegradable, safe preparation, reduced risk of immunological rejection and also biochemically versatile can deliver nonaqueous biomolecules with fewer side effects. For example, they have been successfully applied in transdermal drug delivery systems to enhance skin permeation of biomolecules with high molecular weight and poor water solubility (Qiu et al., 2008). Liposomes are also been used to deliver the genes intended for gene therapies. Cationic lipids which attain amine groups in the polar head are very frequently used for gene delivery, whereas anionic liposome are used in other therapeuticals. Besides, liposome can accumulate at sites of increased vasculature permeability, when their average diameter is in the ultrafilterable range (<200 nm) (Allen and Cullis, 2013). Like other carriers, these liposome have also some unwanted side effects which are the membrane of liposome is generally thin, fragile, and thus inherently not stable (Meng et al., 2009). Liposomes are also limited by their low encapsulation efficiency, rapid leakage of water-soluble drug in the presence of blood components, and poor storage stability (Lim et al., 2008) (Fig. 4.1).

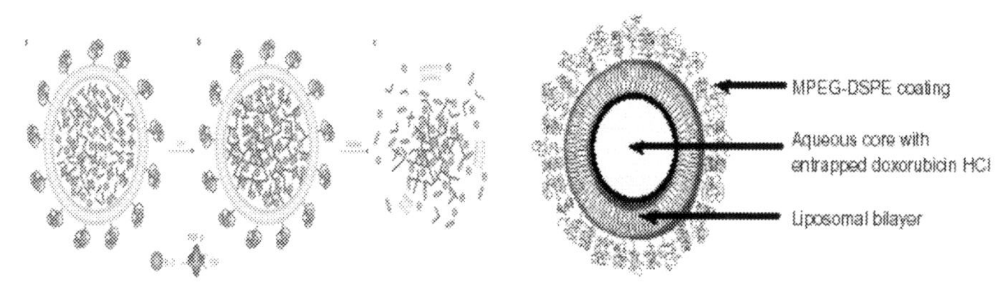

FIGURE 4.1

Schematic presentation of liposomes structures.

4.4.2 Polymeric nanostructures

In the field of therapeuticals delivery system, numerous polymeric nanostructures have been selected as hot topic in the field of biomedical research. Polymer-based bio-nanocarriers can significantly increase the solubility of hydrophobic biomolecules, reduce their tissue toxicity toward normal tissues, prolong the circulation time of biomolecules in blood, facilitate the entry of nanoparticles, and improve the utilization efficiency along with improved bioavailability (Habiba et al., 2015). It is a well-established fact that polymers used for therapeuticals delivery system should be nontoxic and biocompatible. Natural polymers, such as chitosan (Garcia-Fuentes and Alonso, 2012), dextran (Mocanu et al., 2016), heparin (Sakiyama-Elbert, 2011), and hyaluronan (Drobnik, 1991), have been well investigated for therapeuticals delivery system in the past. However, research on using synthetic polymers to build various nanostructures is more prevalent in the field of therapeuticals delivery system. Polyesters, polycarbonates, polyamides, polyphosphazenes, and polypeptides are among the most commonly used synthetic polymers (Li et al., 2013).

4.4.3 Polymeric nanomicelles and nanovesicles

Because of an immense versatility of polymers, nanostructures of different sizes and morphologies have been prepared in the laboratory. As mentioned earlier, amphiphilic molecules are prone to self-assemble into various nanostructures driven by hydrophobic effect. Therefore amphiphilic polymers containing both hydrophilic and hydrophobic blocks have been widely studied for use in therapeuticals delivery system. By controlling the hydrophilic/hydrophobic balance, various nanostructures, such as spherical micelles, cylindrical micelles, and vesicles, can be formed from amphiphilic polymers. According to Won et al. (2002), the weight fraction of the hydrophilic block can play a vital role in controlling the shapes of nanostructures from amphiphilic polymers in a pure water medium. Both polymeric micelles and vesicles are the most common and stable morphological structures of amphiphiles in water (Meng et al., 2009). Polymeric micelles are nanostructures with a

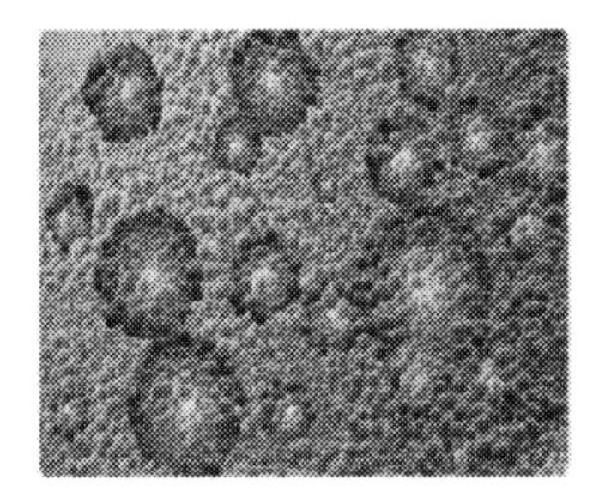

FIGURE 4.2

Picture showing nanomicelles.

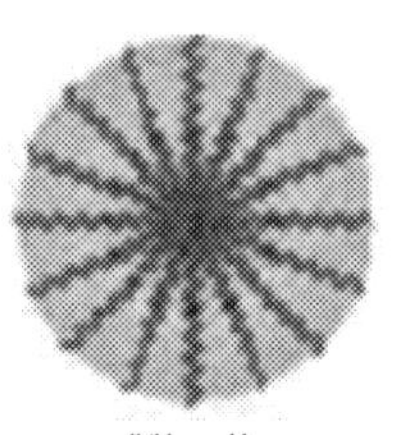

FIGURE 4.3

A model of nanovesicle.

hydrophilic core and a hydrophilic shell both of which have great influence on the distribution of biomolecules. Generally, hydrophilic drug molecules are encapsulated in the core of nanomicelles. Meanwhile, polymeric nanovesicles possess bilayer structures with an aqueous interior core, isolating the core from the external medium (Battaglia and Ryan, 2005). Polymeric vesicles can encapsulate hydrophilic molecules within the aqueous interior and also integrate hydrophobic molecules within the membrane. Therefore polymeric vesicles have the capability to deliver hydrophilic as well as hydrophobic biomolecules such as genes, anticancer biomolecules, and proteins and peptides (Figs. 4.2 and 4.3).

4.4.4 Polymeric nanogels

Polymeric nanomicelles and nanovesicles can only be maintained over the critical micelle concentration (CMC). Below CMC, they will separate into single polymer chains and thus lose the function as biomolecules carriers, and to avoid the dissociation of the self-assembled nanostructures, polymers are linked to obtain nanogels which are more stable in different physiological and physiochemical conditions has been become an important tool in delivery systems of therapeuticals particularly in gene and RNAi delivery. Nanogels have attained high degree of attention due to their high loading capacity and good stability (Li et al., 2013) (Fig. 4.4).

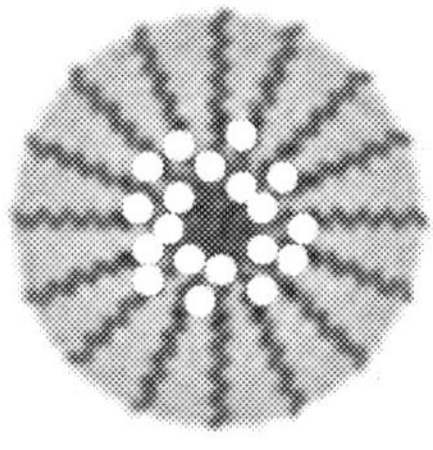

FIGURE 4.4

Pictorial representation of polymeric nanogel.

4.4.5 Polymeric nanocapsules

Void polymeric nanocapsules have also been developed by mini-emulsion polymerization technique. Biomolecules are confined in the cavities of nanocapsules and surrounded by external polymer membranes (Tiarks et al., 2001). Nanocapsules in which the protein of therapeutic interest is encapsulated or dissolved release the protein at the targeted cells, and the protein act onto the defective proteins or genes of the patient's cells by virtue of replacement. Nanocapsules are able to improve the oral bioavailability of proteins and peptides, including insulin, elcatonin, and salmon calcitonin (Prego et al., 2006). Nanocapsules can protect the degradation of biomolecules, especially proteins and peptides which are highly pH and temperature-sensitive, and also reduce systemic toxicity, provide controlled and extended and sustained release, and mask unpleasant taste (Whelan and Whelan, 2001). However, due to the high stability and low permeability of nanocapsules, biomolecules carried by nanocapsules face difficulties both in encapsulation into the capsules after formulation and in the release at target site (Fig. 4.5).

4.4.6 Polymeric dendrimers

Dendrimers are 1–10 nm three-dimensional globular synthetic macromolecules. Apart from these, dendrimers nanostructures with three-dimensional, hyperbranched globular nanopolymeric architectures are extensively used nanostructures in the modern days biomedical research. The attractive features of dendrimers include nanoscale size, narrow polydispersity index, excellent control over molecular structures, and availability of multiple functional groups at the periphery and cavities in the interior (Kesharwani et al., 2014). Dendrimers architecture consists of the core, branches, and many terminal functional groups. The core is an atom or a molecule at the center of the dendrimers with at least two identical chemical functions. From the core, branches with repeated units originate and spread, by having at least one branch junction, to form generations. These branches end with terminal functional groups at the surface of the dendrimers,

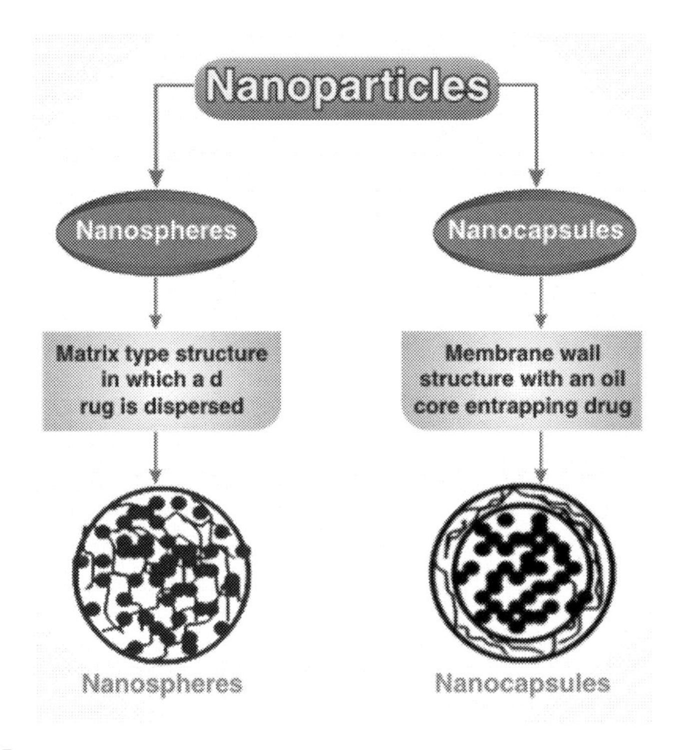

FIGURE 4.5

Classification of nanoparticles into nanospheres and nanocapsules.

which dictate the properties of the dendrimers macromolecule and for these multiple chemical and physical benefits, dendrimers have widely been used in the delivery of different bioactive agents such as oligonucleotides (Kono et al., 1999), enzymes (Dutta et al., 2006), vaccines (Khopade et al., 2002), and genes (Chaplot and Rupenthal, 2014). Biomolecules can be either incorporated into the interior or attached to the surface. Due to their versatility, both hydrophilic and hydrophobic biomolecules can be associated with dendrimers (Ochekpe et al., 2009). The most well-studied dendrimer is polyamidoamine (PAMAM), which is characterized by high solubility and reactivity due to the presence of void internal cavities and multiple functional groups at its periphery (Boas et al., 2006). Dendrimers have become an immense tool for gene delivery as they can interact with DNA, RNA, and oligonucleotides through electrostatic interaction to form complexes that condense the nucleic acid (Ouyang et al., 2011). Hyperbranched dendrimers are more suitable to be used as gene delivery tools than more structured dendrimers as their flexibility allows them to form more compact complexes with DNA (Daneshvar et al., 2013). Under specific physiological and physiochemical conditions, dendrimers form polycations, which bind to the negatively charged nucleic acid. As this dendrimer–nucleic acid complex needs to cross the epithelia to get to its target, it is required to have a positive net charge to enable the cellular uptake of the

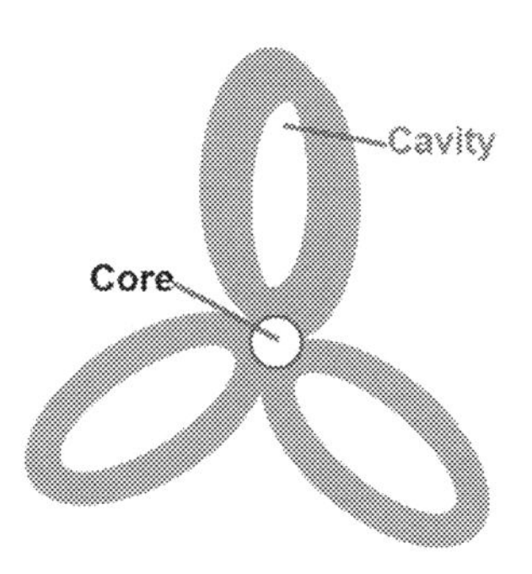

FIGURE 4.6

Schematic presentation of a dendrimers structure.

complex through its binding to the negatively charged cell membrane. Generally, high-generation dendrimers are more toxic than low-generation dendrimers. The major factors affecting the permeability of the dendrimers–gene complex are the surface charge, concentration, generation time, and surface modifications. The positively charged dendrimer–nucleic acid complex binds to the negatively charged cell membrane and is taken up by endocytosis forming an endosome. The endosome destabilizes due to the sponge effect of the dendrimer, releasing the nucleic acid to the cytoplasm. Nucleic acid is then taken up by the nucleus where it is replicated (Klajnert and Bryszewska, 2001) (Fig. 4.6).

4.5 Latest used dendrimers in gene delivery

1. PAMAM: The latest generation PAMAM dendrimers are widely used dendrimers as vectors for gene therapies. PAMAM structure shows a high density of amines in the periphery, which enables the condensation of nucleic acid. On the other hand, the inner amines enable efficient endosomal escape through the proton sponge effect (Tang et al., 2012), which is the resistance of cationic carriers that comprise a secondary or tertiary amine group to endosomal acidification through the absorption of protons. These cationic dendrimers absorb protons to below the physiological pH, which in turn delays the lysosomal fusion to the endosome. This prevents the degradation of nucleic acid and allows the accumulation of counterions like Cl^- in the endosome leading to the endosome rupture and the release of its content into the cytoplasm due to vesicular swelling (Sun et al., 2014). According to Braun, dendrimers with higher generations show better gene transfer than those with lower generations (Shah et al., 2013). However, higher generations of the PAMAM dendrimers show high degree of toxicity due to the increased nonbiodegradability. It has been shown that six generations PAMAM dendrimers are the most efficient for gene delivery (Klajnert and Bryszewska, 2001). Modified PAMAM dendrimers are the most commonly used for the

delivery of DNA and siRNA. Numerous modifications are done in the structure of PAMAM to obtain optimum gene delivery at the targeted site with improved significant reduction in cytotoxicity. Most common modification techniques include "Acetylation" and "internal quaternization" of PAMAM dendrimers that has been shown to reduce cytotoxicity in addition to genotoxicity, the formation of micronuclei, of the dendrimers. These modifications result in a neutral surface dendrimer with cationic charges inside the dendrimer; however, the conformed dendrimers resulted in the formation of condensed spherical siRNA–PAMAM complex, which protects the nucleic acids from degradation and improved their cellular internalization (Kim et al., 2007).

2. Polypropylenimine (PPI): PPI dendrimers are ideally suited for DNA binding and gene delivery, as they comprised 100% protonable nitrogen (Taratula et al., 2009). PPI dendrimers have established itself as a potential candidate for gene delivery due to preferential expression of genes in the liver in targeted liver cancer therapy (Russ et al., 2008). Moreover, the alteration of PPI dendrimers would provide more effective intracellular delivery of the gene. Furthermore, PPI dendrimers have also been used for siRNA delivery where PPI dendrimers were condensed with siRNA to form particles that are caged with dithiol and coated with polyethylene glycol (PEG) exhibited reduced genotoxicity, increased siRNA cellular bioavailability and stability in plasma, which in turn provided efficient gene silencing (Kim et al., 2007; Singha et al., 2011).
3. Polyethylenimine (PEI): PEI dendrimers are water-soluble polymers that can interact with the DNA, because it is positively charged and can protect DNA from degradation, which makes them a great delivery tool for siRNA and DNA (Arima et al., 2013); however, some studies show that PEI is less effective in siRNA delivery due to the reduced electrostatic interaction resulted by the short length of siRNA. PEI exerts the proton sponge effect to release the nucleic acid into the cytoplasm (Luo et al., 2011).
4. Other types of dendrimers: Glyodendrimers, which are dendrimers that are integrated with carbohydrates, have shown a great potential in targeted gene delivery. Cyclodextrins are cyclic oligosaccharides that are composed of a hydrophilic exterior and hydrophobic interior. PEI, especially generation dendrimers, has displayed high transfection efficiency in vitro and in vivo making it ideal for gene delivery (Luo et al., 2012) (Fig. 4.7).

4.6 Polymeric smart nanostructures

Another latest development in nanoresearch is smart nanostructures for gene and other biomolecules delivery. Development of smart nanostructures basically is carried out on different stimuli like pH, redox potential, light which are highly sensitive and exploring these stimuli, the nanostructures are prepared which is a superior approach for delivering and releasing biomolecules to target site at the desired and

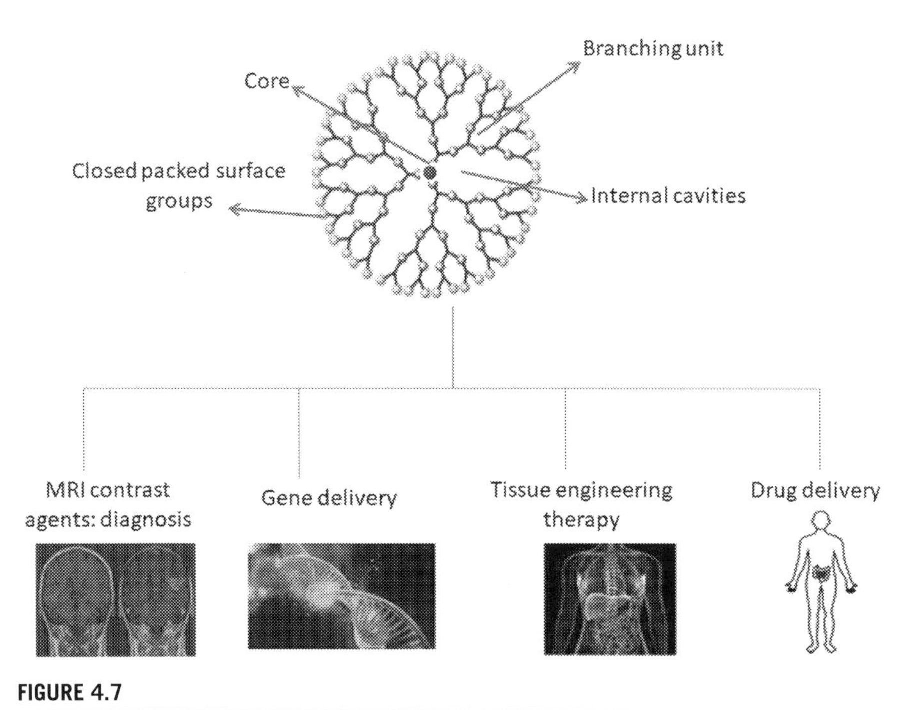

FIGURE 4.7

Latest used dendrimers in gene delivery.

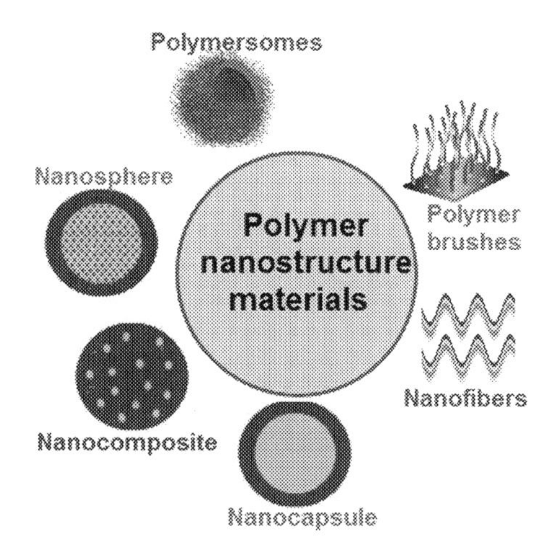

FIGURE 4.8

Types of various polymeric smart nanostructures.

predetermined time. These stimuli, including chemical (e.g., redox, pH), physical (e.g., temperature, light), and biological (e.g., enzymes), have been utilized in the design of smart gene and biomolecules delivery systems (Taniguchi, 1978) (Fig. 4.8).

4.6.1 Ceramic nanostructures

One-dimensional ceramic nanostructures are porous structures of nanoparticles, which are fabricated from biocompatible inorganic compounds, such as silica, calcium phosphate, alumina, and titania. These ceramic nanostructures are considered to be excellent carriers for biomolecules, genes, and proteins and enjoy wide range of therapeutic applications in the biomedical field. Ceramic nanoparticles can be prepared with the desired size, shape, and porosity. Their sizes are less than 100 nm and are able to avoid uptake by the reticuloendothelial system as foreign bodies. Entrapment of essential biomolecules which include proteins, enzymes, genes easily withstand body physiological pH and temperature, hence denaturation does not occur, and their swelling and porosity properties also become intact during their application at the site of action. Another astonishing fact is that the presence of hydroxyl group on the surface of ceramic materials shows natural hydrophilicity (Roy et al., 2003) and these retards the process of oxide particle clearance by the immune system and enhance their circulation time in blood Barbe et al. (2004). The only problem associated with these nanostructures is that they are not biodegradable, so accumulation in the body may show some toxic effects. Ceramic nanofiber composites are considered as an important breakthrough in bio-nanoceramic field as these systems in which biomolecules are entrapped act as local delivery systems at the targeted site. Ceramic nanofiber composites due to their versatility with respect to their composition have widened the scope of exploring myriad applications in biomedical research, particularly in cancer treatment.

4.6.2 Mesoporous silica nanostructures

Mesoporous materials also known as mesoporous molecular sieves are a class of 3D nanostructures with well-defined mesoscale (2–50 nm diameter) pores and surface areas up to 1000 m^2/gm (Barbe et al., 2004). Mesoporous materials are formed by a self-assembly process from combined solutions of sol–gel precursors (metal alkoxides and structure-directing amphiphiles usually block-copolymers or surface-active agents) (Beck and Vartuli, 2006). Mesoporous silica nanoparticles have been the most broadly investigated ceramic nanoparticles for delivery of biomolecules. Mesoporous silica nanoparticles have lots of advantageous properties including monodispersity, high specific surface area, tunable pore size and diameter, high porosity along with versatile functionalization (Slowing et al., 2010; Lu et al., 2008). A large variety of biomolecules have been successfully loaded in mesoporous silica nanoparticles or covalently grafted at mesoporous silica nanoparticles. Mesoporous silica nanoparticles are often functionalized to achieve a better delivery of biomolecules. For example, mannose or galactose functionalized mesoporous silica nanoparticles have been reported to induce a higher cytotoxicity of cancer cells than unfunctionalized ones and target cancer cells more efficiently (Brevet et al., 2009; Gary-Bobo et al., 2012). Silica-based mesoporous materials are used as third-generation bioceramics that facilitate the absorption and local control release of biomolecules at the targeted site. Moreover, these mesoporous materials release biomolecules at a controlled and sustained fashion, which are highly advantageous for the delivery of essential biomolecules.

4.6.3 Calcium phosphate nanostructures

Synthetic calcium phosphate is considered as model biomaterial with excellent biocompatibility. Calcium phosphates materials in nanosize can mimic the dimensions of constituent element of calcified tissues. Synthesis and application of nanostructured calcium phosphate with various morphologies such as nanoparticles, plate-like nanocrystals, nanoneedles, fibers, wires, mesoporous, nanotubes, nanoblades, and powders with 3D structures have been utilized in biomedical arena particularly in gene/biomolecules delivery and human tissue system. Calcium phosphate systems, including hydroxyapatite and tricalcium phosphates, are soluble under acidic conditions (pH $\leq$ 5) during bone remodeling. After cellular uptake, calcium phosphate systems are soluble under the conditions of lysosomal degradation (Sokolova and Epple, 2014). The variable stoichiometry, functionality, and dissolution properties make these nanoparticles suitable for biomolecules delivery. Their chemical similarity to bone and thus biocompatibility as well as variable surface charge density contribute to their controlled release properties (Bose et al., 2011). Among the known calcium phosphate compounds, octacalcium phosphate [$Ca_2(HPO_4)_2(PO_4)_4 \cdot 5H_2O$], amorphous calcium phosphate [$Ca_xH_y(PO_4)_z \cdot nH_2O$, $n = 3-4.5$ and $15-20\% H_2O$], α/β-tricalcium phosphate, and hydroxyapatite are highly utilized materials in biomedical research.

4.6.4 Alumina and titania ceramic nanostructures

Alumina is a chemical compound consisting of aluminum and oxygen (Al_2O_3). The significance of alumina is to create aluminum ion which can take part in catalytic reactions. Moreover, it is thermodynamically stable over wide range of temperature. It is found in so many studies that γ-alumina is more thermodynamically stable than α-alumina when a critical surface area is taken into consideration. Another significant breakthrough in nanomaterials and nanomedicines is the advancement of alumina and titania ceramic nanoparticles for gene and drug deliveries. Development of alumina nanoparticles is carried out due to their mechanical, thermal, and chemical stabilities along with their catalytic natures. Several techniques are available for the preparation of nano-alumina starting from laser ablation technique, sol–gel techniques, metal–organic framework, and hydrothermal and solvothermal techniques to thermal decomposition of an aqueous aluminum nitrate as starting material. These are water dispersible and have highly stable morphology at physiological pH. Moreover, they have tunable porous structure, cost-effective fabrication with low toxicity levels. Alumina nanomaterials are widely used for the delivery of very aqueous soluble drugs and other similar kind of biomolecules. Nano-alumina functionalized with biological fragments, genes, and compounds have shown multiple biomedical applications and localized delivery of therapeuticals. Fluorescent alumina nanoparticles have been capped with natural proteins (Sana et al., 2016). Like alumina nanostructures, agglomerates of radially assembled aluminum hydroxide crumpled nanosheets also exhibit anticancer activity due to their selective adsorption properties and positive charge.

Varied sphere-shaped titania nanostructures including mesoporous spheres, sphere-shaped flaky assemblies, and dendritic particles of uneven diameter and monodispersity in size have been prepared in current years (Chen and Caruso, 2013). Titania nanostructures provide a platform in biomedical application owing to their unique biocompatibility and their capacity to integrate functional moieties to improve biological responses. Moreover, nanostructured silica and its functionalized titania-silica are very important breakthroughs for gene delivery. These nanostructures are very specific and deliberate molecular structures that can interact with the nerve cells and proteins present inside the cell. Other than these nanostructures, zirconia nanoparticles are also capable of delivering gene at specific target site. However, there are concerns about the application of nonbiodegradable ceramic nanoparticles, such as hydroxyapatite, alumina, and titania, because they will accumulate in the body and cause serious toxic effects (Medina et al., 2007).

4.6.5 Metallic nanostructures

Nanostructured metallic materials generally signify the metallic nanoparticles, such as gold, silver, gadolinium, and iron oxide, which have also been studied for targeted gene delivery. Layered double metal hydroxides with two-dimensional structure have been attracted significant interest in searching for new intercalative nanohybrids that perform excellent synergistic effects. Metal nanostructures are considered as novel discoveries in nanomedicine for gene delivery carriers with imaging and targeting a specific system of the body parts. Layered double metal hydroxides nanostructures are manufactured to study the mechanism involved in gene- Layered double metal hydroxides nanostructures, their physiochemical properties, intracellular pathways involved in the whole bioprocess and active targeting in-vitro and in-vivo functions with imaging patterns. In the recent developments in metallic nanostructures, zinc oxide and semiconductor quantum dots have been shown too to have incredible luminescent properties, which together with their low cost, low tissue toxicity, and biocompatibility have twisted these nanostructures into one of the main candidates for bio-imaging. The abilities to produce destructive reactive oxygen species, high catalytic efficiency, strong adsorption capability, and high isoelectric point have been proved to be worthy in the development of smart nanometal nanomaterials for gene and theranostic applications.

4.6.6 Gold and silver nanostructures

Gold nanostructures and nanoparticles (GNN) due to their inimitable properties like tunable surface chemistry, morphology, and optical and electrostatical properties have been recurrently used in gene delivery. Moreover, their favorable optical and chemical properties, including tunable sizes in the range of 0.8–200 nm, easy surface modification with different functional groups, good biocompatibility, and visible light extinction behavior (Xu et al., 2006) have been made gold nanomaterials as special for surface modifications and molecular targeting. Gold nanostructures are highly stable with high degree of immobility in biosystems and they are highly biocompatible with very low tissue toxicity. Surface modified gold nanoparticles are developed as gene delivery vehicles for neoplastic disorders. These nanoparticles exhibit excellent biocompatibility with DNA, RNA, and genes. Gold nanoparticles loaded with specific gene effectively express at the targeted cell and malignant tumor microenvironment. GNN can be conjugated with PEI to deliver genes (Thomas and Klibanov, 2003) and be modified and conjugated with suitable proteins/peptides to target the cell nucleus (Tkachenko et al., 2004). Folate-functionalized Au or Ag nanoparticles have been demonstrated to be able to lower the unwanted toxicity of diminazene aceturate and improve its selectivity and therapeutic efficacy (Adeyemi and Sulaiman, 2015). In many cases, gold nanoparticles are covalently bounded to polymers, greatly enhancing the stability of polymeric nanoparticles for gene and drug deliveries (Aryal et al., 2009). The cytotoxicity of gold nanoparticles is very low (Bechet et al., 2008), and they have served as scaffolds for drug delivery. In contrast, silver nanoparticles are relatively not favored for gene/drug delivery due to their toxicity to eukaryotic cells (Fig. 4.9).

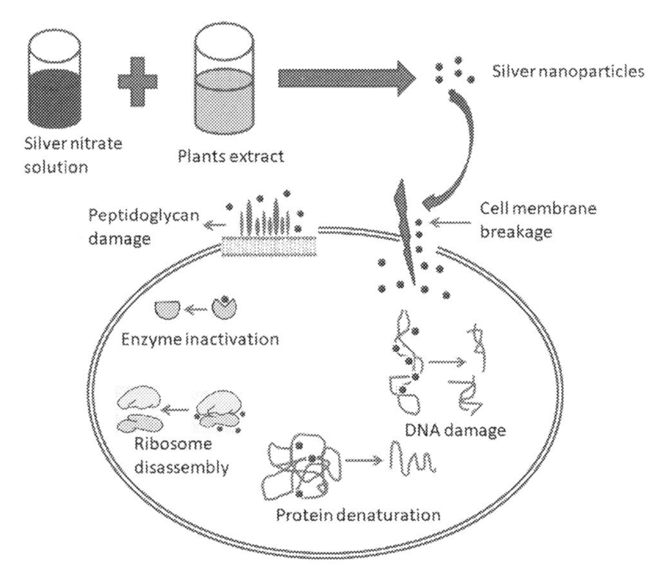

FIGURE 4.9

Schematic presentation of gold and silver nanostructures.

4.6.7 Gadolinium nanostructures

Due to the large neutron capture cross-section area and emission of photons with long flight ranges, gadolinium is a potential agent for neutron capture therapy of tumors (Xu et al., 2006). Gadolinium (III) based nanoparticles have been studied for improved tumor-targeted delivery by the modification of the nanoparticles with folate. The recognition, internalization, and retention of gadolinium nanoparticles in tumor cells were enhanced, indicating a high potential of gadolinium nanoparticles in tumor-targeted delivery (Oyewumi and Mumper, 2002). Gadolinium chelates are widely used contrast agents in gene therapies.

4.6.8 Superparamagnetic oxide nanostructures

Superparamagnetism is one type of magnetism that occurs in ferromagnetic and ferrimagnetic nanostructures. The size of these nanostructures ranges from few nanometers to a couple of tenths of nanometers depending upon the type of materials involved. These nanostructures are single-domain particles and total magnetic moments of such nanostructures are considered as one giant magnetic moment in which magnetic moments of the atoms forming nanostructures contribute. Superparamagnetic oxide nanoparticles such as magnetite (Fe_3O_4) and maghemite (Fe_2O_3) are widely used materials for target delivery by using magnetic force. Drug molecules are conjugated onto the surface-modified magnetic nanoparticles, and then the organic/inorganic superparamagnetic nanohybrids are concentrated at a specific target site within the body by an external, high-gradient magnetic field (Pankhurst et al., 2003). Delivery of biomolecules through magnetic nanoparticles works in a similar fashion to magnetic separation: The biomolecules can be attached to the magnetic particle and then a magnetic force can alter the path of the tagged particles. Once at the right place, the biomolecules can be released from its carrier either via enzymatic activity or physiological changes (pH, osmolality, temperature). Nanoparticles should be considered due to their high likeliness to be influenced in their path. They are more flourishing at withstanding the general flow in the body's circulatory system and biomolecules delivery seems to be more successful in regions with a slow flow and when the magnet can come into close proximity. Magnetic nanoparticles for better therapeutic efficacies are first tagged by means of coating. These coatings can be of organic or inorganic origin. The coating protects the magnetic nanoparticles from extracellular environment and once at their target, it can provide as an attachment point to the targeted entity. In general, there are two types of structural configurations; one is magnetic core with a biocompatible polymer as coating and the other is porous biocompatible polymer, in which the magnetic nanoparticles can diffuse through the pores.

With the fast development of nanobiotechnology in recent times, novel DNA and RNA delivery systems for gene therapy are used instead of viral vectors. These nonviral vectors can be made of a variety of materials including inorganic nanoparticles, especially magnetic and superparamagnetic nanostructures. These nanostructures have multiple advantages over viral vectors, mainly a decreased immune response with flexibility in design allowing them to be functionalized and targeted to specific sites in a biological system with low cytotoxicity.

In gene therapies, the magnetic carriers are coated with the therapeutical gene and transported to the target area. Holding the gene onto the magnetic nanoparticles and carrier at the target for an extended time, the chances rise that the gene can get transfected. Moreover, efficient delivery of genes has been realized by the modification of the magnetic nanoparticles. They can be positively charged by polymers and thus bound to the negatively charged DNA by electrostatic attractions and also protect the DNA (Xiang et al., 2003).

The combination of nanoparticles, gene therapy, and medical imaging has been developed as a new field known as gene theranostics, in which a nanobioconjugate is used to diagnose and treat the particular disease, an individual suffering from. This process generally involves binding between a vector carrying the genetic information and nanoparticles, which provides the signal for imaging. The synthesis of this probe generates a synergic effect, enhancing the efficiency of gene transduction and imaging contrast. Latest approaches regarding the synthesis of nanoparticles for magnetic resonance imaging, gene therapy strategies, and their conjugation and in vivo application are thoroughly studied. Applications of magnetic nanoparticles in gene therapies have been started to develop and it will take more time for better understanding at the molecular level.

4.6.9 Two-dimensional transition metal dichalcogenides

Two-dimensional transition metal dichalcogenides are planar crystals consisting of one or a limited number of Transition Metal Dichalcogenides unit cells. Single-layered "Transition Metal Dichalcogenides" can be described by the formula MX2, where M is the transition metal from groups 4–10 of the periodic table and X is a chalcogen (S, Se, or Te) (Kalantar-Zadeh et al., 2015). Various combinations of transition metals and chalcogens as well as their different arrangements in the two-dimensional crystals can lead to a wide variety of favorable properties (Chhowalla et al., 2013; Butler et al., 2013), making these materials suitable for applications in gene delivery as well as in gene therapies. The genetic material loading capability of two-dimensional MoS2 systems has turned out to be even better than that of graphene oxide due to their surface adsorption effect caused by hydrophobic interactions (Tian et al., 2011; Liu et al., 2014). Their physiochemical properties can also be combined with biomolecules carrying property to deliver specific biomolecules at targeted site (Liu et al., 2014; Yong et al., 2014).

4.6.10 Peptides-based nanostructures

One of the most gifted areas of research in gene delivery is the utilization of peptides as biodegradable, physiologically sensitive, inherently "tunable" and remarkably facile design platform for highly sophisticated gene and nucleic acids delivery systems. Peptides have many distinctive advantages for use in gene and nucleic acids delivery. (1) Biocompatibility and biodegradability construct peptide-based nanostructures suitable for gene and nucleic acids delivery (Castillo-León et al., 2011). (2) Naturally occurring self-assembly motifs present in proteins such as α-helices, β-sheets, and coiled-coils can be used to drive the self-assembly process (Matson et al., 2011). (3) Peptides can structure well-defined nanostructures of any size and shape (Castillo-León et al., 2011). (4) Supplementary peptide functionalization can easily be performed by including various compounds to the peptide structure (Castillo-León et al., 2011). (5) Oligopeptides can be easily produced on a large scale via standard solid-phase synthesis at a relatively low cost. In recent years, a wide range of self-assembled peptides have been put forward for gene and nucleic acids delivery, such as FF, various peptide amphiphiles (PA), and collagen mimetic self-assembled peptides (Jiang et al., 2014). For instance, on the basis of FF, a variety of functional nanostructures have been fabricated, such as nanotubes, spherical vesicles, nanofibrils, nanowires ordered molecular chains, and hybrid nanoparticles (Yan et al., 2010). FF peptide nanotubes have been utilized to load rhodamine and have been found to have the ability to conjugate both hydrophobic and hydrophilic compounds due to their highly hydrophobic aromatic rings and hydrophilic peptide matrix. PA are prone to self-assemble to form nanofibers, micelles and vesicles, nanotapes, nanotubes, and ribbons. The sizes, shapes, and morphologies of nanostructures can be transformed simply by changing the structural elements of the PA (Habibi et al., 2016). As we all know that most anticancer biomolecules are hydrophobic, they suffer from poor water solubility. Besides this, they show tissue toxicity (McNeil, 2009; Soukasene et al., 2011). Chemical attachment of these biomolecules to hydrophilic peptides would create an amphiphilic system necessary for self-assembly, reduce their toxic effects, and improve their efficiency via their incorporation into biomolecules delivering nanocarrier. Peptide-based advanced delivery systems are currently of extensive scientific interest. Rational design of the peptide-based nanostructures can improve their biomolecules/gene/chemicals of therapeutic interests loading capacities. Due to the high internal packing of hydrophobic segments, previous utilization of PA as gene/biomolecules carriers was generally limited by low loading capacity onto nanostructures (about 2%–5%). However, by incorporating multiple short hydrophobic tails, the nanostructure's inner domain has been obviously enlarged and thus the loading efficiency has remarkably increased to 7% (Zhang et al., 2013). Novel nanostructures with various peptide motifs, stimuli-responsive function, and triggered drug and gene delivery at disease sites are constantly emerging. The well-defined nanostructures produced by the self-assembly of peptides are highly promising for gene and nucleic acid delivery (Fig. 4.10).

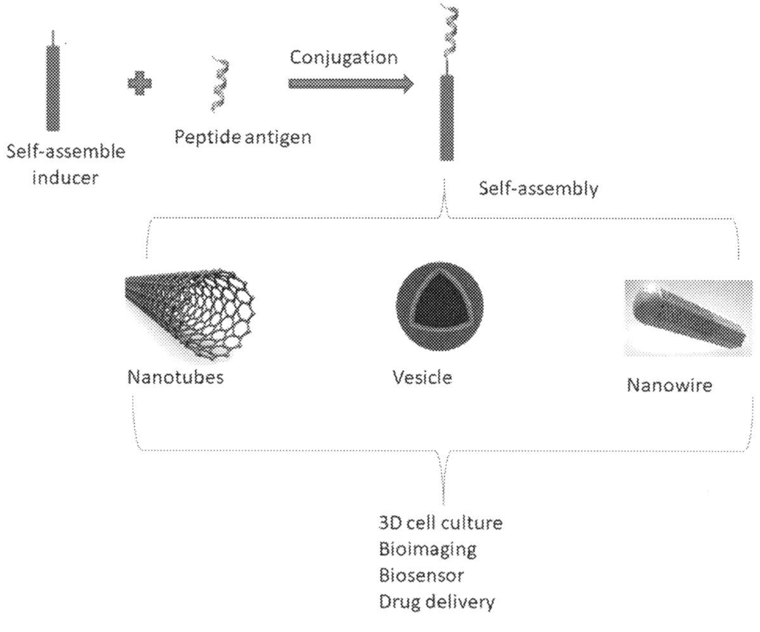

FIGURE 4.10

Peptide-based nanostructures.

4.6.11 Nucleic acid-based nanostructures

As we all know, nucleic acid can be divided into two categories: DNA and RNA. In recent years, nucleic acid nanotechnology has progressed rapidly, especially DNA nanotechnology. A great variety of nucleic acid-based nanostructures with various dimensions, sizes, geometries, and shapes have been well investigated for gene delivery in modern gene therapies.

4.6.11.1 DNA-based nanostructures

DNA-based nanostructures are quite appealing in latest delivery applications for many reasons. They can be decorated with a multitude of functionalities and become multifunctional carriers. They can be easily fabricated by self-assembly. They are of low immunogenicity. They have large flexibility of how biomolecules can be loaded into the DNA carrier. They allow superb control over release (Vries et al., 2013). Oligonucleotides have been successfully applied in the creation of many types of structures such as nanotubes, dendrimer-like DNA nanostructures, polypods, tetrahedra, icosahedra, and many other polyhedral structures (Chang et al., 2011). An aptamer-conjugated DNA icosahedral nanoparticle is used as a carrier of doxorubicin (DOX) for cancer therapy. In the last decade, an approach for constructing various DNA structures, named as DNA origami, has emerged (Chandrasekaran and Zhuo, 2016). It folds a long-stranded bacteriophage through the use of more than 200 complementary staple strands to fold the backbone (Angell et al., 2016). Various nanostructures, both 2D and 3D, such as smiley faces, tetrahedrons, DNA nanotubes, DNA barrels, and DNA "dolphins," have been fabricated through DNA origami (Smith et al., 2011; Zhao et al., 2012; Andersen et al., 2008; Rothemund, 2006; Zhang et al., 2014). DNA tube and DNA triangle, DNA nanotubes, nanoballs, nanobelts, and nanoclews have also been produced by another innovative approach—rolling circle amplification, which develops long-stranded structures with repeating DNA sequences through the use of a circular template and DNA polymerase. They can be used as precise delivery vehicles for biomolecules and genes. Many other unique DNA nanostructures have also been designed for novel delivery of gene and nucleic acids, such as DNA nanofilms and hydrogels. A DNA block copolymer system consisting of polypropylene oxide (PPO) and DNA has been utilized for the delivery of hydrophobic biomolecules. The obtained hybrid particles were about 10 nm with a hydrophobic PPO core to incorporate DOX and a DNA shell functionalized by folate to target cells. There are some obstacles to be checked in the applications of DNA-based nanostructures for smooth delivery of biomolecules. Most of the time it is seen that the expense of the starting materials is high and therefore the in vivo pharmacokinetic bioavailability of the DNA-based structures needs to be enhanced (Fig. 4.11).

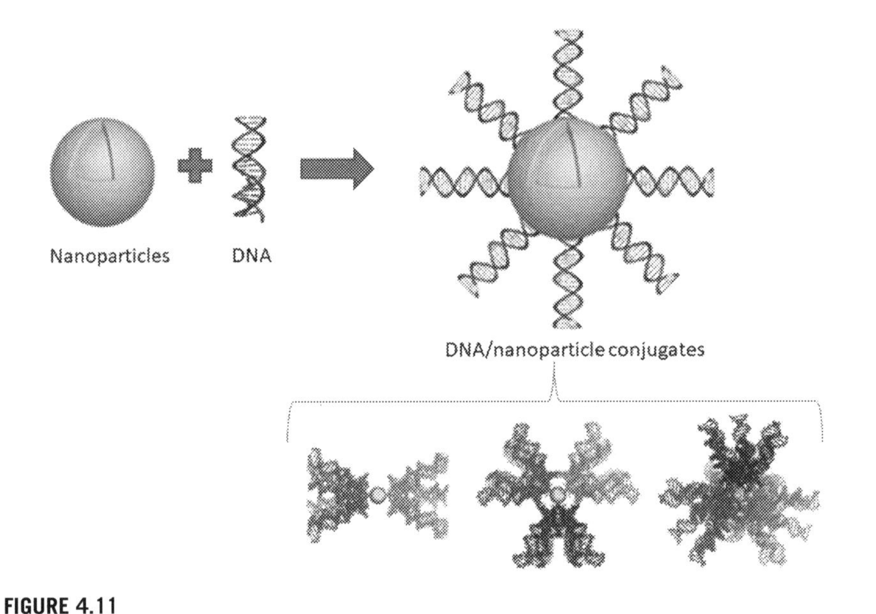

FIGURE 4.11

DNA-based nanostructures.

4.6.11.2 RNA-based nanostructures

Due to the impression that RNA seems unstable, the potential of RNA in modern delivery system has been unobserved for many years. But in recent times, with the development of RNA nanotechnology, RNA-based nanostructures, especially those based on phi29 pRNA, have been utilized in gene and other biomolecules delivery at the targeted site in recent years. According to Heoprich et al. (2003), targeted hammerhead ribozymes delivery has been achieved by using ligand conjugated RNA nanoparticles based on phi29 pRNA. Moreover, RNA nanoparticles can also deliver CpG DNA to macrophages specifically (Khisamutdinov et al., 2014). RNA origami nanostructures have also been reported to produce good delivery of genetic materials and MAbs (monoclonal antibodies). With exceptional thermodynamic stability and plasma stability after chemical modifications, RNA origami is expected to be more favorable than its counterpart DNA origami as a biomolecules carrier for achieving controlled release (Fig. 4.12).

4.6.12 Carbon nanostructures

With the rapid development of carbon nanostructures, many attempts have been made to investigate their applications in gene therapies and gene deliveries in the past. Numerous carbon nanostructures, including CNTs, graphene, and fullerenes, have been utilized for the delivery of genetic materials at the defected gene site. Graphene can be wrapped into spherical structures (zero-dimensional fullerenes), rolled into one-dimensional (1D) structures (CNTs), or stacked into three-dimensional (3D) layered structures (graphite) (Geim and Novoselov, 2007). CNTs, graphene, and fullerenes are equivalent in biochemical nature but vary in wall number, diameter, length, and surface

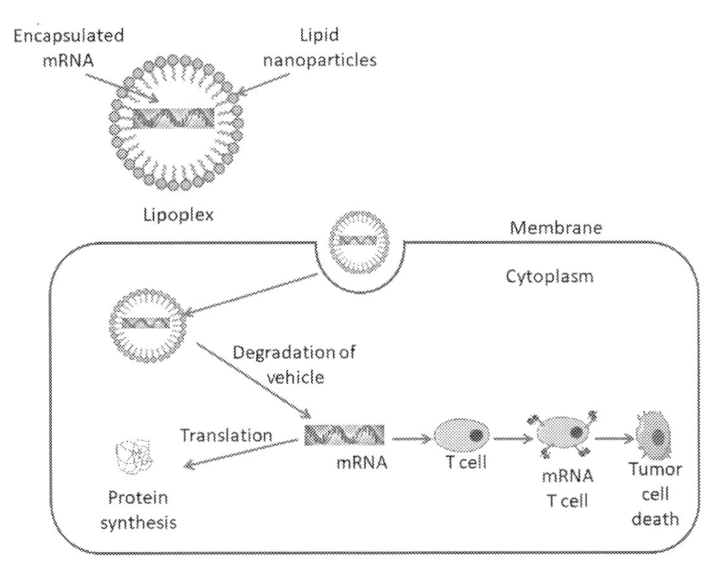

FIGURE 4.12

Representation of RNA based nanostructures.

chemistry. They are all insoluble but they can be modified into water-soluble nanostructures and be opted for biomolecules delivery at the site of action.

4.6.12.1 Graphene

Graphene is an atomic-scale honeycomb lattice made of carbon atoms. So many encouraging properties, like good biocompatibility, low cytotoxicity, and unique physicochemical properties in chemistry, electrics, optics, and mechanics, graphene have been explored as one of the most promising carbon nanostructures for drug delivery. Compared with CNTs, graphene exhibits some important qualities such as low cost, facile fabrication and modification, and a higher DL ratio with two external surfaces (Liu et al., 2013). Thus graphene and its derivatives (e.g., graphene oxide) have been widely explored in the past decade for drug delivery applications.

4.6.12.2 Carbon nanotubes

CNTs have shown promise for the targeted delivery of biomolecules, proteins, and genes because of their favorable properties similar to graphene. More importantly, CNTs offer some interesting advantages over spherical nanoparticles. For instance, their large inner volume allows the loading of small drug molecules while their outer surface can be chemically modified to load proteins and genes for effective drug delivery. In recent years, both single-walled CNTs and MWCNTs have been modified and turned out to be effective in the delivery of biomolecules, proteins, peptides, and nuclear acids (Pantarotto et al., 2004a,b; Zheng et al., 2013) (Fig. 4.13).

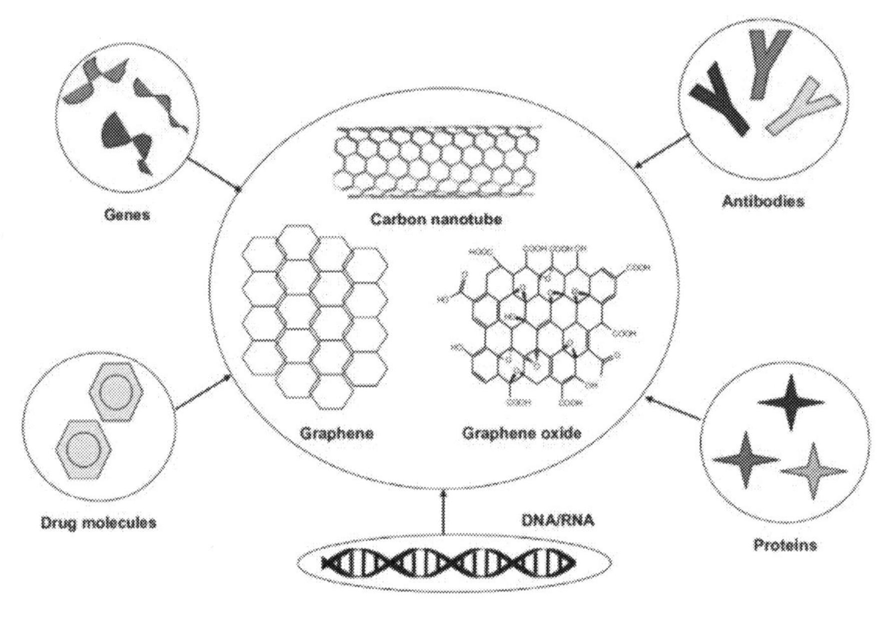

FIGURE 4.13

Schematic presentation of RNA based nanostructures.

4.6.12.3 Fullerenes

As nanomolecular carbon cages, fullerenes can also serve as drug vectors or drug delivery scaffolds with noncovalent linkages or with covalent linkages between the fullerene and a bioactive moiety (Bolskar, 2012). After proper functionalization, such as attaching hydrophilic moieties, fullerenes have turned out to be able to work as drug carriers.

4.6.13 Drug-based nanostructures

As mentioned earlier, drug molecules can also be used as building units to deliver themselves.

Through rational design of the number and type of the biomolecules incorporated, the obtained nanostructures can exhibit various morphologies, such as nanospheres, rods, nanofibers, or nanotubes, to facilitate their delivery to particular sites (Ma et al., 2016).

4.6.13.1 Small molecule biomolecules

Some small molecule biomolecules have shown reversible self-assembly behavior, which can be used to form supramolecular nanostructures of well-defined size and shape (Ma et al., 2016). For example, nanofibers or lozenge-like platelets have been obtained by the self-assembly of folic acid in methanol/water mixtures. As a result of the self-assembly of quinoline alkaloid camptothecin (CPT), 100–400 nm wide helical nanoribbon structures have been fabricated from the injection of an organic solution of CPT into water.

4.6.13.2 Hydrophobic biomolecules

Hydrophobic drug molecules can be conjugated to hydrophilic polymers to form amphiphilic probiomolecules that can spontaneously self-assemble into stable nanostructures. For example, cisplatin and PEG-P (Glu) can form coordination bonds by the coordination between Pt and P(Glu) carboxylate side chains and then self-assemble into micelles (about 28 nm in diameter). In this way, a self-delivery system can be obtained, and it can provide a sustained drug release. With the evolution of self-delivering biomolecules, various supramolecular nanostructures have been formed from the self-assembly of amphiphilic probiomolecules, such as one-dimensional filamentous structures, nanofilaments, nanospheres, and hydrogels.

4.7 Future directions

Although nanogene therapeutics or nanogene theranostics or nanogene deliveries have been revealed to present noteworthy advantages in the treatment of neoplastic disorders which in common man's language known as cancer among a number of diseases in biomedical research, researches are continued to increase its efficacy. Numerous angles of investigation of nanotherapies have been taken into consideration starting from surface area consideration to biomolecules loading concentration and final releasing of such biomolecules at the targeted sites. Toxicity, another consideration also plays a pivotal role in nano-research. Conventional therapeutics in targeted diseases such as cancer, cardiovascular disorders, and HIV-AIDS have shown so many issues starting from their distribution in intracellular and extracellular fluids to toxicity levels at the specific site of action. Moreover, ADME and PK/PD (pharmacokinetic/pharmacodynamics) modeling profiles of conventional therapies from site of application also reveal nontargeting and nonsustained mode of action and pharmacological actions to the site of action. Effects of conventional therapies have been reduced due to its interaction or reaction or degradation with enzyme and other systems of the body. Conventional therapies are clue and answerless in their interaction with normal healthy cells as these also affect and interrupt normal physiological functions of such healthy cells while treating the diseases affected cells.

Nanotherapeuticals is the latest biomolecules delivery system developed in biomedical research domain. Significant breakthroughs have been achieved to address such issues encountered with conventional therapies. Tissue targeting or cell targeting as well as microenvironment of tissues and cells are one of the important breakthroughs in targeted delivery systems with high degree of precision. The delivery system containing nanostructured drug molecules, genes, gene fragments, and other cellular organelles deliver such molecules specifically at the targeted site without affecting nearby cells and tissues. Level of toxicity at cellular level is also highly decreased which has become highly advantageous in targeted therapies. Large surface areas with inclusion of multiple functional groups attached to the nanostructures have shown effective delivery of biomolecules at the specific site of action. Multiple functional groups are bound onto receptors or specific antigens (for cancer, specific malignant antigens, or tumor antigens) allowing the biomolecules to get released at the specific site. Designing of multiple functional groups attachment onto nanostructures has increased the research potential in several ways. Numerous types of molecules with different patterns have been developed to get an ideal structure for targeting the diseases. Modifications of these structures are undertaken too to develop more target friendly delivery systems. Sizes of nanostructures also play a significant role in targeted therapies. Size between 10 nm and 100 nm is ideal for such targeting as elimination of biomolecules become easier compared to conventional therapies.

Gene therapies, the technology of adding or replacing missing or defective genes in diseased cells of a patient has proved to be highly effective for number of diseases including hemophilia, muscular pains, immunological disorders, and certain types of malignancies. Currently, gene therapies include modified viral stains, external electrical fields, or unkind chemical compounds to penetrate cell membranes and deliver genes directly to diseased cells. These technologies have their own limitations; they can be costly, unproductive or cause unwanted stress and toxicity to cells. To overcome these limitations, nanostructures are good alternatives to deliver genetic materials with maximum impact on cell viability and susceptibility and cell metabolism. The nanostructures their biodegradable nature and of infinitesimal sizes have made these technologies more human-friendly. Moreover, their cost-effectiveness has made these structures a very popular one in the recent advancements of gene therapies application. Scientists working in this field of gene therapies have already developed guided nanostructures with or without robotic technology involvement. Nanomotors, a new device in nanogene therapies have been used to enhance disease gene targeting with high degree of precision. Another important development is nanospears, which can deliver therapeutic effectiveness within the body to treat genetic diseases during the exposure of the body to the magnetic field.

Gene therapies and many forms of immunotherapies which are still not fully resolved with respect to the discovering technologies are the most challenging fronts in biomedical research. On many occasions, it is observed that patients' cells are laminated to trace their locations and utilizing the locations of such cells, nanostructures are delivered containing numerous chemical compounds to genetic materials. The methods of development of nanostructured compounds, nanostructured loaded with genetic materials with very low or no tissue toxicities, biocompatibility, good distribution amongst body fluids and good elimination rate with pharmacokinetic parameters are now surfaced out in different laboratories headed by different scientists at different parts of the world. New more approaches are also adopted to address the additional safety issues related to nanostructures and will also help to make these therapies more patient-friendly. The concept of gene editing, model cells, PK/PD modeling, and sample patient cells or cell lines and animal models are already in place so that the scientists can witness some scintillating discoveries related to nano-systems in gene therapies.

References

Adeyemi, O.S., Sulaiman, F.A., 2015. Evaluation of metal nanoparticles for drug delivery systems. J. Biomed. Res. 29 (2), 145–149.

Allen, T.M., Cullis, P.R., 2013. Liposomal drug delivery systems: from concept to clinical applications. Adv. Drug. Delivery Rev. 65 (1), 36–48.

Andersen, E.S., Dong, M., Nielsen, M.M., et al., 2008. DNA origami design of dolphin-shaped structures with flexible tails. ACS Nano 2 (6), 1213–1218.

Angell, C., Xie, S., Zhang, L.F., Chen, Y., 2016. DNA nanotechnology for precise control over drug delivery and gene therapy. Small 12 (9), 1117–1132.

Arima, H., Motoyama, K., Higashi, T., 2013. Sugar-appended polyamidoamine dendrimer conjugates with cyclodextrins as cell-specific non-viral vectors. Adv. Drug. Deliv. Rev. 65, 1204–1214.

Aryal, S., Pilla, S., Gong, S., 2009. Multifunctional nano-micelles formed by amphiphilic gold-polycaprolactone- methoxy poly- (ethylene glycol) (Au-PCL-MPEG) nanoparticles for potential drug delivery applications. J. Nanosci. Nanotechnol. 9 (10), 5701–5708.

Barbe, C., et al., 2004. Silica particles: a novel drug delivery system. J. Adv. Mater. 16 (20), 01–08.

Battaglia, G., Ryan, A.J., 2005. Bilayers and interdigitation inblock copolymer vesicles. J. Am. Chem. Soc. 127 (24), 8757–8764.

Bechet, D., Couleaud, P., Frochot, C., Viriot, M.-L., Guillemin, F., Barberi-Heyob, M., 2008. Nanoparticles as vehicles for delivery of photodynamic therapy agents. Trends Biotechnol. 26 (11), 612–621.

Beck, J.C., Vartuli, J.C., 2006. Recent advances in the sysnthesis, characterization and applications of mesoporous molecular sieves. J. Curr. Opin. Solid. State Mater. Sci. 1 (1), 76–87.

Boas, U., Christensen, J.B., Heegaard, P.M.H., 2006. Dendrimers: design, synthesis and chemical properties. J. Mater. Chem. 16, 3785–3798.

R.D. Bolskar, 2012 Fullerenes for drug delivery. In: Encyclopedia of Nanotechnology, pp. 898–911, Springer, Amsterdam, The Netherlands.

Bose, S., Tarafder, S., Edgington, J., Bandyopadhyay, A., 2011. Calcium phosphate ceramics in drug delivery. J. Miner. 63 (4), 93–98.

Brevet, D., Gary-Bobo, M., Raehm, L., et al., 2009. Mannose-targeted mesoporous silica nanoparticles for photodynamic therapy. Chem. Commun. (12), 1475–1477.

Butler, S.Z., Hollen, S.M., Cao, L., et al., 2013. Progress, challenges, and opportunities in two-dimensional materials beyond graphene. ACS Nano 7 (4), 2898–2926.

M. Çağdaş, A.D. Sezer, S. Bucak, 2014. Liposomes as potential drug carrier systems for drug delivery. In: Application of Nanotechnology in Drug Delivery, InTech.

J. Castillo-León, K.B. Andersen, W.E. Svendsen, 2011. Self-assembled peptide nanostructures for biomedical applications: advantages and challenges. In: Biomaterials Science and Engineering, InTech, Shanghai, China,.

Chandrasekaran, A.R., Zhuo, R., 2016. A 'tile' tale: hierarchical self-assembly of DNA lattices. Appl. Mater. Today 2, 7–16.

Chang, M., Yang, C.-S., Huang, D.-M., 2011. Aptamer-conjugated DNA icosahedral nanoparticles as a carrier of doxorubicin for cancer therapy. ACS Nano 5 (8), 6156–6163.

Chaplot, S.P., Rupenthal, I.D., 2014. Dendrimers for gene delivery—a potential approach for ocular therapy? J. Pharm. Pharmacol. 66 (4), 542–556.

Chen, D., Caruso, R.A., 2013. Recent progress in the synthesis of spherical titania nanostructures and their applications. Adv. Funct. Mater. 23 (11), 1356–1374.

Chhowalla, M., Shin, H.S., Eda, G., Li, L.-J., Loh, K.P., Zhang, H., 2013. The chemistry of two-dimensional layered transition metal dichalcogenide nanosheets. Nat. Chem. 5 (4), 263–275.

Choi, K.Y., Liu, G., Lee, S., Chen, X.Y., 2012. Theranostic nanoplatforms for simultaneous cancer imaging and therapy: current approaches and future perspectives. Nanoscale 4 (2), 330–342.

Chung, E.J., Cheng, Y., Morshed, R., et al., 2014. Fibrin-binding, peptide amphiphile micelles for targeting glioblastoma. Biomaterials 35 (4), 1249–1256.

Connor, E.E., Mwamuka, J., Gole, A., et al., 2005. Gold nanoparticles are taken up by human cells but do not cause acute cytotoxicity. Small 1 (3), 325–327.

Daneshvar, N., Abdullah, R., Shamsabadi, F.T., How, C.W., Mh, M.A., et al., 2013. PAMAM dendrimer roles in gene delivery methods and stem cell research. Cell Biol. Int. 37, 415–419.

Drobnik, J., 1991. Hyaluronan in drug delivery. Adv. Drug. Deliv. Rev. 7 (2), 295–308.

Dutta, T., Aghase, H.B., Vijayarajkumar, P., Joshi, M., Jain, N.K., 2006. Dendrosome-based gene delivery. J. Exp. Nanosci. 1 (2), 235–248.

Garcia-Fuentes, M., Alonso, M.J., 2012. Chitosan-based drug nanocarriers:where dowe stand? J. Control. Rel. 161 (2), 496–504.

Gary-Bobo, M., Hocine, O., Brevet, D., et al., 2012. Cancer therapy improvement with mesoporous silica nanoparticles combining targeting, drug delivery and PDT. Int. J. Pharm. 423 (2), 509–515.

Geim, A.K., Novoselov, K.S., 2007. The rise of graphene. Nat. Mater. 6 (3), 183–191.

Goodman, C.M., McCusker, C.D., Yilmaz, T., Rotello, V.M., 2004. Toxicity of gold nanoparticles functionalized with cationic and anionic side chains. Bioconjug. Chem. 15 (4), 897–900.

Gottarelli, G., Mezzina, E., Spada, G.P., et al., 1996. The self-recognition and self-assembly of folic acid salts in isotropic water solution. Helv. Chim. Acta 79 (1), 220–234.

Habiba, K., Bracho-Rincon, D.P., Gonzalez-Feliciano, J.A., et al., 2015. Synergistic antibacterial activity of PEGylated silver–graphene quantumdots nanocomposites. Appl. Mater. Today 1 (2), 80–87.

Habibi, N., Kamaly, N., Memic, A., Shafiee, H., 2016. Selfassembled peptide-based nanostructures: smart nanomaterials toward targeted drug delivery. Nano Today 11 (1), 41–60.

Han, M., Bae, Y., Nishiyama, N., et al., 2007. Transfection study using multicellular tumor spheroids for screening non-viral polymeric gene vectors with low cytotoxicity and high transfection efficiencies. J. Control. Rel. 121 (1-2), 38–48.

Heoprich, S., Zhou, Q., Guo, S., et al., 2003. Bacterial virusphi29 pRNAas a hammerhead ribozyme escort to destroy hepatitis B virus. Gene Ther. 10 (15), 1258–1267.

Jiang, T., Xu, C.F., Liu, Y., et al., 2014. Structurally defined nanoscale sheets from self-assembly of collagen-mimetic peptides. J. Am. Chem. Soc. 136 (11), 4300–4308.

Kalantar-Zadeh, K., Ou, J.Z., Daeneke, T., Strano, M.S., Pumera, M., Gras, S.L., 2015. Two-dimensional transition metal dichalcogenides in biosystems. Adv. Funct. Mater. 25 (32), 5086–5099.

Kamikawa, Y., Nishii, M., Kato, T., 2004. Self-assembly of folic acid derivatives: induction of supramolecular chirality by hierarchical chiral structures. Chem.—Eur. J. 10 (23), 5942–5951.

D.P. Keith, H. Cui, 2014. Fabrication of drug delivery systems using self-assembled peptide nanostructures. In: Micro and NanofabricationUsing Self-Assembled BiologicalNanostructures, pp. 91–111, Elsevier.

Kesharwani, P., Jain, K., Jain, N.K., 2014. Dendrimer as nanocarrier for drug delivery. Prog. Polym. Sci. 39 (2), 268–307.

Khisamutdinov, E.F., Li, H., Jasinski, D.L., Chen, J., Fu, J., Guo, P., 2014. Enhancing immunomodulation on innate immunity by shape transition among RNA triangle, square and pentagon nanovehicles. Nucleic Acids Res. 42 (15), 9996–10004.

Khopade, A.J., Caruso, F., Tripathi, P., Nagaich, S., Jain, N.K., 2002. Effect of dendrimer on entrapment and release of bioactive from liposomes. Int. J. Pharm. 232 (1–2), 157–162.

Kim, T.I., Baek, J.U., Zhe Bai, C., Park, J.S., 2007. Arginine-conjugated polypropylenimine dendrimer as a non-toxic and efficient gene delivery carrier. Biomaterials 28, 2061–2067.

Klajnert, B., Bryszewska, M., 2001. Dendrimers: properties and applications. Acta Biochim. Pol. 48, 199–208.

Kono, K., Liu, M., Fréchet, J.M.J., 1999. Design of dendritic macromolecules containing folate or methotrexate residues. Bioconj. Chem. 10 (6), 1115–1121.

Kostarelos, K., 2008. The long and short of carbon nanotube toxicity. Nat. Biotechnol. 26 (7), 774–776.

Lee, Y.S., 2008. Self-assembly and Nanotechnology - A Force Balance Approach. Wiley, New York.

Li, Y., Gao, G.H., Lee, D.S., 2013. Stimulus-sensitive polymeric nanoparticles and their applications as drug and gene carriers. Adv. Healthc. Mater. 2 (3), 388–417.

Lim, H.J., Cho, E.C., Shim, J., Kim, D.-H., An, E.J., Kim, J., 2008. Polymer-associated liposomes as a novel delivery system for cyclodextrin-bound drugs. J. Colloid Interface Sci. 320 (2), 460–468.

Lin, R., Cheetham, A.G., Zhang, P., Lin, Y.-A., Cui, H., 2013. Supramolecular filaments containing a fixed 41% paclitaxel loading. Chem. Commun. 49 (43), 4968–4970.

Liu, M., Fréchet, J.M.J., 1999. Designing dendrimers for drug delivery. Pharm. Sci. Technol. Today 2 (10), 393–401.

Liu, J., Cui, L., Losic, D., 2013. Graphene and graphene oxide as new nanocarriers for drug delivery applications. Acta Biomater. 9 (12), 9243–9257.

Liu, T., Wang, C., Gu, X., et al., 2014. Drug delivery with PEGylated MoS2 nano-sheets for combined photothermal and chemotherapy of cancer. Adv. Mater. 26 (21), 3433–3440.

Lock, L.L., Lacomb, M., Schwarz, K., et al., 2013. Self-assembly of natural and synthetic drug amphiphiles into discrete supramolecular nanostructures. Faraday Discuss. 166 (5), 285–301.

Lu, J., Choi, E., Tamanoi, F., Zink, J.I., 2008. Light-activated nanoimpeller- controlled drug release in cancer cells. Small 4 (4), 421–426.

Luo, K., Li, C., Wang, G., Nie, Y., He, B., et al., 2011. Peptide dendrimers as efficient and biocompatible gene delivery vectors: synthesis and in vitro characterization. J. Control. Rel. 155, 77–87.

Luo, K., Li, C., Li, L., She, W., Wang, G., et al., 2012. Arginine functionalized peptide dendrimers as potential gene delivery vehicles. Biomaterials 33, 4917–4927.

Ma, W., Cheetham, A.G., Cui, H., 2016. Building nanostructures with drugs. Nano Today 11 (1), 13–30.

Mastrobattista, E., van der Aa, M.A.E.M., Hennink, W.E., Crommelin, D.J.A., 2006. Artificial viruses: a nanotechnological approach to gene delivery. Nat. Rev. Drug. Discov. 5 (2), 115–121.

Matson, J.B., Zha, R.H., Stupp, S.I., 2011. Peptide self-assembly for crafting functional biological materials. Curr. Opin. Solid. State Mater. Sci. 15 (6), 225–235.

McNeil, S.E., 2009. Nanoparticle therapeutics: a personal perspective. Wiley Interdiscip. Rev. Nanomed. Nanobiotechnol. 1 (1), 264–271.

Medina, C., Santos-Martinez, M.J., Radomski, A., Corrigan, O.I., Radomski, M.W., 2007. Nanoparticles: pharmacological and Journal of Nanomaterials and toxicological significance. Br. J. Pharmacol. 150 (5), 552–558.

Meng, F.H., Zhong, Z.Y., Jan, F.J., 2009. Stimuli-responsive polymersomes for programmed drug delivery. Biomacromolecules 10 (2), 197–209.

Mishra, G.P., Bagui, M., Tamboli, V., Mitra, A.K., 2011. Recent applications of liposomes in ophthalmic drug delivery. J. Drug. Deliv. 2011, 14. Article ID 863734.

Mocanu, G., Nichifor, M., Sacarescu, L., 2016. Dextran based polymeric micelles as carriers for delivery of hydrophobic drugs. Curr. Drug. Deliv. 13 (8).

Ochekpe, N.A., Olorunfemi, P.O., Ngwuluka, N.C., 2009. Nanotechnology and drug delivery part 2: nanostructures for drug delivery. Trop. J. Pharm. Res. 8 (3), 275–284.

Ouyang, D., Zhang, H., Parekh, H.S., Smith, S.C., 2011. The effect of pH on PAMAM dendrimer-siRNA complexation-Endosomal considerations as determined by molecular dynamics simulation. Biophys. Chem. 158, 126–133.

Oyewumi, M.O., Mumper, R.J., 2002. Engineering tumortargeted gadolinium hexanedione nanoparticles for potential application in neutron capture therapy. Bioconj. Chem. 13 (6), 1328–1335.

Pack, D.W., Hoffman, A.S., Pun, S., Stayton, P.S., 2005. Design and development of polymers for gene delivery. Nat. Rev. Drug. Discov. 4 (7), 581–593.

Pan, Y., Neuss, S., Leifert, A., et al., 2007. Size-dependent cytotoxicity of gold nanoparticles. Small 3 (11), 1941–1949.

Pankhurst, Q.A., Connolly, J., Jones, S.K., Dobson, J., 2003. Applications of magnetic nanoparticles in biomedicine. J. Phys. D: Appl. Phys. 36 (13), R167–R181.

Pantarotto, D., Briand, J.-P., Prato, M., Bianco, A., 2004a. Translocation of bioactive peptides across cell membranes by carbon nanotubes. Chem. Commun. 10 (1), 16–17.

Pantarotto, D., Singh, R., McCarthy, D., et al., 2004b. Functionalized carbon nanotubes for plasmid DNA gene delivery. Angew. Chem.-Int. Ed. 43 (39), 5242–5246.

Pernodet, N., Fang, X.H., Sun, Y., et al., 2006. Adverse effects of citrate/gold nanoparticles on human dermal fibroblasts. Small 2 (6), 766–773.

Poland, C.A., Duffin, R., Kinloch, I., et al., 2008. Carbon nanotubes introduced into the abdominal cavity of mice show asbestos-like pathogenicity in a pilot study. Nat. Nanotechnol. 3 (7), 423–428.

Prego, C., Torres, D., Fernandez-Megia, E., Novoa-Carballal, R., Quiñoá, E., Alonso, M.J., 2006. Chitosan-PEG nanocapsules as new carriers for oral peptide delivery: effect of chitosan pegylation degree. J. Control. Rel. 111 (3), 299–308.

Qiu, Y., Gao, Y., Hu, K., Li, F., 2008. Enhancement of skin permeation of docetaxel: a novel approach combining microneedle and elastic liposomes. J. Control. Rel. 129 (2), 144–150.

Raffa, V., Ciofani, G., Nitodas, S., et al., 2008. Can the properties of carbon nanotubes influence their internalization by living cells? Carbon 46 (12), 1600–1610.

Rothemund, P.W.K., 2006. Folding DNA to create nanoscale shapes and patterns. Nature 440 (7082), 297–302.

Roy, I., et al., 2003. Ceramic based nanoparticles entrapping water-insoluble photosensitizing anticancer drugs: a novel drug-carrier system for photodynamic therapy. J. Am. Chem. Soc. 125 (26), 7860–7865.

Russ, V., Günther, M., Halama, A., Ogris, M., Wagner, E., 2008. Oligoethyleniminegrafted polypropylenimine dendrimers as degradable and biocompatible synthetic vectors for gene delivery. J. Control. Rel. 132, 131–140.

Sakiyama-Elbert, S.E., 2011. Drug delivery via heparin conjugates. Compr. Biomater. 4, 333–338.

Sana, M., Ahmad, S.E., Absar, A., 2016. Nanoalumina bioleaching from bauxite ore by *Humicola* sp. Adv. Sci. 8 (4), 298–305.

Shah, V., Taratula, O., Garbuzenko, O.B., Patil, M.L., Savla, R., et al., 2013. Genotoxicity of different nanocarriers: possible modifications for the delivery of nucleic acids. Curr. Drug. Discov. Technol. 10, 8–15.

Singha, K., Namgung, R., Kim, W.J., 2011. Polymers in small-interfering RNA delivery. Nucleic Acid. Ther. 21, 133–147.

Slowing, I.I., Vivero-Escoto, J.L., Trewyn, B.G., Lin, V.S.-Y., 2010. Mesoporous silica nanoparticles: structural design and applications. J. Mater. Chem. 20 (37), 7924–7937.

Smith, D.M., Schüller, V., Forthmann, C., Schreiber, R., Tinnefeld, P., Liedl, T., 2011. A structurally variable hinged tetrahedron framework from DNA origami. J. Nucleic Acids 2011, 9. Article ID 360954.

V. Sokolova, M. Epple, 2014. Bioceramic nanoparticles for tissue engineering and drug delivery. In: Tissue Engineering Using Ceramics and Polymers, pp. 633–647, Elsevier, 2nd ed.

Soppimath, K.S., Aminabhavi, T.M., Kulkarni, A.R., Rudzinski, W.E., 2001. Biodegradable polymeric nanoparticles as drug delivery devices. J. Control. Rel. 70 (1-2), 1–20.

Soukasene, S., Toft, D.J., Moyer, T.J., et al., 2011. Antitumor activity of peptide amphiphile nanofiber-encapsulated camptothecin. ACS Nano 5 (11), 9113–9121.

Sun, Y., Jiao, Y., Wang, Y., Lu, D., Yang, W., 2014. The strategy to improve gene transfection efficiency and biocompatibility of hyperbranched PAMAM with the cooperation of PEGylated hyperbranched PAMAM. Int. J. Pharm. 465, 112–119.

Tang, Y., Li, Y.B., Wang, B., Lin, R.Y., van Dongen, M., et al., 2012. Efficient in vitro siRNA delivery and intramuscular gene silencing using PEG-modified PAMAM dendrimers. Mol. Pharm. 9, 1812–1821.

Taniguchi, N., 1978. Nanotechnology: materials processing with an atomic or molecular size working unit. Kinzoku Hyomen Gijutsu 29, 220–231.

Taratula, O., Garbuzenko, O.B., Kirkpatrick, P., Pandya, I., Savla, R., et al., 2009. Surface-engineered targeted PPI dendrimer for efficient intracellular and intratumoral siRNA delivery. J. Control. Rel. 140, 284–293.

Thomas, M., Klibanov, A.M., 2003. Conjugation to gold nanoparticles enhances polyethylenimine's transfer of plasmid dna into mammalian cells. Proc. Natl Acad. Sci. USA 100 (16), 9138–9143.

Tian, B., Wang, C., Zhang, S., Feng, L., Liu, Z., 2011. Photothermally enhanced photodynamic therapy delivered by nanographene oxide. ACS Nano 5 (9), 7000–7009.

Tiarks, F., Landfester, K., Antonietti, M., 2001. Preparation of polymeric nanocapsules by miniemulsion polymerization. Langmuir 17 (3), 908–918.

Tkachenko, A.G., Xie, H., Liu, Y., et al., 2004. Cellular trajectories of peptide-modified gold particle complexes: comparison of nuclear localization signals and peptide transduction domains. Bioconj. Chem. 15 (3), 482–490.

Vries, J.W.D., Zhang, F., Herrmann, A., 2013. Drug delivery systems based on nucleic acid nanostructures. J. Control. Rel. 172 (2), 467–483.

Whelan, J., Whelan, J., 2001. Nanocapsules for controlled drug delivery. Drug. Discov. Today 6 (23), 1183–1184.

Won, Y.-Y., Brannan, A.K., Davis, H.T., Bates, F.S., 2002. Cryogenic transmission electron microscopy (cryo-TEM) of micelles and vesicles formed in water by poly(ethylene oxide)-based block copolymers. J. Phys. Chem. B 106 (13), 3354–3364.

Xiang, J.-J., Tang, J.-Q., Zhu, S.-G., et al., 2003. IONP-PLL: a novel nonviral vector for efficient gene delivery. J. Gene Med. 5 (9), 803–817.

Xu, Z.P., Zeng, Q.H., Lu, G.Q., Yu, A.B., 2006. Inorganic nanoparticles as carriers for efficient cellular delivery. Chem. Eng. Sci. 61 (3), 1027–1040.

Xu, P.S., Li, S.Y., Li, Q., et al., 2008. Virion-minnicking nanocapsules from pH-controlled hierarchical self-assembly for gene delivery. Angew. Chem. Int. Ed. 47 (7), 1260–1264.

Yan, X., Zhu, P., Li, J., 2010. Self-assembly and application of diphenylalanine- based nanostructures. Chem. Soc. Rev. 39 (6), 1877–1890.

Yong, Y., Zhou, L., Gu, Z., et al., 2014. WS2 nanosheet as a new photosensitizer carrier for combined photodynamic and photothermal therapy of cancer cells. Nanoscale 6 (17), 10394–10403.

Zhang, P., Cheetham, A.G., Lin, Y.-A., Cui, H., 2013. Selfassembled tat nanofibers as effective drug carrier and transporter. ACS Nano 7 (7), 5965–5977.

Zhang, Q., Jiang, Q., Li, N., et al., 2014. DNA origami as an in vivo drug delivery vehicle for cancer therapy. ACS Nano 8 (7), 6633–6643.

Zhao, Y.-X., Shaw, A., Zeng, X., Benson, E., Nyström, A.M., Högberg, B., 2012. DNA origami delivery system for cancer therapy with tunable release properties. ACS Nano 6 (10), 8684–8691.

Zheng, X., Wang, T., Jiang, H., et al., 2013. Incorporation of Carvedilol into PAMAM-functionalized MWNTs as a sustained drug delivery system for enhanced dissolution and drug-loading capacity. Asian J. Pharm. Sci. 8 (5), 278–286.

CHAPTER

5 Dendrimer-based nanoformulations as drug carriers for cancer treatment

Narsireddy Amreddy[1,2], Mahendran Chinnappan[1,2], Anupama Munshi[2,3] and Rajagopal Ramesh[1,2,4]

[1]*Department of Pathology, University of Oklahoma Health Sciences Center, Oklahoma City, OK, United States*

[2]*Stephenson Cancer Center, University of Oklahoma Health Sciences Center, Oklahoma City, OK, United States*

[3]*Department of Radiation Oncology, University of Oklahoma Health Sciences Center, Oklahoma City, OK, United States*

[4]*Graduate Program in Biomedical Sciences, University of Oklahoma Health Sciences Center, Oklahoma City, OK, United States*

5.1 Introduction

According to the American Cancer Society, 1.7 million new cancer patients are expected to be diagnosed in the United States in 2019; further, approximately 606,000 deaths are predicted (American Cancer Society, 2019). Most cancer deaths occur due to drug resistance and metastasis. Early diagnosis can control metastasis, which will make treatments more effective. Different therapeutic modalities although are available to treat cancer have adverse side-effects. Despite advances made in targeted therapy and immunotherapy, these treatments are effective only in few cancer types (Hu-Lieskovan et al., 2014). Chemotherapy has been used extensively to treat all cancer types at various stages. However, conventional chemotherapy has many disadvantages, including poor bioavailability, poor aqueous solubility, rapid clearance, and unfavorable pharmacokinetic properties (Depierre and Westeel, 2007). Multidrug resistance and adverse side effects, such as nephrotoxicity and cardiotoxicity, are significant issues associated with chemotherapy (Gillet and Gottesman, 2010). Gene therapy has also drawn significant attention because of its oncoprotein-targeted therapeutic methodology (Verma et al., 2000). The stability and biodegradability of targeted oncoproteins are the challenges to overcome for having better therapeutic outcomes. To overcome the drawbacks of chemotherapy and gene therapy, carrier-based delivery systems must be developed.

Advances in Polymeric Nanomaterials for Biomedical Applications. DOI: https://doi.org/10.1016/B978-0-12-814657-6.00001-X

Nanoparticle-based cancer therapy have demonstrated promising results. Nanoparticles have unique properties that includes: a size less than 100 nm, easily enter through the cell membrane, can be stabilized in a physiological environment, have prolonged circulation time in the bloodstream, and are rapidly cleared by the kidneys (Desai et al., 1997; Prokop and Davidson, 2008). The surfaces of the nanoparticles can be functionalized with different types of therapeutic and targeting molecules through chemical and physical methods (Cho et al., 2008). Various types of nanoformulations tested for use in different biomedical applications include metallic-, lipid-, polymer and lipid-polymer hybrid-based nanoparticles (Brigger et al., 2012). Each nanoformulation has advantages and disadvantages in terms of drug loading efficiency, drug release kinetics, drug conjugation efficiency, cell uptake and toxicity.

Dendrimers are polymer-based nanoparticles with a size of less than 50 nm and are promising carriers for drug/gene delivery. Dendrimers contain multiple branching units, which are made up of biocompatible monomers, such as amino acids, polymers, and polysaccharides. Dendrimers can be synthesized with different types of peripheral functional groups (−COOH, −SH, −OH, $-NH_2$, −esters), making these nanoparticles useful for biomedical applications (Pedziwiatr-Werbicka et al., 2019). The drug or gene molecules, targeting ligands, and imaging agents can be loaded on dendrimer nanoparticles through chemical and physical methods for multipurpose applications (Fréchet, 2002).

In this chapter, we discuss the various synthesis methods for dendrimer nanoparticles, and their structure and properties are highlighted. We describe the essential properties required when designing dendrimers for biomedical applications especially for their application in cancer diagnosis and therapy.

5.2 Methods for dendrimer synthesis

Dendrimer synthesis involves principles of molecular and polymer chemistry. Molecular synthesis principles include step-by-step controlled synthesis, whereas polymer synthesis involves monomer repetition. Dendrimers can be synthesized with divergent, convergent, mixed divergent/convergent, and orthogonal approaches. Higher generations of dendrimers contain globular, closed packed, and symmetric structures, while lower generations possess open and asymmetric structures. Monodisperse and polydisperse polymers form different types of frameworks such as dendrimers, dendrons, hyperbranched polymers, dendrigrafts, and dendritic-linear hybrids (Abbasi et al., 2014). The size and number of functional groups increase with higher generations of dendrimers. Fig. 5.1 shows a schematic diagram of dendrimer synthesis.

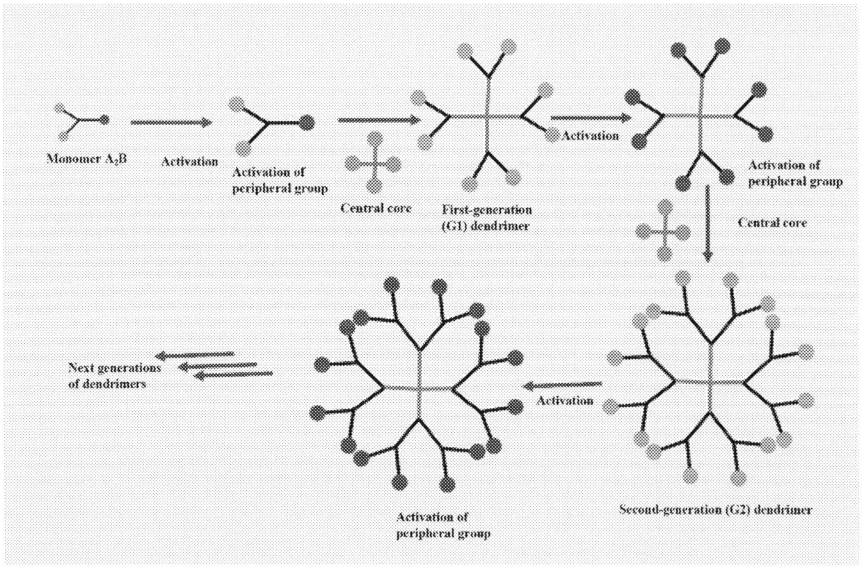

FIGURE 5.1

Schematic representation of different generations of dendrimer synthesis.

5.2.1 Divergent method

The divergent method starts with a multifunctional core and begins conjugation with monomer molecules. The core molecule conjugates with one active, reactive group of monomers creating the first generation of a dendrimer. Subsequently, the inactive groups of monomers in the periphery are activated and continue to conjugate with other monomers to create the second generation. This conjugation continues until the required generation of dendrimers is reached. Usually, higher generation dendrimers are synthesized with this method. The disadvantages of the divergent method, lack of uniform conjugations and dendrimer purity, are lessened with higher generations.

The biocompatible polyamidoamine (PAMAM) and polypropylenimine (PPI) dendrimers have been synthesized by the divergent method. Lee et al. (2006) reported that propargyl-functionalized PAMAM dendrons reacted with a bis(azide) core to achieve more yields of symmetric PAMAM dendrimers in divergent methods by click chemistry. Another group mentioned that the synthesis of amine-functionalized aromatic polyamide dendrimers, trifluoroacetyl used as a protected group with a divergent method. They used the transamidation reduction reaction with hydrazine for the deprotection of amines (Washio et al., 2007). Aoi and coworkers reported using the divergent/convergent joint approach for sugar ball derivatives for surface block dendrimers and hemispherical building blocks (AB type), which can be used for two different functionalities. They used one hemisphere block for cell recognition markers, and the second hemisphere block for other applications (Aoi et al., 1997).

5.2.2 Convergent method

In the convergent method the core group is inactivated, and conjugations happen on the peripheral branches. The layer-by-layer reactions continue until the required generations, called dendrons, are reached. After synthesizing layer-by-layer dendrons the core molecule is activated and joins the dendrons to make dendrimers. In this method the molecular weight difference between required dendrimers and its by-products is high. Thus it is easy to purify the required dendrimers and increase homogeneity. The lower generation dendrimers are more convenient to synthesize using this method. The limitation is that steric hindrance is created when two dendrons are joined (Xu et al., 1994; Grayson and Fréchet, 2001). The most common 5-aminolevulinic acid (ALA) dendrimer was synthesized by conjugating ALA residues through ester linkages. Urbani et al. reported the click chemistry for the synthesis of miktoarm dendrimers and copper (Cu) wire used as a catalyst in the absence of N-based ligand in convergent methods. This Cu wire catalyst strategy gives higher yields of miktoarm (amphiphilic) dendrimer synthesis than in the presence of CuBr/PMDETA complexes, due to the easy removal of excess copper from the final product. They used chemically diverse polymers, such as polystyrene, poly(methyl acrylate), poly(tertbutyl acrylate), and poly(acrylic acid), to synthesize different compositions of miktoarm dendrimers (Urbani et al., 2008).

5.2.3 Orthogonal method

The orthogonal method is another important method of dendrimer synthesis. This method is useful for synthesizing surface multifunctional dendrimers with less steric hindrance and for the synthesis of homogeneous aromatic polyamide dendrons. This approach eliminates the deprotection and activation steps. Another advantage of this approach is that the dendrimers of higher generation can be made from fewer number of reaction and purification steps. Ishida et al. (2000) reported that multiple surface and functional groups were synthesized with aromatic polyamide dendrons by direct condensation method and inserted carbon monoxide in the presence of palladium catalyst. Deb et al. (1997) used the orthogonal approach to synthesize functionalized oligophenylenvinylenes dendrimers with polyvinyl linkages using Heck and Horner–Wadsworth–Emmons chemical reactions.

5.2.4 Metal encapsulated dendrimer synthesis

Metallic-based nanoparticle–encapsulated dendrimer structures have also been synthesized for multipurpose applications. In this approach, metal ions incorporated inside the dendrimer architecture subsequently reduce the metal ions and convert them into uniform size monodisperse metallic nanoparticles. Here, dendrimers act as templates and stabilizing agents for metallic nanoparticle encapsulations. Single and bimetallic nanoparticles can be encapsulated through this route (Crooks et al., 2001).

5.2.5 Dendrimer characterization

The dendrimer structures are purified by size exclusion chromatography, and molecular weight estimation is performed through mass spectrometry techniques, such as matrix-assisted laser desorption/ionization-time of flight and electrospray ionization mass spectrometry. The structure functionality is confirmed with proton and carbon13 nuclear magnetic resonance. The type of functional groups and absorbance properties are studied with Fourier transform infrared spectroscopy and UV–Visible spectroscopy. The hydrodynamic size and shape are measured through dynamic light scattering analysis and transmission electron microscope. The internal structure is confirmed with scattering methods, such as small-angle X-ray, neutron, and laser light scattering.

5.3 Structure and properties of dendrimers

The general terms used in dendrimer chemistry are generation, core, inner shell, pincer, and end groups. The synthesis of a dendrimer begins with one starting center molecule called the core. From the core molecule the different kinds of dendrimers are constructed. Different types of core molecules, such as ammonia, ethylenediamine, and butylenediamine (DAB), are used based on the choice of dendrimer. The generation of dendrimer considers several focal points (layers) from the core molecule toward the periphery. The core molecule generation is considered zero and is represented with "G0"; each layer is considered one generation (Bosman et al., 1999). Fig. 5.2 explains the dendrimer structure and terms used. If a dendrimer has six layers from its core, it is called a sixth-generation dendrimer, abbreviated as G6-dendrimer. The space between any two focal points (layers) is called a "shell." The number of shells depends on dendrimer generation; the dendrimer and internal dendrimer shells are referred to as inner shells, and outer shells are considered the surface of the outer branching point. The pincer contains an outer shell before reaching the surface group. Usually, for each pincer, two surface groups can be conjugated. Then, the total number of pincers is half that of the dendrimer's surface groups. The end group or terminal group (surface group) is crucial for many conjugations. The group that is shown on the surface of the dendrimer is referred to as a terminal group; for example, dendrimers that contain carboxyl functional terminated groups are called "carboxylate-terminated dendrimers."

Dendrimers are designed with different kinds of chemical structures, and each type of dendrimer is synthesized with a particular method. Dendrimers based on amino acids, polymers, and aromatic compounds, such as PAMAM dendrimers, poly-L-lysine (PLL) dendrimers, poly (propylene imine; PPI) dendrimers, poly (aryl ether) dendrimers, poly(aryl alkyne) dendrimers, poly(phenylene)

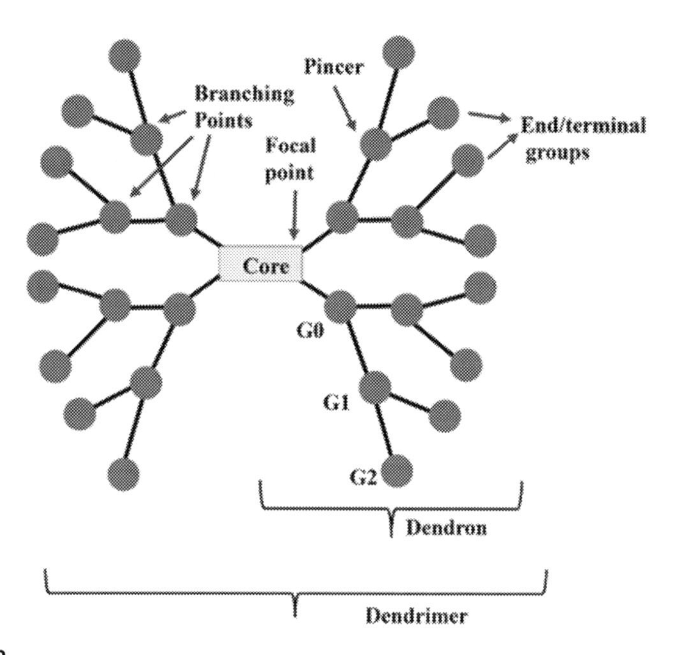

FIGURE 5.2

Schematic representation ofdendrimer components and structure.

dendrimers, poly(alkyl ester) dendrimers, poly(aryl alkene) dendrimers, and poly (alkyl ether) dendrimers, have been reported (Maiti et al., 2004).

The properties of dendrimers are essential for various applications. These properties are influenced by many factors, such as solvent, concentration, salt, and pH. The solvent in the dendrimer solution influences the solubility of dendrimers and therapeutic molecules. Organic solvents are required to solubilize hydrophobic therapeutic molecules. Aqueous solvents are more suitable for solubilizing hydrophilic therapeutics and gene molecules. The solvents can solvate the conformational changes in the dendrimer structure. The lower generation dendrimers have a low solvation effect, whereas higher generation dendrimers show high solvation effect. The concentrations also greatly influence the interactions of the dendrimer with small molecules and larger molecules. The lower concentration dendrimers have more space to interact with other molecules, whereas higher concentration leads to self-assembly and less space to interact. The salt concentrations also impact molecular interactions. High salt concentrations yield more ionic strength and more conformational changes in the dendrimer, and low salt concentrations produce more repulsive forces and profound conformational changes. The pH of the dendrimer solutions affects the charge of the dendrimers. Amine-terminated dendrimers show a positive surface charge at lower pH solutions and interact with negative surface charges (Choudhary et al., 2017).

The interaction of dendrimers with other molecules occurs through covalent conjugations, electrostatic interactions, and hydrogen bonding. Dendrimers covalently conjugate primarily with small molecules and improve the pharmacological properties. These covalent conjugations occur through different kinds of chemistry, such as EDC-NHS and Maleimide-SH. The larger molecules mostly encapsulate through electrostatic interactions. The gene molecules such as siRNA, pDNA, and miRNA possess negative surface charge and thus interact with positive surface charge amino-terminated dendrimers. Hydrogen bonding occurs between the hydrogen-terminated groups, such as both amine groups and amine/carboxylate groups (Klajnert et al., 2007). The higher generations of dendrimers have more of an internal cavity, which helps with hydrogen and coordination bonding. Multivacancy of the dendrimers helps to develop multifunctional dendrimers by interacting with therapeutic, imaging, and targeting molecules. This multifunctional dendrimer improves therapeutic and delivery efficiencies. Self-assembly is another essential type of molecular method that increases the encapsulating capacity of molecules into dendrimers and stability of the complexes. For most successful biomedical applications, pharmacokinetic properties are an important parameter. Pharmacokinetic properties are improving with the biocompatibility of dendrimers and molecules, which have enhanced permeability and retention effects (Galeazzi et al., 2010).

For biomedical applications, PAMAM dendrimer, which is synthesized by the divergent method, is commonly used. Ammonia and ethylenediamine are used as core molecules for PAMAM dendrimers. Ammonia and ethylenediamine contain three and four branching units, respectively. These PAMAM dendrimers can be synthesized for 1–10 generations and form amide bonds by reacting amine groups with esters of methyl acrylate. Terminal groups can be amine, carboxylate, sulfhydryl, or hydroxyl.

PPI-based dendrimers are another class of biocompatible dendrimers. These PPI dendrimers are synthesized by Michael addition reactions between the acetonitrile to a primary amine, followed by reduction of the nitrile group to amines. The core molecule used for PPI dendrimer synthesis is DAB, and the internal structure consists of tertiary propylene amine structures and amine terminal groups (Kaur et al., 2016). Polyethylenimine (PEI) dendrimers are less commonly used dendrimers and are a subclass of PPI dendrimers. PEI dendrimers are synthesized with diamino ethane and diamino propane.

PLL dendrimers, which contain amine-terminated groups and exhibit positive surface charge at physiological pH, are also used for biomedical applications. PLL itself acts as an antitumor agent by inhibiting angiogenesis. A PLL dendrimer–encapsulated docetaxel complex has entered into Phase I clinical trials (DTX; Taxotere) at Starpharma Holdings, Melbourne (Fox et al., 2009).

There are other biocompatible dendrimers that are also being tested for drug delivery and biomedical applications. Neutral surface charge polyester dendrimers, peptide dendrimers, carbohydrate dendrimers, melamine dendrimers, and phosphorus dendrimers are less toxic and used in different types of biomedical applications.

5.4 Dendrimers for biomedical applications

Dendrimers must be biocompatible to avoid toxicity, cross-reactions with tissues and membranes. There are essential parameters that contribute to toxicity, such as biocompatibility of molecules that are being used for dendrimer construction, size, charge, hydrophobic or hydrophilic nature, and surface functional groups. The water-soluble and hydrophilic-based dendrimers show more compatibility for biomedical applications. For the construction of dendrimers, choosing a biocompatible central core molecule, repeated unit, and surface functional groups is essential. The biocompatible core and monomer molecules used in dendrimer synthesis are shown in Fig. 5.3. Amino acid, small molecule, carbohydrate, and PEG-based central core molecules show less toxicity and more compatibility with dendrimers. The repeating unit use with biocompatible polymer or amino acid polymers shows fewer toxic effects. The surface functional groups are essential for dendrimer design, due to their interaction with cell membranes and tissues (Cheng et al., 2011). There are several biocompatible functional groups, including $-NH_2$, $-COOH$, $-SH$, and $-OH$. The amine-terminated dendrimers present a positive surface charge, which strongly interacts with cell membranes and tissues through electrostatic interaction. The higher concentration of positive surface charge results in toxicity due to the proton sponge effect. The carboxylate surface functional groups show a negative surface charge and interact with the membrane through hydrogen bonding, with less toxic effect (Cui et al., 2018). The other neutral surface charge functional groups also show minimal toxic effect.

Higher generation dendrimers contain a more significant number of surface functional groups and a larger size that actively interacts with membranes of biological tissues. These dendrimers tend to form aggregates when interacting with biological molecules, such as proteins, peptides, vitamins, and antibodies. Because of the above, higher generation dendrimers show more toxicity than do corresponding lower generation dendrimers. The use of cleavable linkers through chemical bonds improves the

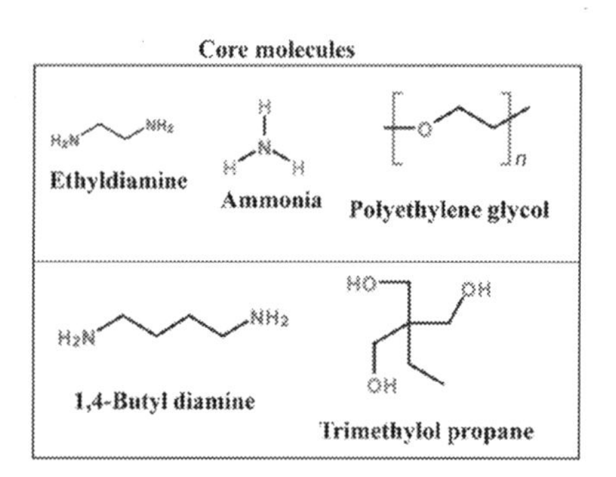

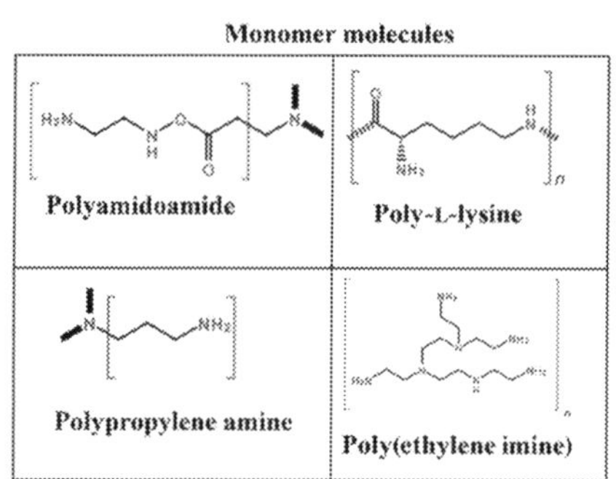

FIGURE 5.3

Core and monomer molecules used in dendrimer synthesis.

biodegradability of the dendrimer, and thus minimizes the toxicity. Most of the organically structured dendrimers are hydrophobic and dissolve in organic solvents. The organic solvents are not compatible for biomedical applications, and hence organic structured dendrimers are not suitable for biomedical applications (Jain et al., 2010).

The surfaces of dendrimers are modified with biodegradable or biocompatible molecules, including PEGylated, acetylated, glycosylated, and amino acid molecules, through chemical conjugations, making the dendrimers more compatible for biomedical applications. The PEGylation on the surface of the dendrimers improves dispersion and biocompatibility and increases the biodistribution and prolonged circulation of dendrimers. PEG modification also increases bioavailability and reduces toxicity. Several reports noted that PEG conjugation could be done with different polymers, including PAMAM, PPI, PLL, and polyester dendrimers (Duncan and Izzo, 2005). PEGylation stabilizes the dendrimer/siRNA or pDNA complexes, and thus increases transfection efficiency.

Acetylation conjugation on the surface of dendrimers enhances hydrophilicity and reduces the hydrophobic nature thereby increasing the drug loading efficiency. Functionalization with acetylation groups reduces the net positive surface charge on the dendrimers resulting in diminished toxicity. The glycosylated modified dendrimers also increase the specificity of uptake and stabilize the complexes that increase drug delivery efficiency.

Sugar molecules, such as maltose, lactose, and glucosylated molecules, can be used to modify dendrimers to reduce cytotoxicity. Cyclodextrin-modified dendrimers also display reduced cytotoxicity and improved therapeutic efficiency. Amino acid functionalization on the surface of dendrimers increases gene transfection efficiency. Modification with lipid molecules increases membrane destruction capacity and toxicity; hence, lipid modification is not biocompatible (Sharma et al., 2011; Yang and John Kao, 2006).

5.5 Dendrimer nanoparticles for cancer therapy

Among different kinds of cancer therapeutic methods, drug and gene therapy have received more attention because of targeted delivery. The critical parameters required for efficient drug delivery include increased bioavailability and high drug accumulation at the tumor site. To increase the solubility of hydrophobic drugs in the physiological environment, pharmacokinetic properties play a role. Another valuable property is specific targeting of tumor tissue to reduce adverse side effects in healthy tissues. To overcome the drawbacks mentioned earlier and for improved therapeutic efficiency, new and efficient drug carriers are warranted. Nanoparticle-based carrier systems hold promise in cancer treatment. Different kinds of nanoparticles, such as metal-, lipid-, and polymer-based nanoparticles, are available. Among these, dendrimer-based polymer nanoparticles are garnering considerable attention due to their multifunctional and biocompatible properties (Baker, 2009; Cheng et al., 2011).

Multiple types of dendrimers are available for biomedical applications. Hydrophobic drug molecules can be covalently conjugated to the dendrimers to increase aqueous solubility. The hydrophilic molecules are loaded onto the dendrimers through covalent, electrostatic, hydrogen bonding, and coordination bonds. The drug molecule conjugation to the dendrimers can be made through specific tumor microenvironment (TME)-cleavable bonds, such as pH-sensitive and glutathione bonds, and photothermal-cleavable bonds. The TME-cleavable linkages enhance the tumor specificity. The gene molecules (siRNA, pDNA, shRNA, and mRNA) are loaded onto the dendrimers through electrostatic interactions. The dendrimer-gene molecule complexes increase the stability of the gene molecule and escape from endosomes to avoid degradability and improve therapeutic efficiency (Castro et al., 2018). Since dendrimers contain multiple peripheral functional groups, they are easy to functionalize with targeting ligands to obtain receptor-mediated uptake to reduce side effects. Dendrimers can also be used for multipurpose applications, such as imaging coupled with targeted delivery. The imaging molecules, such as metallic nanoparticles and fluorescent molecules, can be loaded or coated on dendrimer nanoparticles for imaging and therapeutic applications (Palmerston Mendes et al., 2017). In this section, we discuss the different cancer types and their therapeutic modalities with dendrimer nanoparticles. Fig. 5.4 shows multifunctional dendrimer nanoparticles and their tumor growth inhibition in in vitro and in vivo conditions.

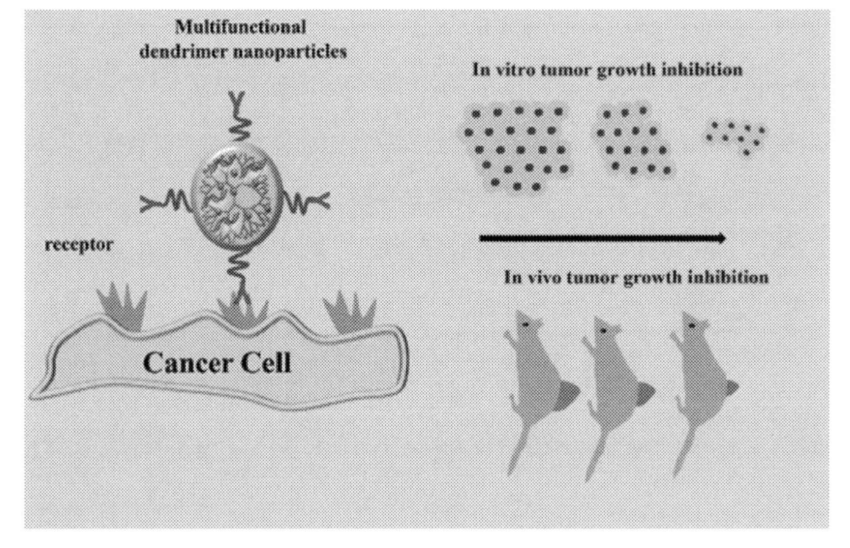

FIGURE 5.4

Schematic diagram representing how multifunctional dendrimer nanoparticles reduce tumor growth.

5.5.1 Lung cancer

Lung cancer is the leading cause of cancer-related deaths in the United States of America (USA) and around the world. Smoking and tobacco use are prominent risk factors for lung cancer. However, lung cancer is also common among those who have never smoked. Irrespective of the early detection and treatment options, the 5-year survival rate for lung cancer is around 10%–15%. Several biomarkers are implicated in lung cancer. These biomarkers include DDR2, FGFR, NTRK1, and PI3KCA; proto-oncogenes, such as B-RAF, MET, RET, EGFR, ROS1, KRAS, and ALK. Several drugs/gene molecules are available to treat lung cancer. Among different types of drug carriers, dendrimer polymer–based nanocarriers are used to treat lung cancer.

Different types of anticancer drug molecules have been encapsulated into dendrimers. The highly hydrophobic anticancer drug paclitaxel (PTX) has low solubility in aqueous conditions. The PTX conjugated to the surface of PEGylated dendrimer and decorated on their surface of the dendrimer with biotin molecules for tumor targeting and was shown to successfully deliver the drug into A549 non–small cell lung cancer (NSCLC) cell line (Rompicharla et al., 2019). Another group attached the PTX to the PEG-dendron through succinic and gallic acid linkers to improve its intracellular uptake and anticancer bioactivity in 2D and 3D cell culture (Correard et al., 2019).

PAMAM dendrimer–based nanoparticles have been attached to multiple therapeutics. Generation-5 PAMAM dendrimers were stabilized on the surface of Ag nanoparticles, followed by encapsulation with 5-fluorouracil (5-FU@DsAgNCs). This 5-FU@DsAgNCs nanocomposite showed an enhanced therapeutic effect on lung (A549) and breast (MCF-7) cancer cell lines (Matai et al., 2015).

Oral inhalation of chemotherapeutics offers advantages toward directed targeting of the nanoformulations and better control over the spatiotemporal availability of the drug. Doxorubicin (Dox) was conjugated to PEG1000-tagged PAMAM in a pH-sensitive manner, and its effects were studied in a pulmonary epithelial (Calu-3) cell line model. The results showed effective killing of the Calu-3 cells due to sustained release of the drug (Zhong et al., 2017). Further, a dry powder inhaler formulation was generated by conjugating Dox with the fourth generation PAMAM dendrimer and produced as a mannitol microparticle for the treatment of lung adenocarcinoma. The dendrimer was designed in such a way that it would only release the drug at a lower pH in the intracellular environment. The researchers observed an inhaled dose and final particle fraction in the lung cells were higher than commercial formulations (Zhong, 2018).

Small molecule inhibitors can also be delivered through dendrimers. Gefitinib targets the epidermal growth factor receptor (EGFR)- tyrosine kinase (TK) and is widely used in NSCLC treatment. It showed enhanced solubility, encapsulation, and controlled delivery with PEGylated PAMAM dendrimers, compared with the inclusion complex of gefitinib with β-cyclodextrin. However, both the inclusion complexation and dendrimer showed reduced hemolytic toxicity and lowered GI 50 values (Shende et al., 2017).

Metal nanoparticles loaded with dendrimer are used for multifunctional purposes. Malekmohammadi et al. (2018) showed curcumin (cu) loaded on reduced graphene oxide nanosheets and immobilized on gold nanoparticles could be conjugated with folic acid molecules on dendritic mesoporous silica-coat. This targeted Cur-AuNPs@GFMS nanocomposite showed enhanced drug delivery and improved therapeutic efficiency compared to nontargeted nanocomposites (Malekmohammadi et al., 2018). Other laboratories have used fourth-generation PAMAM dendrimer to coat iron oxide nanoparticles (G4@IONPs). Injection of these G4@IONPs into BALB/c mice resulted in the enrichment of the iron particles in the liver, kidney, and lung tissues (Salimi et al., 2018).

Gene delivery with dendrimers is also a promising method for lung cancer treatment. Dendrimers have been used as a nonviral system to deliver shRNA for silencing the Bcl-xL protein expression. PAMAM dendrimers with 10-bromodecanoic acid and 10C-PEG modification carrying Bcl-XL shRNA efficiently transfected A549 cells and markedly reduced Bcl-xL expression while concomitantly increasing apoptotic cell death (Ayatollahi et al., 2017). Another study used a peptide attached to PAMAM dendrimers to deliver plasid DNA to NSCLC cells in vivo. (Holt and Daftarian, 2018). Chondroitin sulfate (CS)-modified PAMAM dendrimer has been tested for delivering the micro-RNA (miR)-34a. Intraveneous (i.v.) injection of CS-PAMAM/miR-34a into a A549 lung tumor-bearing greatly reduced tumor growth and induced tumor cell apoptosis (Chen et al., 2017). Wang et al (2015a,b) conjugated S6 aptamer to PAMAM dendrimer, for delivering miR-34a miRNA to lung cancer cells. Their study showed addition of the aptamer improved the cellular uptake and transfection efficiency. Masuda et al, (2016) tested anti-muc1 aptament conjugated sixth-generation glutamic acid–modified dendritic PLL system (KG6E) as drug delivery vehicle in MUC1 overrexpressing A549 lung cancer cells. They showed the anti-MUC1 apt/KG6E dendrimer efficiently targeted and was internalized by A549 cells compared to scrambler apt/KG6E system (Masuda et al., 2016). Our group reported PAMAM dendrimer that are decorated on their surface with folic acid specifically targeted folate-receptor-α overexpressing lung cancer cells and successfully co-delivered cisplatin and HuR-targeted siRNA. The tumor-targeted drug delivery resultsed in enhanced antitumor activity compared to nontargeted dendirmers.

5.5.2 Breast cancer

Breast cancer is one of the leading causes of cancer-related mortality among women. Multiple risk factors, which include prolonged physical inactivity, hormone replacement therapy, hormone modified contraceptives, and unhealthy lifestyle, have been associated with breast cancer. Metastasis results in an increased death rate. Significant areas of metastasis are observed in the bone, liver, brain, and especially in the lungs; the latter organ affected in 60% of patients diagnosed with breast cancer. Early diagnosis of the disease will play a critical role in the treatment option for effectively controlling breast cancer. Several biomarkers have been identified to help with early diagnosis, disease origin, and targeted therapy. These biomarkers include mammaglobin, GCDFP-15, GATA3 ER,HER-2, hormone receptors, and proliferation markers, such as Ki-67, cyclin D & E, CD31, CD34, factor VII, and podoplanin. Chemotherapy is common in breast cancer treatment. However, treatment-related toxicity is common indicating improved drug delivery system that can reduced toxicity will aid in effectively controlling breast cancer.

Although nanomaterial-based drugs are available for breast cancer treatment, their nonspecificity and biocompatibility must be improved. A new cell mimetic strategy generating nano-prodrug assembly of Dox on DNA tetrahedron dendrimer, liposomes, and macrophage membrane called Dox-MPK@MDL was reported by Li et al., (2019). The study showed that the release of prodrug from Dox-MPK@MDL was pH dependent and had excellent biocompatibility, increased serum half-life, and specficically targeted metastatic tumor cells (Li et al., 2019).

Multiple strategies have been attempted to improve on the shortcomings observed with classical chemotherapy methods. Cancer cells have been reported to be highly active in glucose metabolism. A study focused on targeting breast cancer cells with docetaxel-carrying PAMAM dendrimers with glucose modification (PAMAM-dox-glc) was performed. The efficiency of the dendrimer complex in inducing the cellular toxicity was evaluated using GLUT1 inhibitors, which abrogated the PAMAM-dox-glc-stimulated cellular cytotoxicity (Sztandera et al., 2019). Tumor inhibition has also been reported using the sonochemotherapy method. A nanocarrier system comprising carboxyl-terminated PAMAM dendrimer conjugated with hyaluronic acid, fluorochrome indocyanine green (ICG), and Dox hydrochloride was evaluated in the CD44-overexpressing 4T1 C breast cancer cell line both, in vitro and in vivo. A combination of ultrasonic treatment with the nanocarrier administration resulted in significant inhibition of tumor growth in vivo (Wu et al., 2019).

Overexpression of HER-2 on the surface of the cancer cells is associated with increased proliferation and cancer. Conjugation of macromolecular dendrimers with an antibody capable of targeting these receptors enables effective targeted delivery of the anticancer therapeutics. PAMAM dendrimers conjugated with trastuzumab have been used to carry docetaxel and PTX. Evaluation of their cellular uptake and internalization showed enrichment in PAMAM-doc-trastuzumab and PAMAM-PTX-trastuzumab compounds compared with free trastuzumab, PTX, or docetaxel in a study with HER-2-negative MCF-7 and HER-2-positive SKBR-3 cells (Marcinkowska et al., 2019). In another study, CXCR4-targetged drug delivery was investigated. LFC131 peptide targets CXCR4 receptors that are overexpressed and involved in breast cancer metastasis. LFC131 peptide was conjugated to Dox-carrying PAMAM dendrimers and tested for their ability to prevent breast tumors from metastasizing to other organs. The study results showed LFC131-drug carrying dendrimer treatment inhibited breast cancer cell migration and metastasis (Chittasupho et al., 2017)

5.5.3 Osteosarcoma (bone cancer)

Among primary bone cancer types, osteosarcoma is the most common and occurs mainly in children and adolescents. Osteosarcoma appears more often in males than in females. Multiple therapeutic modalities, for example, chemotherapy, surgery, and radiation, are used. If patients are appropriately treated, the survival rate is around 70%. Bone is one of the major organs to which cancers from other sites, such as blood, breast, and prostate cancer metastasize. Due to the lack of targeting, chemotherapy causes toxicity and less biodistribution to the site of bone cancer. Nanoparticle-based delivery systems have exciting results for osteosarcoma-targeted therapy.

Nanocarriers designed to target the bone tumor using ligands, namely, alendronate and pamidronate, have not been entirely successful due to the lack of higher selectivity toward the bone. Carboxy-terminated dendrimers with platinum nanoparticles have been observed to be enriched in bone tumor regions compared with healthy bones. A combination of photothermal therapy with this dendrimer administration resulted in the suppression of bone tumors (Yan et al., 2019). Gene therapy targeting the tumor necrosis factor–related apoptosis-inducing ligand (TRAIL) gene has shown to be a promising strategy for multiple cancers. However, the lack of an efficient vector has been a limiting factor. Triazine-modified dendrimer macromolecule G5-DAT66 has been demonstrated to be effective in vitro using the MG-63 osteosarcoma cell line and in vivo in a mouse model bearing osteosarcoma (Wang et al., 2015a,b). A polysaccharide-derived nanomaterial delivery vehicle for the siRNA of elevated astrocyte gene-1 (AEG-1) was created by click conjugation of azide chitosan with propargyl focal point PLL dendron, followed by folic acid tagging, and was named Cs-g-PLLD-FA/siAEG-1. Cs-g-PLLD-FA/siAEG-1 was able to effectively inhibit tumor growth and lung metastasis in mice (Can et al., 1998).

5.5.4 Glioblastoma (brain cancer)

The most common type of brain cancer in adults is glioblastoma, which grows rapidly and spreads quickly. Glioblastoma creates its own blood vessels to obtain a blood supply and hence quickly spreads to healthy brain tissues. The overall 5-year survival rate is about 5.6%. Although a complete cure is not available, treatments are available to improve survival rates and reduce complications. Targeted drug delivery is one of the best methods to cross the blood–brain barrier (BBB) and deliver drugs to the brain. Nanoparticle-based targeted drug delivery methods are one of the better alternatives used to treat brain cancers.

The application of gene therapy to brain-related complications, such as cancer, Alzheimer's, or Parkinson's disease, is difficult because of the lack of efficient drug delivery vehicles. A recent study demonstrated the use of lactoferrin-tagged generation 3-diaminobutyric PPI (DAB) dendrimer for the delivery of plasmid DNA. The study showed that the dendrimer increased uptake of DNA up to 2.1-fold by brain cells and increased transgene expression up to 6.4-fold (Somani et al., 2015).

Another study aimed at improving the effectiveness of Dox, one of the first drugs available for glioblastoma, in penetrating the BBB and reducing its hemolytic property and short half-life. Dendrimer-cationized-albumin (dCatAlb) was encrusted with Dox-containing PLGA nanoparticles (dCatAlb-pDNP). The nanoformulation was shown to have improved characteristics of pH-dependent release of the Dox, reduced hemolytic activity, increased uptake and cytotoxicity by inducing apoptosis in U87MG cells and bEND.3 model (Muniswamy et al., 2019).

5.5.5 Melanoma (skin cancer)

Melanoma is a type of skin cancer that is aggressive and fast-growing. The overall incidence of melanoma are higher in men. However, the incidence appears to be higher in women who are less then 50 years of age compared to men of the same age groups. The 5-year survival rate is around 90%. Melanoma often penetrate into the inner deep layers of skin and easily spreads to other organs. Targeted chemotherapy, surgery, and radiation therapeutics are used for melanoma treatment. These treatment methods have poor bioavailability and side effects.

Dual targeting of macrophages and cancer cells has been recommended for effective treatment of aggressive melanoma using photodynamic therapy. Cowpea mosaic virus (CPMV) has been reported to target the immunosuppressive subgroup of macrophages and cancer cells selectively. A recent report utilized a hybrid of the noninfectious CPMV nanoparticle and dendron along with photosensitizer to potentially remove the cancer cells and macrophages for improved melanoma treatment (Wen et al., 2016). Nanoparticle and dendrimer hybrid nanocarriers have attempted to improve the stability and controlled release of chemotherapeutic drug. A study focused on the controlled release of PTX used the PAMAM dendrimer with dithiocarbamate and crosslinked with arginine gold nanoparticles. The hybrid nanoparticle and dendrimer-mediated controlled release of the drug was observed to be much more efficient than that of the free drug, as shown in B16F10 cells and in an in vivo model (Jeong et al., 2016). A temozolomide (TMZ)-encapsulated PAMAM—based drug delivery system was shown to enhance the sensitivity of human melanoma cells, namely, A375 cells, to TMZ (Jiang et al., 2017). Dendrimers have been employed to assess the tumor damage caused by ionizing radiation. A recent study analyzed the effects on the tumor tissues of mice with G4 PAMAM dendrimers conjugated with dodecane tetraacetic acid (DOTA) and radiolabeled with (177)Lu. The results showed increased amounts of Fe, Mg, Rb, S, and Zn and reduced amounts of Br, Ca, Cl, K, and Na. These observations can be considered as an indicator of tumor tissue damage caused by the ionizing radiation from the dendrimers (Kovacs et al., 2015).

5.5.6 Liver cancer

The most common type of liver cancer is hepatocellular carcinoma (HCC). Primary liver cancer forms from the liver cell (hepatocyte). People who have liver diseases, congenital disabilities, cirrhosis, and hepatitis infection are more likely to develop liver cancers. The cancer that spreads from other organs to the liver is called metastatic cancer. Most liver cancers are secondary, or metastasized cancers. Chemotherapy is an important therapeutic approach to treat liver cancer, but it causes drug resistance and toxicity. Dendrimer nanoparticle–based delivery of chemotherapeutic drugs or gene molecules could yield better therapeutic outcomes.

HCC is a complicated form of liver cancer that continues to lack an effective diagnosis and targeted therapy due to the nonavailability of potential biomarkers and is largely metastatic. Asialoglycoprotein receptors are observed to be expressed in higher concentration in HCC. Galactosamine (Gal) is mainly used in targeted therapy for HCC due to its increased binding capacity to asialoglycoprotein. PAMAM dendrimers conjugated with Gal, curcumin derivative (CDF), and a near infra-red dye named S0456 were evaluated in HCC cell lines. The results showed that CDF is a potential anticancer therapeutic, compared with Dox, sorafenib, and cisplatin (Yousef et al., 2018). Multifunctional dendrimer formulations using PAMAM dendrimer generation 4, 5, and 6 conjugated to polydopamine-anchored magnetic nanoparticles (Fe_3O_4) were tested as a liver cancer treatment. The results showed an improved anticancer effect of the multifunctional dendrimer formulations compared with the individual components (Jędrzak et al., 2019).

mRNA replacement–based treatment options have been shown to be promising for liver disorders. The potential of this method remains diminished due to the lack of efficient mRNA carrier systems. mRNA-loaded lipid nanoparticle–based dendrimer has been explored as an effective way to treat children born with defective fumarylacetoacetate hydrolase (FAH). The double knockout C57BL/6 mouse model of FAH has been shown to maintain an equivalent concentration of total bilirubin, alanine transaminase, and aspartate transaminase and remained at healthy weight throughout the treatment course, indicating the effectiveness of the treatment method (Cheng et al., 2018).

5.5.7 Pancreatic cancer

Pancreatic cancer is one of the fastest-growing cancers, with late prognosis and the lowest survival rate among all other cancers. The pancreas produces enzymes and hormones that are involved in metabolic reactions, such as digestion. The American Cancer Society (ACS) report revealed that only 23% of patients survive 1 year after diagnosis, and the 5-year survival rate is about 8.2%. Pancreatic ductal adenocarcinoma (PDAC), which forms in the epithelial ducts, is a predominant (80%) type of pancreatic cancer. Available treatment methods are surgery, radiation, and chemotherapy. Only a few patients are eligible for surgery due to late diagnosis. Chemotherapy has poor drug accumulation in pancreatic cancer cells because the TME has dense stroma and weak vasculature. Delivering therapeutics to pancreatic cancer remains a challenge because of the low penetration of the drugs and increased drug resistance.

Nanoparticle-based targeted therapies offer a promising approach to overcome these drawbacks. A recent study encapsulated gold nanoparticles (Au DENPs) in dendrimer for the codelivery of gemcitabine and miR-21 inhibitor, named Gem-Au DENPs/miR-21i. The Gem-Au DENPs/miR-21i formulation was promoted by the ultrasound-targeted microbubble destruction (UTMD) method. The results showed an increased cellular uptake of Gem-Au DENPs/miR-21i, which can be enhanced by using UTMD. The codelivery of Gem and miR-21 was also enhanced by using UTMD in vitro and in a xenograft pancreatic tumor model (Lin et al., 2018). In addition, PAMAM generation-3 dendrimers have been complexed with nucleic acid–binding polymers (NABP) for use in pancreatic cancer. PAMAM-G3/NABP effectively reduced nucleic acid–mediated activation of Toll-like receptors (TLRs) and tumor invasion in vitro in pancreatic cancer. The nanocarrier formulation has also been demonstrated to be effective in curbing the pro-invasive signals of microvesicles by directly binding to them (Naqvi et al., 2018).

5.6 Conclusion and future perspectives

Dendrimers have a highly defined structure with uniform size. Dendrimer nanoparticles are synthesized with biocompatible monomers, such as amino acids, polysaccharides, and polyesters. Multiple therapeutic moieties can be conjugated covalently and electrostatically. Hydrophobic, hydrophilic, and amphiphilic molecules also can be conjugated or loaded with dendrimers. The targeting ligands, antibodies, peptides, and aptamers can be functionalized on the surface of dendrimers. Multiple surface functional groups can be conjugated for imaging and therapeutic applications.

Dendrimer-nanoparticle formulations with anticancer agents efficiently improve the therapeutic efficiency and can override some of the limitations encountered with conventional chemotherapy. Since dendrimers can diffuse into tissues and can carry numerous types of therapeutics, they can be used to treat different cancers. Herein, we have provided examples of dendrimer formulations to treat different cancer types. However, readers are informed that the examples provided are not exhaustive and additional reading is recommended.

Although dendrimer-based nanoparticles are well studied in drug delivery applications for cancer therapy, there are still several areas in drug delivery that need to be addressed for increasing the therapeutic efficacy. Strategies to reduce toxicity and increase biodistribution, pharmacokinetics, circulation time, and drug accumulation in tumors need to be addressed for improving the patient's quality of life (QOL) and in acheving in disease free long-term patient survival. Finally, methods to scale-up the nanoformulations and demonstrate safety and efficacy is a prerequisite for clinical translation.

Acknowledgments

The work was supported in part by grants (R01 CA167516 & R01CA233201) received from the National Institutes of Health (NIH), an Institutional Development Award (IDeA) from the National Institute of General Medical Sciences (P20 GM103639) of the National Institutes of Health, MERIT Review Grant (101BX003420A1) from the Department of Veterans Affairs, Oklahoma Center for the Advancement of Science and Technology (OCAST; HR18−088), Department of Defense (DOD; W81XWH-19-1-0647 and W81XWH-18-1-0637), a pilot grant from the Stephenson Cancer Center funded by the NCI Cancer Center Support Grant (P30 CA225520) (AM), OUHSC Department of Radiation Oncology Research Development Funds (AM), and by funds received from the Stephenson Cancer Center Seed Grant (RR), Presbyterian Health Foundation Seed Grant (RR, AM), Presbyterian Health Foundation Bridge Grant (RR, AM), and Jim and Christy Everest Endowed Chair in Cancer Developmental Therapeutics (RR) at the University of Oklahoma Health Sciences Center. Rajagopal Ramesh is an Oklahoma TSET Research Scholar and holds the Jim and Christy Everest Endowed Chair in Cancer Developmental Therapeutics.

References

Abbasi, E., Aval, S.F., Akbarzadeh, A., Milani, M., Nasrabadi, H.T., Joo, S.W., et al., 2014. Dendrimers: synthesis, applications, and properties. Nanoscale Res. Lett. 9, 247. Available from: https://doi.org/10.1186/1556-276X-9-247.

American Cancer Society, 2019. Cancer Facts & Figures.

Amreddy, N., Babu, A., Panneerselvam, J., Srivastava, A., Muralidharan, R., Chen, A., et al., 2018. Chemo-biologic combinatorial drug delivery using folate receptor-targeted dendrimer nanoparticles for lung cancer treatment. Nanomedicine 14, 373−384. Available from: https://doi.org/10.1016/j.nano.2017.11.010.

Aoi, K., Itoh, K., Okada, M., 1997. Divergent/convergent joint approach with a half-protected initiator core to synthesize surface-block dendrimers. Macromolecules 30, 8072−8074. Available from: https://doi.org/10.1021/ma961397n.

Ayatollahi, S., Salmasi, Z., Hashemi, M., Askarian, S., Oskuee, R.K., Abnous, K., et al., 2017. Aptamer-targeted delivery of Bcl-xL shRNA using alkyl modified PAMAM dendrimers into lung cancer cells. Int. J. Biochem. Cell Biol. 92, 210−217. Available from: https://doi.org/10.1016/j.biocel.2017.10.005.

Baker, J.R., 2009. Dendrimer-based nanoparticles for cancer therapy. Hematol. Am. Soc. Hematol. Educ. Program 708−719. Available from: https://doi.org/10.1182/asheducation-2009.1.708.

Bosman, A.W., Janssen, H.M., Meijer, E.W., 1999. About dendrimers: structure, physical properties, and applications. Chem. Rev. 99, 1665−1688. Available from: https://doi.org/10.1021/cr970069y.

Brigger, I., Dubernet, C., Couvreur, P., 2012. Nanoparticles in cancer therapy and diagnosis. Adv. Drug Deliv. Rev. 64 (Suppl.), 24−36. Available from: https://doi.org/10.1016/j.addr.2012.09.006.

Can, S., Zhu, Y.S., Cai, L.Q., Ling, Q., Katz, M.D., Akgun, S., et al., 1998. The identification of 5 alpha-reductase-2 and 17 beta-hydroxysteroid dehydrogenase-3 gene defects in male pseudohermaphrodites from a Turkish kindred. J. Clin. Endocrinol. Metab. 83, 560–569. Available from: https://doi.org/10.1210/jcem.83.2.4535.

Castro, R.I., Forero-Doria, O., Guzmán, L., 2018. Perspectives of dendrimer-based nanoparticles in cancer therapy. An. Acad. Bras. Cienc. 90 (2 Suppl. 1), 2331–2346. Available from: https://doi.org/10.1590/0001-3765201820170387.

Chen, W., Liu, Y., Liang, X., Huang, Y., Li, Q., 2017. Chondroitin sulfate-functionalized polyamidoamine as a tumor-targeted carrier for miR-34a delivery. Acta Biomater. 57, 238–250. Available from: https://doi.org/10.1016/j.actbio.2017.05.030.

Cheng, Y., Zhao, L., Li, Y., Xu, T., 2011. Design of biocompatible dendrimers for cancer diagnosis and therapy: current status and future perspectives. Chem. Soc. Rev. 40, 2673–2703. Available from: https://doi.org/10.1039/c0cs00097c.

Cheng, Q., Wei, T., Jia, Y., Farbiak, L., Zhou, K., Zhang, S., et al., 2018. Dendrimer-based lipid nanoparticles deliver therapeutic FAH mRNA to normalize liver function and extend survival in a mouse model of hepatorenal tyrosinemia type I. Adv. Mater. 30, e1805308. Available from: https://doi.org/10.1002/adma.201805308.

Chittasupho, C., Anuchapreeda, S., Sarisuta, N., 2017. CXCR4 targeted dendrimer for anticancer drug delivery and breast cancer cell migration inhibition. Eur. J. Pharm. Biopharm. 119, 310–321. Available from: https://doi.org/10.1016/j.ejpb.2017.07.003.

Cho, K., Wang, X., Nie, S., Chen, Z.G., Shin, D.M., 2008. Therapeutic nanoparticles for drug delivery in cancer. Clin. Cancer Res. 14, 1310–1316. Available from: https://doi.org/10.1158/1078-0432.CCR-07-1441.

Choudhary, S., Gupta, L., Rani, S., Dave, K., Gupta, U., 2017. Impact of dendrimers on solubility of hydrophobic drug molecules. Front. Pharmacol. 8, 261. Available from: https://doi.org/10.3389/fphar.2017.00261.

Correard, F., Roy, M., Terrasson, V., Braguer, D., Estève, M.A., Gingras, M., 2019. Delaying anticancer drug delivery by self-assembly and branching effects of minimalist dendron-drug conjugates. Chemistry 25, 9586–9591. Available from: https://doi.org/10.1002/chem.201801092.

Crooks, R.M., Zhao, M., Sun, L., Chechik, V., Yeung, L.K., 2001. Dendrimer-encapsulated metal nanoparticles: synthesis, characterization, and applications to catalysis. Acc. Chem. Res. 134, 181–190. Available from: https://doi.org/10.1021/ar000110a.

Cui, Y., Liang, B., Wang, L., Zhu, L., Kang, J., Sun, H., et al., 2018. Enhanced biocompatibility of PAMAM dendrimers benefiting from tuning their surface charges. Mater. Sci. Eng. C Mater Biol. Appl. 93, 332–340. Available from: https://doi.org/10.1016/j.msec.2018.07.070.

Deb, S.K., Maddux, T.M., Yu, L., 1997. A simple orthogonal approach to poly(phenylenevinylene) dendrimers. J. Am. Chem. Soc. 119, 9079–9080. Available from: https://doi.org/10.1021/ja971790o.

Depierre, A., Westeel, V., 2007. Preoperative chemotherapy in non-small cell lung cancer: advantages, disadvantages, level of evidence. Rev. Mal. Respir. 24 (8 Pt 2), 6S59–63S59.

Desai, M.P., Labhasetwar, V., Walter, E., Levy, R.J., Amidon, G.L., 1997. The mechanism of uptake of biodegradable microparticles in Caco-2 cells is size dependent. Pharm. Res. 14, 1568–1573.

Duncan, R., Izzo, L., 2005. Dendrimer biocompatibility and toxicity. Adv. Drug Deliv. Rev. 57, 2215–2237.

Fox, M.E., Guillaudeu, S., Fréchet, J.M., Jerger, K., Macaraeg, N., Szoka, F.C., 2009. Synthesis and in vivo antitumor efficacy of PEGylated poly(L-lysine) dendrimer-camptothecin conjugates. Mol. Pharm. 6, 1562–1572. Available from: https://doi.org/10.1021/mp9001206.

Fréchet, J.M.J., 2002. Dendrimers and supramolecular chemistry. PNAS 99, 4782–4787. Available from: https://doi.org/10.1073/pnas.082013899.

Galeazzi, S., Hermans, T.M., Paolino, M., Anzini, M., Mennuni, L., Giordani, A., et al., 2010. Multivalent supramolecular dendrimer-based drugs. Biomacromolecules 11, 182–186. Available from: https://doi.org/10.1021/bm901055a.

Gillet, J.P., Gottesman, M.M., 2010. Mechanisms of multidrug resistance in cancer. Methods Mol. Biol. 596, 47–76. Available from: https://doi.org/10.1007/978-1-60761-416-6_4.

Grayson, S.M., Fréchet, J.M., 2001. Convergent dendrons and dendrimers: from synthesis to applications. Chem. Rev. 101, 3819–3868. Available from: https://doi.org/10.1021/cr990116h.

Holt, G.E., Daftarian, P., 2018. Non-small-cell lung cancer homing peptide-labeled dendrimers selectively transfect lung cancer cells. Immunotherapy 10, 1349–1360. Available from: https://doi.org/10.2217/imt-2018-0078.

Hu-Lieskovan, S., Robert, L., Moreno, B.H., Ribas, A., 2014. Combining targeted therapy with immunotherapy in BRAF-mutant melanoma: promise and challenges. J. Clin. Oncol. 32, 2248–2254. Available from: https://doi.org/10.1200/JCO.2013.52.1377.

Ishida, Y., Jikei, M., Kakimoto, M., 2000. Rapid synthesis of aromatic polyamide dendrimers by an orthogonal and a double-stage convergent approach. Macromolecules 33, 3202–3211. Available from: https://doi.org/10.1021/ma991700v.

Jain, K., Kesharwani, P., Gupta, U., Jain, N.K., 2010. Dendrimer toxicity: let's meet the challenge. Int. J. Pharm. 394, 122–142. Available from: https://doi.org/10.1016/j.ijpharm.2010.04.027.

Jędrzak, A., Grześkowiak, B.F., Coy, E., Wojnarowicz, J., Szutkowski, K., Jurga, S., et al., 2019. Dendrimer based theranostic nanostructures for combined chemo- and photothermal therapy of liver cancer cells in vitro. Colloids Surf. B Biointerfaces 173, 698–708. Available from: https://doi.org/10.1016/j.colsurfb.2018.10.045.

Jeong, Y., Kim, S.T., Jiang, Y., Duncan, B., Kim, C.S., Saha, K., et al., 2016. Nanoparticle-dendrimer hybrid nanocapsules for therapeutic delivery. Nanomedicine (Lond.) 11, 1571–1578. Available from: https://doi.org/10.2217/nnm-2016-0034.

Jiang, G., Li, R., Tang, J., Ma, Y., Hou, X., Yang, C., et al., 2017. Formulation of temozolomide-loaded nanoparticles and their targeting potential to melanoma cells. Oncol. Rep. 37, 995–1001. Available from: https://doi.org/10.3892/or.2016.5342.

Kaur, D., Jain, K., Mehra, N.K., Kesharwani, P., Jain, N.K., 2016. A review on comparative study of PPI and PAMAM dendrimers. J. Nanopart. Res. 18, 146. Available from: https://doi.org/10.1007/s11051-016-3423-0.

Klajnert, B., Pastucha, A., Shcharbin, D., Bryszewska, M., 2007. Binding properties of polyamidoamine dendrimers. J. Appl. Polym. Sci. 103, 2036–2040.

Kovacs, L., Tassano, M., Cabrera, M., Zamboni, C.B., Fernández, M., Anjos, R.M., et al., 2015. Development of (177)Lu-DOTA-dendrimer and determination of its effect on metal and ion levels in tumor tissue. Cancer Biother. Radiopharm. 30, 405–409. Available from: https://doi.org/10.1089/cbr.2014.1675.

Lee, J.W., Kim, B.K., Kim, H.J., Han, S.C., Shin, W.S., Jin, S.H., 2006. Convergent synthesis of symmetrical and unsymmetrical PAMAM dendrimers. Macromolecules 39, 2418–2422. Available from: https://doi.org/10.1021/ma052526f.

Li, Y., Yan, T., Chang, W., Cao, C., Deng, D., 2019. Fabricating an intelligent cell-like nano-prodrug via hierarchical self-assembly based on the DNA skeleton for suppressing lung metastasis of breast cancer. Biomater. Sci. 7, 3652–3661. Available from: https://doi.org/10.1039/c9bm00630c.

Lin, L., Fan, Y., Gao, F., Jin, L., Li, D., Sun, W., et al., 2018. UTMD-promoted co-delivery of gemcitabine and miR-21 inhibitor by dendrimer-entrapped gold nanoparticles for pancreatic cancer therapy. Theranostics 8, 1923–1939. Available from: https://doi.org/10.7150/thno.22834.

Maiti, P.K., Çağın, T., Wang, G., Goddard, W.A., 2004. Structure of PAMAM dendrimers: generations 1 through 11. Macromolecules 37, 6236–6254. Available from: https://doi.org/10.1021/ma035629b.

Malekmohammadi, S., Hadadzadeh, H., Farrokhpour, H., Amirghofran, Z., 2018. Immobilization of gold nanoparticles on folate-conjugated dendritic mesoporous silica-coated reduced graphene oxide nanosheets: a new nanoplatform for curcumin pH-controlled and targeted delivery. Soft Matter 14, 2400–2410. Available from: https://doi.org/10.1039/c7sm02248d.

Marcinkowska, M., Stanczyk, M., Janaszewska, A., Sobierajska, E., Chworos, A., Klajnert-Maculewicz, B., 2019. Multicomponent conjugates of anticancer drugs and monoclonal antibody with PAMAM dendrimers to increase efficacy of HER-2 positive breast cancer therapy. Pharm. Res. 36, 154. Available from: https://doi.org/10.1007/s11095-019-2683-7.

Masuda, M., Kawakami, S., Wijagkanalan, W., Suga, T., Fuchigami, Y., Yamashita, F., et al., 2016. Anti-MUC1 aptamer/negatively charged amino acid dendrimer conjugates for targeted delivery to human lung adenocarcinoma A549 cells. Biol. Pharm. Bull. 39, 1734–1738.

Matai, I., Sachdev, A., Gopinath, P., 2015. Multicomponent 5-fluorouracil loaded PAMAM stabilized-silver nanocomposites synergistically induce apoptosis in human cancer cells. Biomater. Sci. 3, 457–468. Available from: https://doi.org/10.1039/c4bm00360h.

Muniswamy, V.J., Raval, N., Gondaliya, P., Tambe, V., Kalia, K., Tekade, R.K., 2019. 'Dendrimer-cationized-albumin' encrusted polymeric nanoparticle improves BBB penetration and anticancer activity of doxorubicin. Int. J. Pharm. 555, 77–99. Available from: https://doi.org/10.1016/j.ijpharm.2018.11.035.

Naqvi, I., Gunaratne, R., McDade, J.E., Moreno, A., Rempel, R.E., Rouse, D.C., et al., 2018. Polymer-mediated inhibition of pro-invasive nucleic acid DAMPs and microvesicles limits pancreatic cancer metastasis. Mol. Ther. 26, 1020–1031. Available from: https://doi.org/10.1016/j.ymthe.2018.02.018.

Palmerston Mendes, L., Pan, J., Torchilin, V.P., 2017. Dendrimers as nanocarriers for nucleic acid and drug delivery in cancer therapy. Molecules 22, 1401. Available from: https://doi.org/10.3390/molecules22091401.

Pedziwiatr-Werbicka, E., Milowska, K., Dzmitruk, V., Ionov, M., Shcharbinb, D., Bryszewska, M., 2019. Dendrimers and hyperbranched structures for biomedical applications. Eur. Polym. J. 119, 61–73. Available from: https://doi.org/10.1016/j.eurpolymj.2019.07.013.

Prokop, A., Davidson, J.M., 2008. Nanovehicular intracellular delivery systems. J. Pharm. Sci. 97, 3518–3590. Available from: https://doi.org/10.1002/jps.21270.

Rompicharla, S.V.K., Kumari, P., Bhatt, H., Ghosh, B., Biswas, S., 2019. Biotin functionalized PEGylated poly(amidoamine) dendrimer conjugate for active targeting of paclitaxel in cancer. Int. J. Pharm. 557, 329–341. Available from: https://doi.org/10.1016/j.ijpharm.2018.12.069.

Salimi, M., Sarkar, S., Fathi, S., Alizadeh, A.M., Saber, R., Moradi, F., et al., 2018. Biodistribution, pharmacokinetics, and toxicity of dendrimer-coated iron oxide nanoparticles in BALB/c mice. Int. J. Nanomed. 13, 1483–1493. Available from: https://doi.org/10.2147/IJN.S157293.

Sharma, A., Gautam, S.P., Gupta, A.K., 2011. Surface modified dendrimers: synthesis and characterization for cancer targeted drug delivery. Bioorg. Med. Chem. 19, 3341–3346. Available from: https://doi.org/10.1016/j.bmc.2011.04.046.

Shende, P., Patil, S., Gaud, R.S., 2017. A combinatorial approach of inclusion complexation and dendrimer synthesization for effective targeting EGFR-TK. Mater. Sci. Eng. C Mater Biol. Appl. 76, 959–965. Available from: https://doi.org/10.1016/j.msec.2017.03.184.

Somani, S., Robb, G., Pickard, B.S., Dufès, C., 2015. Enhanced gene expression in the brain following intravenous administration of lactoferrin-bearing polypropylenimine dendriplex. J. Controlled Release 217, 235–242. Available from: https://doi.org/10.1016/j.jconrel.2015.09.003.

Sztandera, K., Działak, P., Marcinkowska, M., Stańczyk, M., Gorzkiewicz, M., Janaszewska, A., et al., 2019. Sugar modification enhances cytotoxic activity of PAMAM-doxorubicin conjugate in glucose-deprived MCF-7 cells—possible role of GLUT1 transporter. Pharm. Res. 36, 140. Available from: https://doi.org/10.1007/s11095-019-2673-9.

Urbani, C.N., Bell, C.A., Whittaker, M.R., Monteiro, M.J., 2008. Convergent synthesis of second generation AB-type miktoarm dendrimers using "Click" chemistry catalyzed by copper wire. Macromolecules 41, 1057–1060. Available from: https://doi.org/10.1021/ma702707e.

Verma, I.M., Naldini, L., Kafri, T., Miyoshi, H., Takahashi, M., Blömer, U., et al., 2000. Gene therapy: promises, problems and prospects. Genes and Resistance to Disease. Springer, Berlin, Heidelberg, pp. 147–157.

Wang, H., Zhao, X., Guo, C., Ren, D., Zhao, Y., Xiao, W., et al., 2015a. Aptamer-dendrimer bioconjugates for targeted delivery of miR-34a expressing plasmid and antitumor effects in non-small cell lung cancer cells. PLoS One 10, e0139136. Available from: https://doi.org/10.1371/journal.pone.0139136.

Wang, Y., Li, L., Shao, N., Hu, Z., Chen, H., Xu, L., et al., 2015b. Triazine-modified dendrimer for efficient TRAIL gene therapy in osteosarcoma. Acta Biomater. 17, 115–124. Available from: https://doi.org/10.1016/j.actbio.2015.01.007.

Washio, I., Shibasaki, Y., Ueda, M., 2007. Facile synthesis of amine-terminated aromatic polyamide dendrimers via a divergent method. Org. Lett. 97, 1363–1366. Available from: https://doi.org/10.1021/ol0702425.

Wen, A.M., Lee, K.L., Cao, P., Pangilinan, K., Carpenter, B.L., Lam, P., et al., 2016. Utilizing viral nanoparticle/dendron hybrid conjugates in photodynamic therapy for dual delivery to macrophages and cancer cells. Bioconjug. Chem. 27, 1227–1235. Available from: https://doi.org/10.1021/acs.bioconjchem.6b00075.

Wu, P., Sun, Y., Dong, W., Zhou, H., Guo, S., Zhang, L., et al., 2019. Enhanced antitumor efficacy of hyaluronic acid modified nanocomposites combined with sonochemotherapy against subcutaneous and metastatic breast tumors. Nanoscale 11, 11470–11483. Available from: https://doi.org/10.1039/c9nr01691k.

Xu, Z., Kahr, M., Walker, K.L., Wilkins, C.L., Moore, J.S., 1994. Phenylacetylene dendrimers by the divergent, convergent, and double-stage convergent methods. J. Am. Chem. Soc. 116, 4537–4550. Available from: https://doi.org/10.1021/ja00090a002.

Yan, Y., Gao, X., Zhang, S., Wang, Y., Zhou, Z., Xiao, J., et al., 2019. A carboxyl-terminated dendrimer enables osteolytic lesion targeting and photothermal ablation of malignant bone tumors. ACS Appl. Mater. Interfaces 11, 160–168. Available from: https://doi.org/10.1021/acsami.8b15827.

Yang, H., John Kao, W., 2006. Dendrimers for pharmaceutical and biomedical applications. J. Biomater. Sci. Polym. Ed. 17, 1–2.

Yousef, S., Alsaab, H.O., Sau, S., Iyer, A.K., 2018. Development of asialoglycoprotein receptor directed nanoparticles for selective delivery of curcumin derivative to hepatocellular carcinoma. Heliyon 4, e01071. Available from: https://doi.org/10.1016/j.heliyon.2018.e01071.

Zhong, Q., 2018. Co-spray dried mannitol/poly(amidoamine)-doxorubicin dry-powder inhaler formulations for lung adenocarcinoma: morphology, in vitro evaluation, and aerodynamic performance. AAPS PharmSciTech 19, 531–540. Available from: https://doi.org/10.1208/s12249-017-0859-1.

Zhong, Q., Humia, B.V., Punjabi, A.R., Padilha, F.F., da Rocha, S.R.P., 2017. The interaction of dendrimer-doxorubicin conjugates with a model pulmonary epithelium and their cosolvent-free, pseudo-solution formulations in pressurized metered-dose inhalers. Eur. J. Pharm. Sci. 109, 86–95. Available from: https://doi.org/10.1016/j.ejps.2017.07.030.

CHAPTER

Polymer nanomaterials in bioimaging

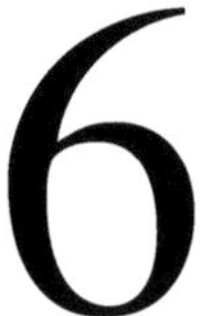

Morteza Sasani Ghamsari

Photonics and Quantum Technologies Research School, Nuclear Science and Technology Research Institute, Tehran, Iran

6.1 Introduction

The first captured X-ray image by Wilhelm Roentgen in 1896 signaled the dawn of a era in the history of medical diagnosis. Since the inception of X-ray technology for medical imaging, many noninvasive diagnostic techniques for evaluating heart activity have been developed (Sharma et al., 2006). In recent years, these methods have been successfully applied to fields ranging from clinical diagnosis to research in cellular biology and drug discovery. Among them, the visual representation technique and the process in which the interior of the body are viewed for clinical analysis and medical intervention or visualization of the function of some organs or tissues has gained popularity for medical diagnostics and treatments. There are several medical imaging processes that are used to obtain images of the human body to assist in the diagnosis and treatment of patients. The most common imaging techniques are computerized tomography, magnetic resonance imaging, nuclear medicine imaging, X-ray, and ultrasound imaging (Janib et al., 2010). Depending on the imaging technique and preprocessing parameters, structural and/or functional information at different scales and accuracy levels can be revealed. The selection of medical imaging modality is directed by the type of data required, such as in vivo phenomena or biological entities and tissues that are required from the employed technique. Analyzing imaging techniques via a step-by-step approach is an appropriate way to develop an efficient and relevant diagnostic process (Wallyn et al., 2019). When the imaging processes are involved with the complex chain of acquiring, processing, and visualizing structural or functional images of living objects or systems to extract and process the image-related data, the use of biomarkers helps to image specific targets or pathways, and is called bioimaging (Raghavendra and Pullaiah, 2018). In real time, the visualization method of noninvasive biological processes is also known as bioimaging. In a broader sense, bioimaging also refers to the method used for the visualization of biological material that has been fixed for observation. This kind of observation method aims to gain information on the biological objectives without physical interference. It should be noted that molecular imaging is defined as in vivo characterization and measurement of biologic processes at the cellular and molecular

Advances in Polymeric Nanomaterials for Biomedical Applications. DOI: https://doi.org/10.1016/B978-0-12-814657-6.00011-2

levels (Weissleder and Mahmood, 2001). However, bioimaging interacts with life processes as little as possible. Moreover, it is often used to provide detailed information from the 3D observation of a specimen. Using bioimaging resources, the observation of subcellular structures and entire cells over tissues can be done. To extract image-related data using the bioimaging process, different sources, such as light, fluorescence, electrons, ultrasound, X-ray, magnetic resonance, and positrons, are used for imaging which differ in terms of sensitivity and resolution, complexity, time of data acquisition, and financial cost. Among these, photon-based procedures for extraction of image-related data have been greatly developed for bioimaging as they offer high spatial and temporal resolution as well as a clear image due to the drastic modulation of the fluorescence signal and high sensitivity, high selectivity, convenience, diversity, and nondestructive character of imaging probes (Lee et al., 2018; Terai and Nagano, 2008; Chen and Yin, 2014). Chen and Yin reviewed the mechanism of fluorescence-based techniques, strategies in designing and development, preparation methods, widely used in biological imaging that generated due to image-related data from fluorescent probes, that are exploited to label the target with specific chemical structures. Recently, fluorescent nanostructure probes (organic, inorganic, and organic/inorganic hybrid), such as fluorescent proteins, organic dyes, metal complexes, semiconductor nanocrystals, and upconversion nanophosphors, have gained increased attention because of their inherent unique properties such as sensitivity, signal stability, and multiplexing capability, however their performance can be improved by enhancing their chemical and optical properties, surface modification, and conjugation with biomolecules and/or fluorophores (Chen and Yin, 2014). The intrinsic ability of the polymeric nanoparticles for functionalization with the multiple functionalities of imaging probes or targeting ligands is too high. In addition, their nature makes them as a versatile building block for nanomedicine. They encapsulate and load a variety of therapeutic agents considerably and able to enhance in vivo concentration ratio of the packaged small-molecule contrast agents to a target organ/site. Therefore, they provide facilities and practical strategies for developing multimodal medical imaging that can compensate disadvantages of one imaging modality from another (Yao et al., 2014; Elsabahy et al., 2015). It is also pointed out that multimodality imaging can be achieved by carrying multiple types of contrast agents in the polymer nanoparticle package coincidentally. In this chapter, the applications of polymers in various imaging modalities are considered. Generally, the focus continues on organic fluorescent imaging probes and their practical applications. The recent progress that has been achieved in bioimaging with the employment of polymeric fluorescent imaging agents is summarized.

6.2 NIR optical bioimaging

Noninvasive fluorescent imaging, as mentioned above, has high imaging sensitivity and can be used for the early detection of disease owing to the cellular or molecular level information it imparts (Li et al., 2018b). Among the fluorescent imaging methods, near-infrared (NIR) fluorescence imaging provides a platform for in vivo imaging and imaging-guided surgery with deep penetration and high spatiotemporal resolution due to the high sensitivity and use of NIR fluorophores comprised of nanostructured materials, as well as NIR light which is an effective tool for deep-tissue imaging (Lin et al., 2019). However, in vivo biological imaging, with the retention and accumulation of NIR nanomaterial fluorophores (NIR-II fluorophores) in the body, raises concerns due to potential immunogenic responses and this limits its commercially availability and/or clinical applications (Zhu et al., 2018b) (Fig. 6.1). Visible fluorescence imaging is not as effective as NIR fluorescence because of the low penetration depth inside the body, being strongly absorbed by biological chromophores (hemoglobin) and rendering deep tissue imaging and strong auto-fluorescence of biologically important molecules such as collagen, NADPH, fatty acids, flavins, and porphyrins (Reineck and Gibson, 2017). NIR light is strongly absorbed by biological components such as water and lipids, easily penetrates significantly deeper into biological matter, and reduces scattering of light and autofluorescence from excited elastin, collagen, and other biological fluorophores. Therefore bioimaging in the second near-infrared (NIR-II, 1000−1700 nm) window has also gained a lot of interest due to its advantages such as higher spatial resolution (micrometer scale) at

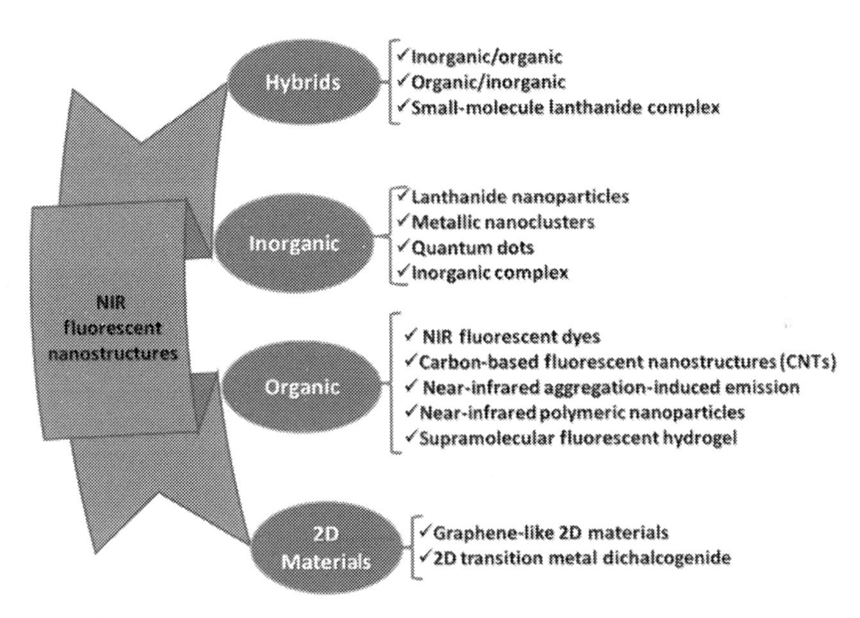

FIGURE 6.1

Classification of NIR fluorescent nanostructures (FNSs) based on their different chemical structural compositions.

subcentimeter depths, tumor identification, vascular visualization, and molecular imaging, however, it generally suffers from long-term toxicity concerns and relatively low fluorescence quantum yield (Wu et al., 2019). NIR probes include organic NIR fluorescent dyes, small-molecule lanthanide complexes and nanoparticles, NIR polymeric nanoparticles, NIR aggregation-induced emission (AIE) active probes, ratiometric fluorescent probes, and supramolecular assembled nanoparticles (Fig. 6.1).

Previously, the most active NIR fluorophores were limited to inorganic fluorescent probes such as rare earth materials and quantum dots (QDs). In comparison with inorganic probes, organic NIR fluorescent probes are very attractive ideal probes for clinical bioimaging as they show selective accumulation, intense emission, high photostability, and high quantum yields (Haque et al., 2017). It seems that different factors including the photobleaching, aggregation and high plasma protein binding, false-positive signals due to endocytosis, nonuniversal nature, etc. are associated with both the probe and the receptor contributing in to the lack of processability of these characteristics by probes. Moreover, despite the fact that probe conjugation (with a recognized moiety) process reduces possible side effects, it happens at the cost of probe sensitivity due to the functional-group tolerance limitations (Gao et al., 2014).

6.2.1 Conjugated polymer nanoparticles

As mentioned earlier, the organic optical nanoagents are preferred for NIR bioimaging due to their excellent fluorescence brightness, good photostability, high radiative rate, facile surface functionalization, and low cytotoxicity. Recently, organic semiconducting agents composed completely from organic and biologically inert π-conjugated semiconducting polymer nanoparticles (SPNs) and semiconducting molecule nanoparticles have emerged as alternative candidates due to the low photostability of traditional NIR organic dyes (Zhu et al., 2012; Jiang and Pu, 2018). Conjugated polymers (CPs) show good biocompatibility, and their ability for facile in situ surface modification has rendered them extremely useful for a number of biological applications such as cell imaging and tracking, and tumor imaging. The absorption coefficients of organic semiconducting agents are often too large and their size controllability is high relative to other inorganic optical agents. Therefore their optical properties can be tuned by controlling their size and surface functionalization (Pu and Liu, 2011; Zhu et al., 2018a; Wang et al., 2018a). However, many attempts have been made to improve the performance of NIR polymeric fluorophores. For example, the synthesis of CPs with tunable band gap in the NIR-II channel using donor−acceptor (D−A) alternating copolymerization was proposed to result in good photostability (Ding et al., 2018; Ding et al., 2019; Li et al., 2018a). It has been also reported that a smaller band gap copolymer can be achieved by more electron-donating donors and electron-withdrawing acceptors. In addition, band gap narrowing in a longer copolymer can be received with greater delocalization of π-electrons (Wang et al., 2011).

Hong et al. reported a bright NIR-II fluorescent copolymer pDA that realized a biocompatible probe with high quantum yield (QY $\approx$ 1.7%) (Hong et al., 2014). Diketopyrrolopyrrole-based SPNs (PDFT1032) have been constructed for in vivo imaging and image-guided tumor surgery in the second NIR window as it is an electron-withdrawing acceptor that has a low band gap through D–A alternating copolymerization. This finding demonstrated that PDFT1032 can be used for several important biomedical applications in the NIR-II window (Shou et al., 2018). Nevertheless, many barriers remain that significantly limit the optical-based bioimaging methods. As has been discovered, the fluorescence signals strongly interfere with the autofluorescence and background noises originating from the intrinsic heterogeneity and inherent complexity of biological samples. Therefore, to make the precise identification of biological targets, highly fluorescent and strongly light-responsive sources are needed (Zhang et al., 2018). To overcome this barrier, one approach is to combine a fluorophore with a photochromic moiety (Yildiz et al., 2009). Photochromism is simply defined as a light-induced reversible change of color and therefore a reversible transformation between two molecular forms with discrete molecular properties occurs when photochromic molecules respond to the light signal. The ability of light-triggered organic molecules to reversibly undergo changes in spectral absorption provides photoswitching performance (Bouas-Laurent and Dürr, 2001; Helmy et al., 2014; Andreasson and Pischel, 2015; Aiken et al., 2018). The use of reversible photoswitching moieties as light-activated molecular switches has been impacted on the wide range of applications. The simple light-induced chemical and physical changes in the switching species can result in an array of desirable outputs at the nanoscale, such as bioimaging. Accordingly, the light response of the photoswitchable nanoprobes, whose fluorescence emissions alternate between two colors or a bright-to-dark state, is a key determinant in light-activated imaging. The detectability as well as the capability of signal identification of these kind of nanoagents could be enhanced using the generation of switchable fluorescence signals. Consequently, target signals can be easily and accurately identified and distinguished using autofluorescence and other interferences (Li et al., 2019a; Qi et al., 2018b). Among photochromic molecules, spiropyran (SP), diarylethene, and azobenzene and their derivatives are among those used for the construction of photoswitchable nanoprobes (Li et al., 2019c; Qi et al., 2018b; Beharry et al., 2011). Li and others have carried out a series of pioneering works in developing imaging techniques with improved resolution and brightness. They used SP and its derivative-based photoswitchable nanoparticles to develop photoactuated unimolecular logical switching-attained reconstruction microscopy and the improvement of the photoswitching-enabled Fourier transform (PFT) fluorescence microscopy technique was also considered (Li et al, 2011; Tian et al., 2009). Nevertheless, the photoswitching capability cannot be supported by the majority of fluorescent chromophores. Consequently, a single NP with integration of the fluorescence-emitting and photochromic moieties must be constructed to form a Förster resonance energy transfer (FRET) pair photoswitchable nanoprobe based on FRET

(Beharry et al., 2011; Kuo et al., 2016). Chen and co-workers reported an efficient method to produce a nanosized platform for the delivery of an optimized ratio of the two components by the means of a host–guest strategy for maximizing the combination therapy efficacy of cancer treatment. The tunability of the ratio between photosensitizer and reactive oxygen species (ROS)-sensitive prodrugs is considered as the key feature of this host–guest strategy (Chen et al., 2019a). In one study, the accumulation process was tracked by NIR imaging to maximize the efficacy of photodynamics and chemotherapy. Liu et al. studied eight dithienylethene (DTE) groups integrated onto one polyhedral oligomeric silsesquioxane (POSS) core to revive a novel super molecular photoswitch. A higher contrast on/off photoswitching performance and quicker responsive speed than with free DTE molecules at the same molar concentration of photochromic units was observed by the POSS-DTE_8 molecules after being doped into CP nanoparticles (CPNs) due to increased molecular interaction of the ring-open form and lowered energy of the ring-closed form of the DTE units on the POSS core and subsequent energy transfer between the photoswitch and fluorophores (Liu et al., 2018a). Wang and co-workers developed an efficient approach to make a fluorescent polymer both photoswitchable and stimuli-responsive as a smart material for photoresponsive polymer illuminants and offering a new platform for multifunctional molecular switching and multiresponsive materials by rationally introducing a photochromic bisthienylethene derivative and fluorescent 4-dicyanomethylene-2,6-distyryl-4H-pyran derivative units in the side chains via copolymerization using facile one-step miniemulsion polymerization (Wang et al., 2019b). Mutoh et al. reported photoactivatable fluorescence based on negative photochromism, where the absorption spectrum of the compound after irradiation was blue-shifted relative to that before irradiation. In their study, a naphthalimide unit was introduced as a green fluorophore to the negative photochromic binaphthyl-bridged imidazole dimer. They found that the Förster resonance energy transfer fluorescence leads to efficient quenching of the naphthalimide unit in the initial colored isomer (fluorescence quantum yield: $\Phi_{fluo} = 0.01$ due to the formation of the transient isomer). Accordingly, the turn-on mode fluorescence switching can suitably be obtained through negative photochromic molecules formation which gives an attractive insight into the development of reversible fluorescence switching molecules (Mutoh et al., 2019). A series of synthesized Pdots with narrow-band emissions ($\leq$29 nm) and large Stokes shifts ($\geq$200 nm) can be obtained by designing the π-bridges taking into consideration three points: (1) the existence of absorption ranging from 400 to 600 nm; (2) the enhanced steric effect of the semiconducting polymers to alleviate the aggregation-induced quenching; and (3) an improvement of the energy transfer from the donor to the acceptor (Yue et al., 2017).

The second strategy that was employed to improve the performance of CPs for NIR bioimaging is the AIE that can exhibit a high emission quantum yield and high luminescence. However, the fluorescence quantum yield of dyes is decreased or even completely quenched in increased concentrations or in an aggregation state (Wan et al., 2015; Zhang et al., 2014). This phenomenon is known as the notorious aggregation-caused quenching (ACQ) effect, and is due to the large conjugated planar structure of dye molecules that induces strong intermolecular p−p interactions and carries out fluorescence quenching and photobleaching (Yuan et al., 2010; Wan et al., 2016). In 2001, Luo et al. found that silacyclopentadiene (siloles)-based molecules could emit intense fluorescence at a high concentration or aggregation state which is precisely opposite to ACQ. This abnormal phenomenon is defined as AIE (Luo et al., 2001; Lv et al., 2016). Therefore the polymers with AIE ability have attracted increasing research attention for their potential application in bio-imaging (Tang et al., 2014; Pal et al., 2018; Fu et al., 2019; Jin et al., 2019). Wang et al. summarized the recent progress in exploring high-tech applications of AIE luminogens (AIEgens) as highly luminescent, photostable, and biocompatible biological sensors, chemical probes, optoelectronic devices, and intelligent materials. Their discussion focused on mechanistic analysis, classifying the electronic interactions involved into three categories: (1) through-bond, (2) through-space, and (3) through-bond and -space conjugations. They demonstrated that fluorescence imaging can be employed as a powerful tool for cancer diagnosis and medicinal therapy using the AIE effect and restriction of intramolecular motion (RIM) [intramolecular rotation (RIR) and restriction of intramolecular vibration (RIV)] plays a critical role in the AIE effect (Wang et al., 2015). As was found, the propeller-shaped molecules, such as HPS and tetraphenylethene (TPE), are AIE active due to the RIR process and the RIV process is activated when the aggregation of the large π-conjugated system formed by the shell-like molecules that their phenyl rings and alkene rods are connected through covalent bonds (Mei et al., 2014). The AIE dots are generally fabricated by encapsulating AIEgens into lipid or BSA shells through a nanoprecipitation route (Ding et al., 2013). Long and others fabricated AIE-active fluorescent organic nanoparticles (FONs) via a "one pot" mercaptoacetic acid-locking imine reaction using mercaptoacetic acid as the "lock" molecule which occurred when an AIE-active dye (named CHO-An-CHO) was covalently conjugated with NH_2-terminated polymers (PEG-PABA). These final polymers (denoted as PEG-PABA-An-CHO) possessed amphiphilic properties and could self-assemble into PEG-PABA-An-CHO FONs with excellent water dispersibility and displayed enhanced luminescence in aqueous solution due to the aggregation of the AIE feature of CHO-An-CHO (Long et al., 2017). Feng et al. successfully developed ultra-bright organic dots with AIE (AIE dots), exhibiting high fluorescence, super photostability, excellent cellular retention and biocompatibility, and excellent cell labeling on all tested human cell lines and superior tracing performance for cellular imaging and cell tracking (Feng et al., 2014). Qian et al. developed a smart nano-delivery system, STD-NM, that was designed to present the AIE characteristics, that could open a new avenue in precise tumor imaging and specific cancer therapeutics (Qian et al., 2019). Yang et al. reported the design and synthesis of highly NIR emissive organic nanodots with AIE characteristics that showed a rather high quantum yield of 33% in aqueous media and studied the regenerative mechanism of adipose-derived stem cells in the treatment of radiation-induced skin injury (Qian et al., 2019). Liu and co-workers developed simple, well-designed, and universal novel hydrazine hydrate cross-linked amphiphilic poly (PEG-co-FHMA) copolymers using reversible addition-fragmentation chain transfer polymerization to construct PEG-co-FHMA copolymers that provide AIE-active hydrophobic moiety (Liu et al., 2019b). Thus this work opens up a new avenue for preparing cross-linked biocompatible fluorescent polymers for biomedical applications. Recently, the preparation of an AIE-active FL probe (AIE-FR-TPP) was reported that was prepared by conjugation of a far-red/near-infrared (FR/NIR)-emitting AIE fluorogen with the mitochondria-targeting group able to be used as a multifunctional fluorophore for mitochondrial imaging and photodynamic therapy (PDT), that can selectively light up the cellular mitochondria with low working concentration, short staining time, and good biocompatibility (Zou et al., 2018). Gao et al. summarized the current status of the development of aggregation-induced emission luminogens (AIEgens)-based conventional fluorophores for cancer theranostics (Gao and Zhong Tang, 2017).

Additionally, red AIE nanoparticles have also received new attention for biomedical applications. Che and others designed and synthesized three AIE-active red-emissive BODIPY derivatives using AIEgen and amphipathic polymeric with long-wavelength absorption and emitting bright red light with a high fluorescence quantum yield in aqueous media, which hold great potential for monitoring biological processes due to their strong fluorescence signals, ultrafast staining procedure, and long-term tracing abilities, that have also been used for hypochlorite detection and bioimaging in live cells (Che et al., 2019; Wang et al., 2018b). Ni and others synthesized NIR afterglow luminescent nanoparticles with AIE characteristics that emit rather high NIR afterglow luminescence persisting over 10 days and provide ultrahigh tumor-to-liver signal ratio and low afterglow background noise (Ni et al., 2019).

Gao and co-workers reported recent advances in fluorescent bioprobes with AIE characteristics used in specific biomedical applications including for bacteria imaging and suppression, targeted cellular/intracellular organelle imaging and ablation, and also in vivo blood vessel imaging and disease theranostics. The key point that can be found from their summation is a limitation of AIEgens. Despite the thrilling progress achieved over the past decade, they concluded that AIEgens are not good at building fluorescence "turn-on" nanoprobes. They stated that sophisticated molecular design and modification needs to be achieved when the combined strengths of AIE, high signal-to-background ratio (SBR), and EPR effect are considered for the AIEgen nanoprobe, for example, to employ photo-induced electron transfer (PET) to quench AIEgen fluorescence in the nanoprobe and then cancel PET after responding to a disease microenvironment (Gao et al., 2018). Furthermore, much research has explained that the recent investigations into AIEgens for in vivo diagnosis and therapy include long-term tracking, 3D angiography, multimodality imaging, disease theranostics, and activatable sensing for in vivo biomedical applications (Qi et al., 2018a). The fluorescent molecules with propeller-shaped structures can present either restricted intramolecular motion or intramolecular rotation in the aggregated form. The highly twisted molecular conformation is due to the intermolecular $\pi-\pi$ stacking interaction. On the basis of the intramolecular motions and also the intramolecular rotation effect, a large number of fluorescence probes, such as 9,10-distyrylanthracene derivatives, TPE derivatives have been developed that have AIE characteristics generated from various physical and chemical reactions (cleaving the covalent bond of the probe, the release of hydrophobic AIEgens that aggregate and subsequently switch-up fluorescence in aqueous media due to either RIM or RIR) (Xu et al., 2019). The limitations of AIEgens can be overcome by selection of the excitation/emission methods, using nonlinear optics phenomenon, including multiphoton absorption, harmonic generation, and the upconversion process which enables AIEgens to be useful in a broader range of biomedical applications (Gu et al., 2018). Moreover, the integration of AIE-based photosensitizers and different therapeutic modalities in one platform will provide an excellent method to further improve cancer treatment efficiency.

6.2.2 Dye-doped semiconducting polymer dots

Semiconducting polymer dots (Pdots) are a special subset of CPNs. To qualify as Pdots, the CPNs should satisfy three criteria. First, the nanoparticle size should be less than about 30 nm to be consistent with the concept of a "dot." Second, the nanoparticle should contain more than 50% of semiconducting polymers to ensure high single-particle brightness. Finally, the interior of the nanoparticle should be hydrophobic. Therefore nanoparticles that do not satisfy these three criteria are referred to as CPNs. The functionalization and bioconjugation of Pdots make them useful tools for biological applications including cellular labeling through endocytosis, immunofluorescence labeling, bio-orthogonal labeling by click chemistry, in vivo imaging, and single-particle tracking using Pdots, and sensors and drug/gene delivery systems (Yu et al., 2017). The main problem with such probes is that they suffer from serious issues of self-quenching and reabsorption phenomena and the leakage of dye from Pdots in the long term has limited their biological applications and so to overcome this novel NIR-emissive Pdots must be developed. This effort resulted in the design of NIR BODIPY-based and squaraine-based semiconducting polymers with the NIR emitting unit forming part of the backbone of the semiconducting polymer (Rong et al., 2013). Recently, to solve the above-mentioned challenge, several strategies have been developed. For example, the embedded poly(9,9-dioctylfluorene-co-benzothiadiazole) (PFBT) P-dots by the NIR dye silicon 2,3-naphthalocyanine bis(trihexylsilyloxide) were introduced by efficient energy transfer from PFBT to NIR dye for improvement of the fluorescence intensity and brightness of the NIR dye. In order to prevent leakage of the encapsulated dyes from the P-dot matrices, the amphiphilic, nonfluorescent polymer PS-PEG-COOH was used [PS = polystyrene and

PEG = poly(ethylene glycol)] (Jin et al., 2011). This greatly reduces the single-particle brightness of the resulting P-dots and limits their biological applications. The photophysical properties of Pdots are affected by potential leakage of the embedded polymers, therefore the prepared Pdots with the established photophysical properties must be achieved. This means that for the synthesis of polymers with different emission wavelengths and controlled properties, many attempts and time-consuming works are required. Squaraine-based semiconducting polymer dots (Pdots) with large Stokes shifts and narrow-band emissions in the NIR region containing fluorene and squaraine units have been developed that showed very bright and narrow-band NIR emissions by the exciton diffusion and likely through-bond energy transfer (Wu et al., 2015). A new class of SPN − QD hybrid with high brightness, narrow emission, NIR fluorescence, and excellent cellular targeting capability has been synthesized for effective and specific cellular and subcellular labeling without any noticeable nonspecific binding (Chan et al., 2012a). The multicolor narrow emissive Pdots based on different boron dipyrromethene (BODIPY) units employ the intraparticle energy transfer to provide highly bright, narrow, and multiple-wavelength emission semiconducting polymers using BODIPY loading (Rong et al., 2013). Ke and others have systematically investigated the effect of π-bridges on the fluorescence quantum yields of the donor–bridge–acceptor-based Pdots. The design and synthesis of this type of Pdot exhibited narrow-band emissions, ultrahigh brightness, and large Stokes shifts in the NIR region (Ke et al., 2017). Tang et al. reported a new and relatively generic design strategy using a bio-erasable intermolecular D–A interaction to construct activatable NIR-II fluorescence probes. They constructed an organic semiconducting nanoprobe, through blending a biomarker-sensitive organic semiconducting non-fullerene acceptor with a biomarker-inert semiconducting polymer donor in an amphiphilic polymer-coated single nanoparticle to suppress NIR-II fluorescence of the donor via a intermolecular D–A interaction (Tang et al., 2019). Chan and others developed photoswitchable Pdots by conjugating photochromic SP molecules onto poly[9,9-dioctylfluorenyl-2,7-diyl(-co-1,4-benzo-{2,1′-3}-thiadiazole)] (PFBT) (Chan et al., 2012b). The BODIPY-based donor/D–A system achieved highly efficient long-wavelength-excitable NIR polymer dots with narrow and strong absorption features to achieve ultrabright, green laser-excitable Pdots with narrow-band NIR emission by introducing a BODIPY-based assistant polymer donor as D_1. In comparison with the binary D_2–A Pdots, the D_1/D_2–A Pdots showed improved fluorescence quantum yield (Φ_f) (as high as 40.2%) and absorption cross-section (σ) (Chen et al., 2019b). The Stokes shifts of reported BODIPY-based probes were studied with different substituents such as phenyl groups and methoxy groups on the specific position of BODIPY (expand the Stokes shift of BODIPY-based probes) (Zhu et al., 2019). Liu and co-workers synthesized and characterized an enzyme-activatable NIR fluorescent probe, GP-DM, for determining the activity of dipeptidyl peptidase IV for early detection of pathologies, individual tailoring of drug therapy, and image-guided tumor resection (Liu et al., 2018b).

6.3 Two-photon imaging

The simultaneous absorption of two photons by the same molecule is an optical characteristic that was analyzed theoretically in the 1930s (Goppert-Mayer, 1931). Soon after the invention of the laser, this kind of optical effect was experimentally demonstrated in 1961(Kaiser and Garrett, 1961). In comparison with one-photon absorption (1PA), two-photon absorption (2PA) involves the simultaneous interaction of two photons and is only observed in the particular interaction of materials with focused pulsed lasers (intense laser beams), so that 2PA increases with the square of the light intensity, whereas 1PA depends linearly on the intensity. Consequently, a very high instantaneous photon density can be generated by 2PA. Most of the applications for 2PA result from this intensity dependence. Absorption of two photons with half the energy or twice the wavelength (2PA) is equivalent to the given excited state by using the corresponding one-photon transition which provides a wide range of applications (Pawlicki et al., 2009). Over the past few decades, two-photon absorbance (TPA) as a nonlinear optical phenomenon has gained a lot of interest at both the theoretical and experimental levels and has been applied in various biological applications including bioimaging, PDT, and especially fluorescence microscopy (Chen et al., 2016). On the basis of TPA, a microscopy procedure was developed by Webb and co-workers in 1990 called two-photon fluorescence microscopy (TPM) (Denk et al., 1990). Currently, fluorescence microscopy plays a critical role in biology and biomedical sciences and is used as an essential tool to visualize bioimaging. Systematically, TPM has achieved great progress and hence, it is now used in a wide range of bioimaging studies. Imaging and analysis of the dynamic processes in living cells and tissues are the most common applications of TPM: tracking organelle (mitochondria, lysosomes, vacuoles, etc.) dynamics, visualizing drug delivery, imaging cancer and neural tissue, studying the vasculature, heart, eye and brain, and detecting small molecules among others (Chen et al., 2016). To extend and increase the extensive use of two-photon fluorescence microscopy (2PFM) in the biomedical field, new probes that undergo efficient 2PA are needed which could be done by normalizing the 2PA action cross-section by introducing polyethylene glycol (PEG), anionic acid groups, cationic ammonium salt, and PAMAM dendrimers for characterizing bioimaging two-photon fluorescence (2PF) probes, by the photodecomposition quantum yield (Yao and Belfield, 2012). He et al. reported the nonlinear optical properties of small phosphorescent polymer dots (Pdots) with strong red-emitting phosphorescence (620 nm). They used an fs pump-probe experiment to analyze the emission decay time of phosphorescent polymer dots (Pdots) and found that the singlet excited state lifetime of the Pdots has a value of 164 ps. Their finding confirmed that the Pdots exhibit large 2PA action cross-section ($\eta\delta_{max} = 15$ GM) and moderate phosphorescence quantum yield ($\eta = 1.36\%$). Due to the efficient two-photon (TP) excited energy transfer, the potential of these Pdots for use in TP time-resolved phosphorescent microscopy has been experimentally demonstrated (He et al., 2015). Qi and co-workers inspired the development in the preparation and characterization of efficient NIR fluorophores applied for deep-tissue biomedical imaging. TP fluorescence microscopic imaging is a power tool to realize deep-tissue and high-resolution imaging as confirmed by Qi et al. The crab-shaped AIEgen was considered for their study and it was established that this kind of AIEgen can possess a planar core structure and several twisting phenyl/naphthyl rotators. The crab-shaped AIEgen affords both high fluorescence quantum yield and efficient TP activity (Qi et al., 2018c). Ultrabright red luminogens with AIE features, D–A structures, and intense charge transfer effects have been developed that showed emission quenching. Such AIE dots with high brightness, high quantum efficiency, a large Stokes shift, and good biocompatibility were prepared using the nanoprecipitation procedure. The 2PA cross-section of the AIE dots was high and they can be utilized as highly efficient photostable fluorescent probes that made them suitable fluoroprobes for in vivo deep-tissue imaging by a TP technique (Qin et al., 2018). Lee et al. proposed a newly generated bright blue fluorescent dextran, named HCD-70K, that monitors the blood vessels using blue and intercompatible typical fluorescent materials. The HCD-70K can flow within the blood vessel and gives data about the whole structure of the blood vessel. On the basis of the metal-free bio-orthogonal click chemistry, hydroxy-coumarin dye was used to fabricate the DBCO-functionalized dextran-70K and can provide a promising opportunity for efficient vascular visualization in various research areas (Hyeon Lee et al., 2019). Niu and others developed two highly photostable AIEgens based on the cyanostilbene core, with a large Stokes shift (>180 nm), high fluorescence quantum yield (12.8%–13.7%), good 2PA cross-section (up to 88 GM), and high resistance to photobleaching under one-photon and TP continuous irradiation, for in vitro and ex vivo bioimaging to visualize and track specific organelle-associated dynamic changes in live systems (Niu et al., 2019). Xia et al. employed the fluorescence emission spectra and DFT/TDDFT calculations to design and study a series of compounds (W_1–W_8) based on triphenylamine with the $-C=N-$ or $-NH-$ group. In all compounds, the forming of D-π-A or D-π-D features has been designed for different purposes. In their structure, the donor and acceptor were connected by a carbon–carbon double bond and then the oxygen or pyridine nitrogen atom was introduced to obtain the cave-like structure. For instance, probes W_1–W_2 featured convenient detection for glutathione using hydrolysis and W_3–W_4 utilized displacement to probe glutathione possessing sensitivity. Their findings demonstrated that the photophysical properties of probes are strongly dependent on the structural variations and those successfully applied to the determination of glutathione in living cells due to the low cytotoxicity and good cell permeability (Xia et al., 2019). Sun et al. designed a ratiometric TP fluorescent probe for a dual-response of mitochondrial SO_2 derivatives with potential to regulate the various physiological processes; sulfur dioxide (SO_2) can relax blood vessels and increase antioxidative capacity, as well as maintain redox equilibrium, based on a carbazole framework to support a platform for dual-detection of mitochondrial SO_2

derivatives and viscosity, with low cell cytotoxicity and can be successfully applied to detect HSO_3^- in living cells and in vivo (Sun et al., 2019). Zhao and others developed a novel near-infrared and TP ratiometric fluorescent probe (NIR-SO2-TP) that was used for optical sensing of SO_2. A coumarin-benzopyrylium π-conjugated platform was used to synthesize the newly fluorescent probe with high selectivity, rapid response time, lower detection limit, and a large Stokes shift (185 nm) (Zhao et al., 2019). As is known, mitochondria are the powerhouses of cells and can be produced by adenosine triphosphate. However, monitoring of the ROSs such as ClO^- in mitochondria is one of the necessary functions for immunity. However, there are limitations to the monitoring and visualizing of ClO^- in mitochondria. In comparison with one-photon microscopy, TP microscopy offers several advantages for detection of ClO^- in mitochondria (Feng et al., 2018).

Huang et al. designed a probe (Lyso-DCHO) utilizing a carbazole-based two-dimensional intramolecular charge transfer system to detect cysteine (Cys) with a ratiometric signal (119 nm emission shift). Due to the good localization of Lyso-DCHO in lysosomes with good biocompatibility and high selectivity, a dual-channel fluorescence response toward Cys in lysosomes was achieved when the probe was excited by the TP excitation (Huang et al., 2019). In addition, TP semiconducting polymer dots with dual emission and ability for ratiometric fluorescent sensing and bioimaging were developed by a number of researchers for detection of the Golgi apparatus in live tissue and visualizing of hydrogen polysulfide in mitochondria (Bao et al., 2019; Han et al., 2019). Zhang et al. addressed a novel class of engineered Sec-responsive fluorescent nanoprobes that were excited by the combination of two photons and used FRET mechanisms to provide a direct and selective procedure for sensing and imaging of biological Sec over abundant competing biothiols (Zhang et al., 2019a). Wang and others presented two new TP fluorescence probes that exhibited almost no mitochondrial membrane potential damage based on diethylamine coumarin skeleton with specific targeting of mitochondria (Wang et al., 2019a). Zhuang and others prepared two new AIEgens, which were designed and synthesized on the basis of a rigid $D-\pi-A$ skeleton and two photons absorption characteristics. Both showed strong AIE with emission enhancement. A large 2PA cross-section of synthesized AIEgens and their good biocompatibility and ability for highly specific targeting of mitochondria in living cells led to revealing of great potential in clinical applications of TP cell and tissue bioimaging and image-guided and mitochondria-targeted photodynamic cancer therapy (Zhuang et al., 2019). Recently, a curcumin (Cur)-loaded oxidation-responsive mPEG-b-PLG (Se)-TP polymeric micelle system with great AIE active and TP imaging properties was synthesized for simultaneous antitumor treatment and bioimaging (He et al., 2019). Xiang and co-workers synthesized and characterized two biocompatible and photostable organic dots fabricated by encapsulating TPE derivatives within a DSPE-PEG matrix that showed absorption peaks at wavelengths of 425 and 483 nm and their emission peaks at the visible region with green and red fluorescence at 560 and 645 nm and providing high fluorescence quantum yields of 64% and 22%, respectively, can be used to stain living cells for one- and two-photon fluorescence bioimaging as well as targeting of integrin $\alpha_v\beta_3$-overexpressing breast cancer cells (Xiang et al., 2015). These results demonstrate that the present fluorescent organic dots are promising candidates for living cell and tissue imaging. Wang and others synthesized ultrasmall single-chain CP dots with bright NIR-I emission for NIR-II excited deep in vivo TP intact brain imaging, displaying the absorption of light with the main peak at $\approx$600 nm and emitting bright fluorescence at the NIR-I region ($\approx$725 nm) with a quantum yield of 20.6 $\pm$ 1.0%. In addition, they believed that the received value of a TP cross-section (σ2) of CPdots1 is one of the largest values for the organic NIR fluorophores and its 2PA cross-section (σ2) value is equal to 1.21×10^3 GM at 1200 nm, where 1 GM is 10^{-50} cm^4 s/photon. The femtosecond (fs) laser excitation of CPdots1 leads to bright 2PF. The broad absorption of CPdots1 provides a high SBR of 2PF images of brain blood vessels, and therefore these images can be compared when CPdots1 are excited using a fully tunable fs-laser system. Due to the more reduced scattering and less absorption of light in the NIR-II region by brain tissue, in vivo 2PF imaging with a depth of 1010 μm and a high SBR of 35 was realized for a mouse brain blood vessel network with craniotomy. A 3D reconstruction of the brain blood vessel network was achieved with a vertical depth of 400 μm through intact skull with the assistance of bright NIR-I emission and NIR-II 2PA (Wang et al., 2019c).

6.4 Supramolecular imaging

Supramolecular polymers are one of the novel classes of dynamic and noncovalent polymers that display specific structural and physicochemical properties such as the ability to undergo reversible changes of structure, shape, and function in response to diverse external stimuli, inherent degradable polymer backbones, smart responsiveness to various biological stimuli, and the ease of incorporation of multiple biofunctionalities (e.g., targeting and bioactivity), making them promising candidates for use in widespread applications ranging from academic research to industrial fields such as drug delivery, gene transfection, protein delivery, bioimaging and diagnosis, tissue engineering, and biomimetic chemistry (Dong et al., 2015). Therefore it is expected that the functionalized supramolecular polymers indicate the great potential of applications in the biomedical field. In addition, as a novel class of smart materials, supramolecular polymers can exhibit AIE properties and become highly emissive in the aggregate state. AIE characteristics of supramolecular polymers bring new opportunities and challenges for their biological applications in fluorescent sensors, bio-imaging agents, and organic electronic devices, and, owing to their ability for environmental adaptation and self repair, they can be used in drug delivery and biomimetic systems. The formation of aggregated supramolecular polymers with bright emissions and good quantum yields at high concentration (AIE properties) gives new vitality to luminescent materials to promote the emission of AIE fluorophores. The main driving forces for fabricating fluorescent supramolecular polymers with AIE properties result from their intermolecular noncovalent interactions that have an important influence on the fluorescence properties of the chromophores (multiple hydrogen bonding interactions, metal coordination bonds, $\pi-\pi$ stacking interactions, electrostatic interactions, and host–guest interactions) (Li et al., 2019a). Yu and others innovatively developed a theranostic supramolecular polymer using β-cyclodextrin as the host and camptothecin as the guest linked by a glutathione-cleavable disulfide bond by supramolecular polymerization and exhibited a high level of factor and its lactone ring opening in a physiological environment which is favorable for intravenous formulation and maintenance of therapeutic efficacy. Several preparation procedures including orthogonal self-assembly driven by $\pi-\pi$ stacking interaction, host – guest complexation, and hydrogen bonds can be employed for the synthesis of supramolecular nanoparticles. Improving the delivery of the obtained supramolecular polymers to tumor sites and rapidly excreting them from the body after drug release thus can be achieved, effectively avoiding systemic toxicity, especially long-term immunotoxicity. In vivo investigations demonstrate that this supramolecular nanomedicine possesses superior antitumor performance and antimetastasis capability (Yu et al., 2018). A new NIR-controlled supramolecular engineering strategy has been developed to provide in vivo assembly and NIR-II (1000–1700 nm) light regulated disassembly of lanthanide upconversion nanoparticles using second NIR window nanoprobes as well as to enhance the retention of NIR-II nanoprobes in the tumor area via host–guest interactions of azobenzene and β-cyclodextrin. In addition, the controllable disassembly of nanoprobes using an NIR-laser provides a reduction in the bioimaging background as well as acceleration of the reticuloendothelial system clearance rate which can also be used in other nano- to microscale contrast agents to improve the bioimaging signal-to-noise ratio and reduce long-term cytotoxicity (Zhao et al., 2018). Liu and co-workers developed a water-soluble two-dimensional supramolecular organic framework via self assembly of cucurbit[8]uril and a three-arm flat linker molecule, which contains a benzene ring as the core and three Brooker's merocyanine (BM) analogs as arms that can be used for deoxyribonucleic acid (DNA) affinity and live-cell imaging due to AIE properties. The formation of a 2D SOF was received by the strong host–guest interactions between BM and CB[8]. The AIE enhancement effect in H_2O was indicated by 2D SOF. In addition, DNA-induced photoluminescence enhancement was observed for the monomer. As a result, this AIEgen-based 2D SOF could feature not only as a cell visualizer but also as a tracker for the nucleus in biological imaging due to the dynamic assembly process (Liu et al., 2019a). Li et al. prepared a novel photoresponsive, water-soluble supramolecular dendronized polymer through a γ-cyclodextrin-coumarin host–guest interaction, which has good biocompatibility and is lysosome-targetable for bioimaging for breast cancer cell diagnosis. Due to the addition of coumarin cyclo and cleavage reactions, this supramolecular polymer can be further converted into its covalent polymer and noncovalent polymer when it is irradiated by the different light energies and the photo-stimulation response material may have application prospects in organelle-targeting applications (Li et al., 2019b).

In addition to the other numerous bioimaging tools like paramagnetic agents, radio-labeled probes, and acoustically active nanostructures; supramolecular fluorescent hydrogel (SFH) has also been developed and gained great interest because of its 3D cross-linked structure, excellent biodegradability and biocompatibility, and smart responses to physiological stimuli. Therefore the exploration of SFH with the combined advantages of fluorescence and supramolecular hydrogels is highly desirable for bio-imaging applications with the insights into both physiological and pathological processes in a real-time and sensitive manner (Mehwish et al., 2019). Zhang et al. summarized the recently emerged light-responsive supramolecular polymers. The characteristics such as light-regulated morphology transformation, tunable fluorescent emission, switchable self-healing ability, muscle-like actuation, and programmed shape memory can be observed in this set of smart optical materials (Zhang et al., 2019b). It seems that the light response of this kind of supramolecular polymer, even in an orthogonal multistimuli or multiproton controllable mode, can provide great potential for future smart optical material applications (Fig. 6.2).

6.5 Photoacoustic imaging

As a new imaging modality, photoacoustic imaging (PAI) shows great promise in biomedical applications due to its tissue penetration depths and high resolution (Wang et al., 2019d). It is a burgeoning biomedical structural and functional imaging technique which utilizes ultrasonic signals as an information carrier that captures information about optical absorption properties relevant to physiology and pathology inside tissues. The PAI method is based on different processes that can be given as: (1) the light energy must be absorbed by tissue after being irradiated by visible light or NIR light; (2) the induced photoacoustic signals are produced by the adiabatic expansion of absorber that; (3) the signals were detected by the transducers; and (4) a data acquisition card stores up information for image reconstruction analysis (Wu et al., 2014). Over three decades, various PAI techniques such as photoacoustic spectroscopy, photoacoustic tomography (PAT), photoacoustic microscopy, and photoacoustic endoscopic imaging have been developed (Xu and Wang, 2006). PAI is a powerful preclinical tool that has many promising applications and can be used for different purposes. There are several kinds of contrast agent that vary in principles, materials, shapes, and sizes used in different imaging modalities. On the basis of photoacoustic effects, an ideal contrast agent such as SPNs, metallic, oxide, and semiconducting nanoparticles must significantly increase contrast, effectively improve imaging depth or accuracy,

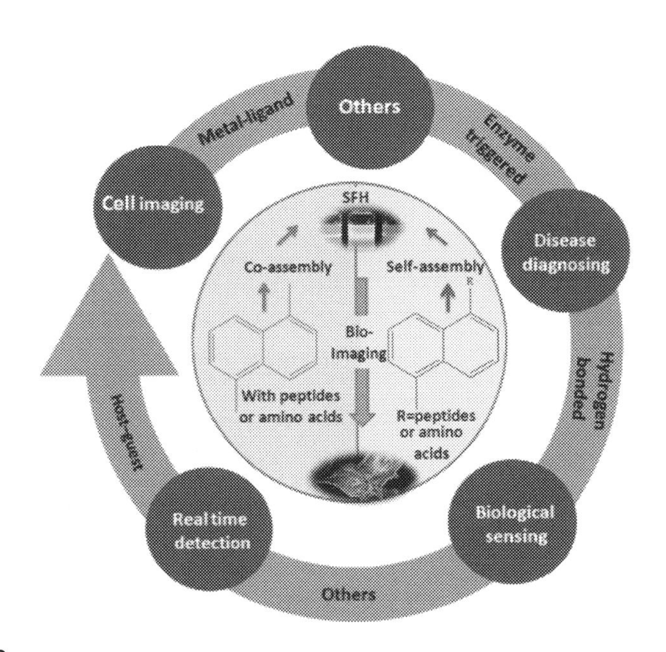

FIGURE 6.2

Overview of representative families of SFH based on different interactions with their applications as bio-imaging tools (Mehwish et al., 2019). *SFH*, Supramolecular fluorescent hydrogel.

Reproduced by permission of The Royal Society of Chemistry.

and provide specific molecular information (Wu et al., 2014; Lyu et al., 2019; Yoo et al., 2018). In Fig. 6.3, the advanced nanomaterials as exogenous contrast agents for PAI and PAI applications in nanomedicine are shown. However, unlike inorganic and metallic nanomaterials, CP fluorescent nanoparticles have been studied for only a few years, and so researchers need to explore them further (Wu et al., 2014). Although the bioimaging capabilities of polymers have been studied for a few years, their applications to PAI and PTT are much more recent. Previously, Kim et al. reviewed the recent progress on the application of organic nanoformulations as PAI contrast agents (biocompatible and biodegradable organic agents such as liposomal agents, colored microbubbles, and polymeric agents). They concluded that intensive systemic studies must be performed to (1) reduce phototoxicity, (2) improve photostability, (3) achieve appropriate clearance efficiency, and (4) develop large-scale manufacturing processes to achieve fast clinical translation and commercialization of organic PAI contrast agents. They believed that rigorous studies need to be performed by carefully considering chemical compositions, shapes, sizes, and surface modifications of the nanoparticles to certify their biodistribution and pharmacokinetics and to demonstrate their specific clinical applications (Kim et al., 2016). It seems that the possibility to

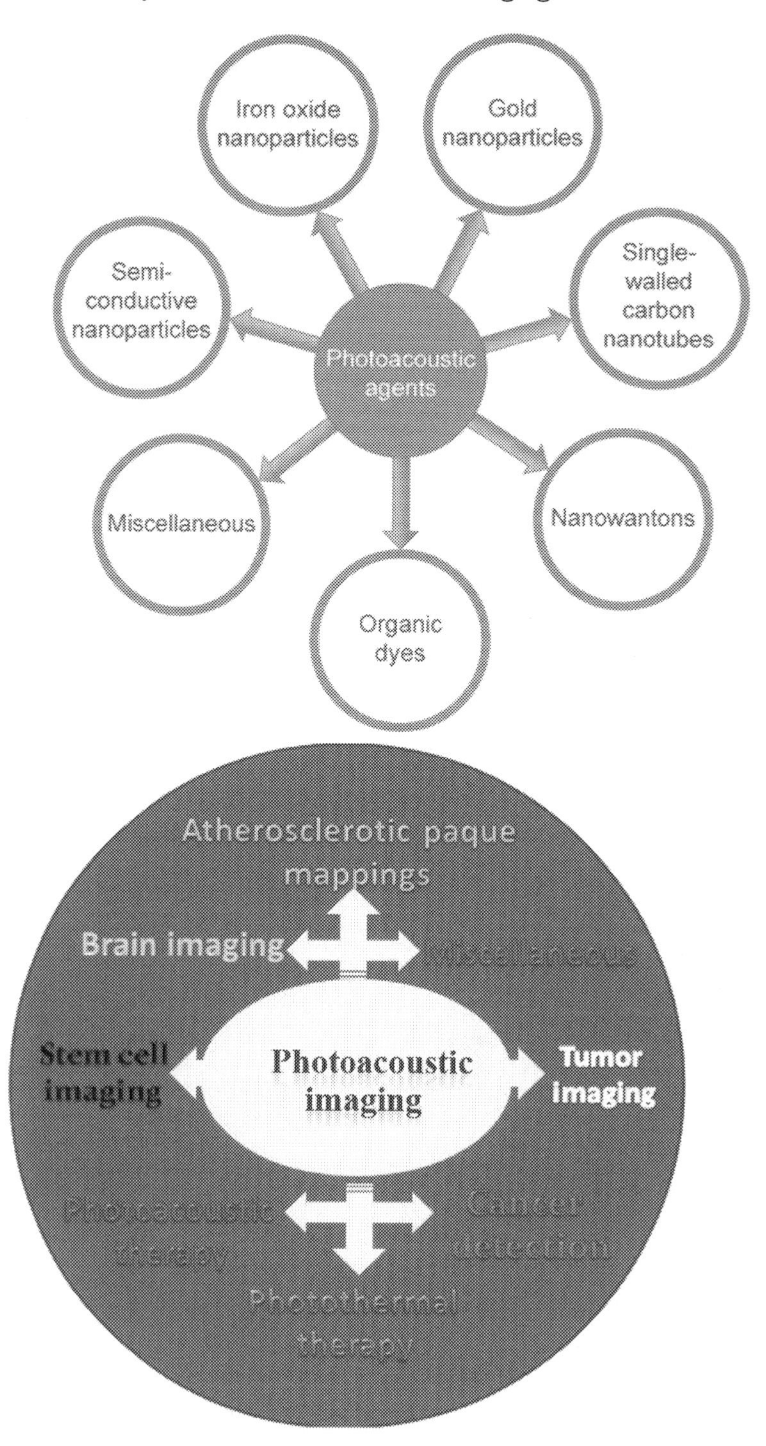

FIGURE 6.3

(Left) Advanced nanomaterials as exogenous contrast agents for photoacoustic imaging (PAI) (Wu et al., 2014). (Right) Domains of biomedical applications of photoacoustic imaging in nanomedicine.

bypass the biodegradability of these agents is exploring the transurethral or oral administration methods. In Table 6.1, physical properties, optical properties, and multimodal imaging capabilities of organic polymeric nanoparticles are shown (Kim et al., 2016). Weber et al. critically reviewed the physical, chemical, and biochemical characteristics of the existing photoacoustic contrast agents, highlighting key applications and present challenges for molecular PAI. They described the exogenous contrast agents and believed that these agents are still in the early stages of exploration, mostly having been demonstrated only in single proof-of-concept studies. They emphasized that a better understanding of the photophysical and biological properties of the promising classes needs to receive high impact in preclinical molecular imaging and to enable their routine use (Weber et al., 2016).

In addition, other approaches to molecular imaging indicate that the field could make good progress by focusing development and commercial efforts on contrast agents that prove successful in rigorous studies of biocompatibility and achieve biological validation in realistic animal models of disease (Weber et al., 2016). As emerging concepts in molecular PAI, they introduced smart (or "activatable") contrast agents that elicit a prescribed signal change, such as a shift in the peak absorption wavelength, in response to a biological stimulus of interest. Yoo and co-workers briefly introduced state-of-the-art multiscale imaging systems and summarized recent progress on exogenous bio-compatible and -degradable agents consisting of CP cores and hydrophilic polymer shells (polysaccharides, phospholipids, and DNA), which are generally formed via nanoprecipitation or nanoemulsion techniques, providing the photophysical properties of a semiconducting polymer can be translated into detectable ultrasonic signals in response to laser pulses and address biomedical applications and clinical practice (Yoo et al., 2018). The presence of the peripheral surfactant polymer leads to stabilization of the overall structure under physiological conditions (Fig. 6.4). In addition, the biocompatible nanostructured organic materials include particles, hydrogels, micelles, vesicles, polymersomes, and conventional hydrophilic polymers as potential candidates to play a key role in PAI (Yoo et al., 2018). Theses polymers have been incorporated into contrast agents through controlled polymerization, copolymerization, or postpolymerization modification (Fig. 6.5).

It has pointed out by Yoo and co-workers that the functional polymers with special topologies or architectures with the chemically removable groups (e.g., labile groups, stimuli-responsive groups, or self-immolative groups) have interestingly shown biodegradability when exposed to bio-related signals such as pH, enzymes, temperature, and biogenic chemicals. Liu et al. outlined the basic PAI principles and focused on the application of organic-dye-based PA probes for molecular detection and in vivo imaging. Finally, they evaluated their application prospects while considering the potential challenges in the biomedical fields (Liu et al., 2019c). Jiang et al. reported the first series of metabolizable NIR-II PA agents based on SPNs. Such completely organic nanoagents consist of π-conjugated yet oxidizable optical polymer as PA generators and hydrolyzable

Table 6.1 Physical properties, optical properties, and multimodal imaging capabilities of organic polymeric nanoparticles (Kim et al., 2016).

		Excitation λ (nm)	PA sensitivity	FL quantum yield (%)	Size (nm)	Shape	Multimodal imaging capability
Semiconducting polymer NPs	SPN1	660	$\lesssim$5 μg/mL	0.100	$\approx$46	Spherical	PA, FL
	SPN2	635	$\lesssim$5 μg/mL	0.005			–
	SPN3	712	$\lesssim$5 μg/mL	0.010			–
	SPN4	748	$\lesssim$2 μg/mL	0.001			–
PFTTQ polymer NPs		800	$\lesssim$50 μg/mL	$\approx$0	$\approx$50	Spherical	–
Melanin NPs		680	$<$0.625 μM	$\approx$0	$\approx$10	Spherical	PA, PET, MRI
Nanonaps		707 or 860	$<$133 μg/mL	$\approx$0	$\approx$20	Spherical	PA, PET
HAS-BPOx-IR825		600	$<$128 μg/mL	0.33	$\approx$80	Spherical	PA, FL
PPy NPs		808	$<$10 μg/mL	$\approx$0	$\approx$46	Spherical	–

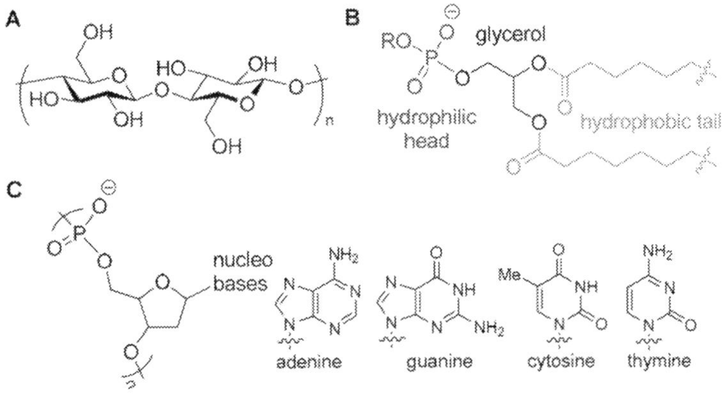

FIGURE 6.4

Chemical structures of (A) cellulose, (B) phospholipid, and (C) deoxyribonucleic acid (DNA) (Yoo et al., 2018).

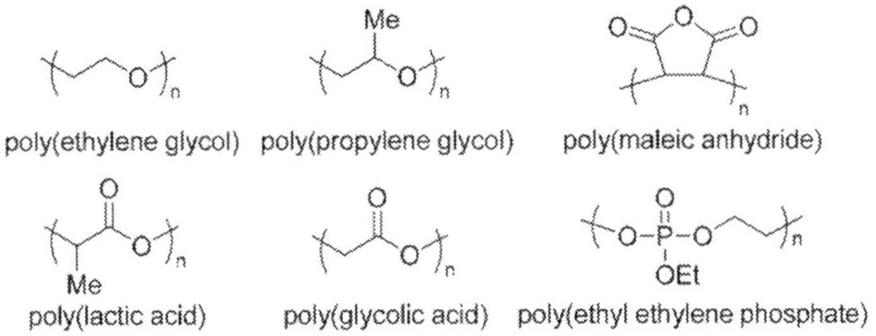

FIGURE 6.5

Typical synthetic polymeric components incorporated into various nanostructures for PA agents via controlled polymerization, copolymerization, or postpolymerization modification (Yoo et al., 2018).

amphiphilic polymers as a particle matrix to provide water solubility. Due to the presence of myeloperoxidase and lipase abundant in phagocytes, the obtained SPNs are readily degraded and transfer from nonfluorescent nanoparticles (30 nm) into NIR fluorescent ultrasmall metabolites (≈ 1 nm). In addition, these nanoagents can be effectively cleared out via both hepatobiliary and renal excretions after systematic administration (Jiang et al., 2019). Erfanzadeh and Zhu stated that in order to facilitate clinical applications of PAI and encourage its application in low-resource settings, research on low-cost PAI with inexpensive optical sources has gained attention. In their article, the advances made in PAI with low-cost sources were reviewed. They concluded that the designed PAI systems in ORPAM, ARPAM, and PAT configurations with various wavelengths, resolutions, and imaging depths have shown potential for clinical and preclinical applications if they used the low-cost pulsed sources (Erfanzadeh and Zhu, 2019).

References

Aiken, S., Edgar, R.J.L., Gabbutt, C.D., Mark Heron, B., Hobson, P.A., 2018. Negatively photochromic organic compounds: exploring the dark side. Dye. Pigm 149, 92–121.

Andreasson, J., Pischel, U., 2015. Molecules with a sense of logic: a progress report. Chem. Soc. Rev. 44, 1053–1069.

Bao, B., Yang, Z., Liu, Y., Xu, Y., Gu, B., Chen, J., et al., 2019. Two-photon semiconducting polymer nanoparticles as a new platform for imaging of intracellular pH variation. Biosens. Bioelectron. 126, 129–135.

Beharry, A.A., Wong, L., Tropepe, V., Woolley, G.A., 2011. Fluorescence imaging of azobenzene photoswitching in vivo. Angew. Chem., Int. Ed. 50, 1325–1327.

Bouas-Laurent, H., Dürr, H., 2001. Organic photochromism. Pure Appl. Chem. 73, 639–665.

Chan, Y.-H., Elena Gallina, M., Zhang, X., Wu, I.-C., Jin, Y., Sun, W., et al., 2012a. Reversible photoswitching of spiropyran-conjugated semiconducting polymer dots. Anal. Chem. 84, 9431–9438.

Chan, Y.-H., Ye, F., Elena Gallina, M., Zhang, X., Jin, Y., Wu, I.-C., et al., 2012b. Hybrid semiconducting polymer dot-quantum dot with narrow-band emission, near-infrared fluorescence, and high brightness. J. Am. Chem. Soc. 134, 7309–7312.

Che, W., Zhang, L., Li, Y., Zhu, D., Xie, Z., Li, G., et al., 2019. Ultrafast and noninvasive long-term bioimaging with highly stable red aggregation-induced emission nanoparticles. Anal. Chem. 91, 3467–3474.

Chen, M., Yin, M., 2014. Design and development of fluorescent nanostructures for bioimaging. Prog. Polym. Sci. 39, 365–395.

Chen, Y., Guan, R., Zhang, C., Huang, J., Ji, L., Chao, H., 2016. Two-photon luminescent metal complexes for bioimaging and cancer phototherapy. Coord. Chem. Rev. 310, 16–40.

Chen, H., Zeng, X., Phoebe Tham, H., Fiona Phua, S.Z., Cheng, W., Zeng, W., et al., 2019a. NIR-light-activated combination therapy with a precise ratio of photosensitizer and prodrug using a host–guest strategy. Angew. Chem. 131, 7723–7728.

Chen, L., Chen, D., Jiang, Y., Zhang, J., Yu, J., DuFort, C.C., et al., 2019b. A BODIPY-based donor/donor–acceptor system: towards highly efficient long-wavelength-excitable near-IR polymer dots with narrow and strong absorption features. Angew. Chem. Int. Ed. 58, 7008–7012.

Denk, W., Strickler, J.H., Webb, W.W., 1990. Two-photon laser scanning fluorescence microscopy. Science 248, 73–76.

Ding, D., Li, K., Liu, B., Zhong Tang, B., 2013. Bioprobes based on AIE fluorogens. Acc. Chem. Res. 46, 2441–2453.

Ding, F., Zhan, Y., Lu, X., Sun, Y., 2018. Recent advances in near-infrared II fluorophores for multifunctional biomedical imaging. Chem. Sci. 9, 4370–4380.

Ding, F., Fan, Y., Sun, Y., Zhang, F., 2019. Beyond 1000 nm emission wavelength: recent advances in organic and inorganic emitters for deep-tissue molecular imaging. Adv. Healthc. Mater. 8, 1900260.

Dong, R., Zhou, Y., Huang, X., Zhu, X., Lu, Y., Shen, J., 2015. Functional supramolecular polymers for biomedical applications. Adv. Mater. 27, 498–526.

Elsabahy, M., Heo, G.S., Lim, S.-M., Sun, G., Wooley, K.L., 2015. Polymeric nanostructures for imaging and therapy. Chem. Rev. 115, 10967–11011.

Erfanzadeh, M., Zhu, Q., 2019. Photoacoustic imaging with low-cost sources: a review. Photoacoustics 14, 1–11.

Feng, G., Yong Tay, C., Xiang Chui, Q., Liu, R., Tomczak, N., Liu, J., et al., 2014. Ultrabright organic dots with aggregation-induced emission characteristics for cell tracking. Biomaterials 35, 8669–8677.

Feng, Y., Li, S., Li, D., Wang, Q., Ning, P., Chen, M., et al., 2018. Rational design of a diaminomaleonitrile-based mitochondria-targeted two-photon fluorescent probe for hypochlorite in vivo: Solvent-independent and high selectivity over Cu^{2+}. Sens. Actuators B Chem. 254, 282–290.

Fu, W., Yan, C., Guo, Z., Zhang, J., Zhang, H., Tian, H., et al., 2019. Rational design of near-infrared aggregation-induced-emission active probes: in situ mapping of amyloid-β plaques with ultrasensitivity and high-fidelity. J. Am. Chem. Soc. 141, 3171–3177.

Gao, M., Zhong Tang, B., 2017. Aggregation-induced emission probes for cancer theranostics. Drug. Discov. Today 22, 1288–1294.

Gao, S., Chen, D., Li, Q., Ye, J., Jiang, H., Amatore, C., et al., 2014. Near-infrared fluorescence imaging of cancer cells and tumors through specific biosynthesis of silver nanoclusters. Sci. Rep. 4, 4384.

Gao, H., Zhang, X., Chen, C., Li, K., Ding, D., 2018. Unity makes strength: how aggregation-induced emission luminogens advance the biomedical field. Adv. Biosys 2, 1800074.

Goppert-Mayer, M., 1931. Elementary processes with two quantum jumps. Ann. Phys. 401, 273–294.

Gu, B., Yong, K.-T., Liu, B., 2018. Strategies to overcome the limitations of AIEgens in biomedical applications. Small Methods 2, 1700392.

Han, Q., Ru, J., Wang, X., Dong, Z., Wang, L., Jiang, H., et al., 2019. Photostable ratiometric two-photon fluorescent probe for visualizing hydrogen polysulfide in mitochondria and its application. ACS Appl. Bio Mater. 2, 1987–1997.

Haque, A., Haque Faizi, M.S., Ahmad Rather, J., Khan, M.S., 2017. Next generation NIR fluorophores for tumor imaging and fluorescence-guided surgery: a review. Bioorg. Med. Chem. 25, 2017–2034.

He, T., Hu, W., Shi, H., Pan, Q., Ma, G., Huang, W., et al., 2015. Strong nonlinear optical phosphorescence from water-soluble polymer dots: towards the application of two-photon bioimaging. Dye. Pigm 123, 218–221.

He, H., Zhuang, W., Ma, B., Su, X., Yu, T., Hu, J., et al., 2019. Oxidation-responsive and aggregation-induced emission polymeric micelles with two-photon excitation for cancer therapy and bioimaging. ACS Biomater. Sci. Eng. 5, 2577–2586.

Helmy, S., Leibfarth, F.A., Oh, S., Poelma, J.E., Hawker, C.J., Read de Alaniz, J., 2014. Photoswitching using visible light: a new class of organic photochromic molecules. J. Am. Chem. Soc. 136, 8169–8172.

Hong, G., Zou, Y., Antaris, A.L., Diao, S., Wu, D., Cheng, K., et al., 2014. Ultrafast fluorescence imaging *in vivo* with conjugated polymer fluorophores in the second near-infrared window. Nat. Commun. 5, 4206.

Huang, Y., Ren, Q., Li, S., Feng, Y., Zhang, W., Fang, G., et al., 2019. A dual-emission two-photon fluorescent probe for specific-cysteine imaging in lysosomes and in vivo. Sens. Actuators B Chem. 293, 247–255.

Hyeon Lee, S., Ho Choe, Y., Hyung Kang, R., Rim Kim, Y., Hee Kim, N., Kang, S., et al., 2019. A bright blue fluorescent dextran for two-photonin vivo imaging of blood vessels. Bioorg. Chem. 89, 103019.

Janib, S.M., Moses, A.S., MacKay, J.A., 2010. Imaging and drug delivery using theranostic nanoparticles. Adv. Drug. Deliv. Rev. 62, 1052–1063.

Jiang, Y., Pu, K., 2018. Multimodal biophotonics of semiconducting polymer nanoparticles. Acc. Chem. Res. 51, 1840–1849.

Jiang, Y., Kumar Upputuri, P., Xie, C., Zeng, Z., Sharma, A., Zhen, X., et al., 2019. Metabolizable semiconducting polymer nanoparticles for second near-infrared photoacoustic imaging. Adv. Mater. 31, 1808166.

Jin, Y., Ye, F., Zeigler, M., Wu, C., Chiu, D.T., 2011. Near-infrared fluorescent dye-doped semiconducting polymer dots. ACS Nano 5, 1468–1475.

Jin, G., He, R., Liu, Q., Lin, M., Dong, Y., Li, K., et al., 2019. Near-infrared light-regulated cancer theranostic nanoplatform based on aggregation-induced emission luminogen encapsulated upconversion nanoparticles. Theranostics 9, 246–264.

Kaiser, W., Garrett, C.G.B., 1961. Two-photon excitation in CaF_2:Eu^{2+}. Phys. Rev. Lett. 7, 229–231.

Ke, C.-S., Fang, C.-C., Yan, J.-Y., Tseng, P.-J., Pyle, J.R., Chen, C.-P., et al., 2017. Molecular engineering and design of semiconducting polymer dots with narrow-band, near-infrared emission for in vivo biological imaging. ACS Nano 11, 3166–3177.

Kim, J., Park, S., Lee, C., Kim, J.Y., Kim, C., 2016. Organic nanostructures for photoacoustic imaging. ChemNanoMat 2, 156–166.

Kuo, C.-T., Thompson, A.M., Elena Gallina, M., Ye, F., Johnson, E.S., Sun, W., et al., 2016. Optical painting and fluorescence activated sorting of single adherent cells labelled with photoswitchable Pdots. Nat. Commun. 7, 11468.

Lee, M.H., Sharma, A., Chang, M.J., Lee, J., Son, S., Sessler, J.L., et al., 2018. Fluorogenic reaction-based prodrug conjugates as targeted cancer theranostics. Chem. Soc. Rev. 47, 28–52.

Li, A.D.Q., Zhan, C., Hu, D., Wan, W., Yao, J., 2011. Photoswitchable nanoprobes offer unlimited brightness in frequency-domain. J. Am. Chem. Soc. 133, 7628–7631.

Li, J., Rao, J., Pu, K., 2018a. Recent progress on semiconducting polymer nanoparticles for molecular imaging and cancer phototherapy. Biomaterials 155, 217–235.

Li, Y., Li, X., Xue, Z., Jiang, M., Zeng, S., Hao, J., 2018b. Second near-infrared emissive lanthanide complex for fast renal-clearable in vivo optical bioimaging and tiny tumor detection. Biomaterials 169, 35–44.

Li, B., He, T., Shen, X., Tang, D., Yin, S., 2019a. Fluorescent supramolecular polymers with aggregation induced emission properties. Polym. Chem. 10, 796–818.

Li, H., Wu, J., Yin, J.-F., Wang, H., Wu, Y., Kuang, G.-C., 2019b. Photoresponsive, water-soluble supramolecular dendronized polymer with specific lysosome-targetable bioimaging application in living cells. Macromol. Rapid Commun. 40, 1800714.

Li, M., Zhao, J., Chu, H., Mi, Y., Zhou, Z., Di, Z., et al., 2019c. Light-activated nanoprobes for biosensing and imaging. Adv. Mater. 45, 1804745.

Lin, J., Zeng, X., Xiao, Y., Tang, L., Nong, J., Liu, Y., et al., 2019. Novel near-infrared II aggregation-induced emission dots for in vivo bioimaging. Chem. Sci. 10, 1219–1226.

Liu, R., Yang, Y., Cui, Q., Xu, W., Peng, R., Li, L., 2018a. A diarylethene-based photoswitch and its photomodulation of the fluorescence of conjugated polymers. Chem. Eur. J. 24, 17756–17766.

Liu, T., Ning, J., Wang, B., Dong, B., Li, S., Tian, X., et al., 2018b. Activatable near-infrared fluorescent probe for dipeptidyl peptidase IV and its bioimaging applications in living cells and animals. Anal. Chem. 90, 3965–3973.

Liu, H., Zhang, Z., Zhao, Y., Zhou, Y., Xue, B., Han, Y., et al., 2019a. A water-soluble two-dimensional supramolecular organic framework with aggregation-induced emission for DNA affinity and live-cell imaging. J. Mater. Chem. B 7, 1435–1441.

Liu, Y., Mao, L., Yang, S., Liu, M., Huang, H., Wen, Y., et al., 2019b. Fabrication and biological imaging of hydrazine hydrate cross-linked AIE-activefluorescent polymeric nanoparticles. Mater. Sci. Eng. C 94, 310–317.

Liu, Y., Teng, L., Liu, H.-W., Xu, C., Guo, H., Yuan, L., et al., 2019c. Recent advances in organic-dye-based photoacoustic probes for biosensing and bioimaging. Sci. China Chem. 62, 1275–1285.

Long, Z., Liu, M., Jiang, R., Wan, Q., Mao, L., Wan, Y., et al., 2017. Preparation of water soluble and biocompatible AIE-active fluorescent organic nanoparticles via multicomponent reaction and their biological imaging capability. Chem. Eng. J. 308, 527–534.

Luo, J., Xie, Z., Lam, J.W., Cheng, L., Chen, H., Qiu, C., et al., 2001. Aggregation-induced emission of 1-methyl-1, 2, 3, 4, 5-pentaphenylsilole. Chem. Commun. 1740–1741.

Lv, Q., Wang, K., Xu, D., Liu, M., Wan, Q., Huang, H., et al., 2016. Synthesis of amphiphilic hyperbranched AIE active fluorescent organic nanoparticles and their application in biological application. Macromol. Biosci. 16, 223–230.

Lyu, Y., Li, J., Pu, K., 2019. Second near-infrared absorbing agents for photoacoustic imaging and photothermal therapy. Small Methods 3, 1900553.

Mehwish, N., Dou, X., Zhao, Y., Feng, C.-L., 2019. Supramolecular fluorescent hydrogelators as bio-imaging probes. Mater. Horiz. 6, 14–44.

Mei, J., Hong, Y., Lam, J.W.Y., Qin, A., Tang, Y., Zhong Tang, B., 2014. Aggregation-induced emission: the whole is more brilliant than the parts. Adv. Mater. 26, 5429–5479.

Mutoh, K., Miyashita, N., Arai, K., Abe, J., 2019. Turn-on mode fluorescence switch by using negative photochromic imidazole dimer. J. Am. Chem. Soc. 141, 5650–5654.

Ni, X., Zhang, X., Duan, X., Zheng, H.-L., Xue, X.-S., Ding, D., 2019. Near-infrared afterglow luminescent aggregation-induced emission dots with ultrahigh tumor-to-liver signal ratio for promoted image-guided cancer surgery. Nano Lett. 19, 318–330.

Niu, G., Zhang, R., Gu, Y., Wang, J., Ma, C., Kwok, R.T.K., et al., 2019. Highly photostable two-photon NIR AIEgens with tunable organelle specificity and deep tissue penetration. Biomaterials 208, 72–82.

Pal, K., Sharma, V., Sahoo, D., Kapuria, N., Koner, A.L., 2018. Large Stokes-shifted NIR-emission from nanospace-induced aggregation of perylenemonoimide-doped polymer nanoparticles: imaging of folate receptor expression. Chem. Commun. 54, 523–526.

Pawlicki, M., Collins, H.A., Denning, R.G., Anderson, H.L., 2009. Two-photon absorption and the design of two-photon dyes. Angew. Chem. Int. Ed. 48, 3244–3266.

Pu, K.-Y., Liu, B., 2011. Fluorescent conjugated polyelectrolytes for bioimaging. Adv. Funct. Mater. 21, 3408–3423.

Qi, J., Chen, C., Ding, D., Zhong Tang, B., 2018a. Aggregation-induced emission luminogens: union is strength, gathering illuminates healthcare. Adv. Healthc. Mater. 7, 1800477.

Qi, J., Chen, C., Zhang, X., Hu, X., Ji, S., Kwok, R.T.K., et al., 2018b. Light-driven transformable optical agent with adaptive functions for boosting cancer surgery outcomes. Nat. Commun. 9, 1848.

Qi, J., Sun, C., Li, D., Zhang, H., Yu, W., Zebibula, A., et al., 2018c. Aggregation-induced emission luminogen with near-infrared-II excitation and near-infrared I emission for ultra deep Intravital two-photon microscopy. ACS Nano 12, 7936–7945.

Qian, Y., Wang, Y., Jia, F., Wang, Z., Yue, C., Zhang, W., et al., 2019. Tumor-microenvironment controlled nanomicelles with AIE property for boosting cancer therapy and apoptosis monitoring. Biomaterials 188, 96–106.

Qin, W., Zhang, P., Li, H., Lam, J.W.Y., Cai, Y., Kwok, R.T.K., et al., 2018. Ultrabright red AIEgens for two-photon vascular imaging with high resolution and deep penetration. Chem. Sci. 9, 2705–2710.

Raghavendra, P., Pullaiah, T., 2018. Advances in Cell and Molecular Diagnostics. Academic Press, London.

Reineck, P., Gibson, B.C., 2017. Near-Infrared fluorescent nanomaterials for bioimaging and sensing, Adv. Optical Mater., 5. p. 1600446.

Rong, Y., Wu, C., Yu, J., Zhang, X., Ye, F., Zeigler, M., et al., 2013. Multicolor fluorescent semiconducting polymer dots with narrow emissions and high brightness. ACS Nano 7, 376–384.

Sharma, P., Brown, S., Walter, G., Santra, S., Moudgil, B., 2006. Nanoparticles for bioimaging. Adv. Colloid Interface Sci. 123–126, 471–485.

Shou, K., Tang, Y., Chen, H., Chen, S., Zhang, L., Zhang, A., et al., 2018. Diketopyrrolopyrrole-based semiconducting polymer nanoparticles for in vivo second near-infrared window imaging and image-guided tumor surgery. Chem. Sci. 9, 3105–3110.

Sun, C., Cao, W., Zhang, W., Zhang, L., Feng, Y., Fang, M., et al., 2019. Design of a ratiometric two-photonfluorescent probe for dual-response of mitochondrial SO_2 derivatives and viscosity in cells and in vivo. Dye. Pigm 171, 107709.

Tang, F., Wang, C., Wang, J., Wang, X., Li, L., 2014. Fluorescent organic nanoparticles with enhanced fluorescence by self-aggregation and their application to cellular imaging. ACS Appl. Mater. Interfaces 6, 18337–18343.

Tang, Y., Li, Y., Lu, X., Hu, X., Zhao, H., Hu, W., et al., 2019. Bio-Erasable intermolecular donor–acceptor interaction of organic semiconducting nanoprobes for activatable NIR-II fluorescence imaging. Adv. Funct. Mater. 29, 1807376.

Terai, T., Nagano, T., 2008. Fluorescent probes for bioimaging applications. Curr. Opin. Chem. Biol. 12, 515–521.

Tian, Z., Wu, W., Wan, W., Li, A.D.Q., 2009. Single-chromophore-based photoswitchable nanoparticles enable dual-alternating-color fluorescence for unambiguous live cell imaging. J. Am. Chem. Soc. 131, 4245–4252.

Wallyn, J., Anton, N., Akram, S., Vandamme, T.F., 2019. Biomedical imaging: principles, technologies, clinical aspects, contrast agents, limitations and future trends in nanomedicines. Pharm. Res. 36, 78.

Wan, Q., Wang, K., He, C., Liu, M., Zeng, G., Huang, H., et al., 2015. Stimulus responsive cross-linked AIE-active polymeric nanoprobes: fabrication and biological imaging application. Polym. Chem. 6, 8214–8221.

Wan, Q., Liu, M., Xu, D., Mao, L., Tian, J., Huang, H., et al., 2016. Fabrication of aggregation induced emission active luminescent chitosan nanoparticles via a "one-pot" multicomponent reaction. Carbohydr. Polym. 152, 189–195.

Wang, Y., Peng, Q., Hou, Q., Zhao, K., Liang, Y., Li, B., 2011. Tuning the electronic structures and optical properties of fluorene-based donor–acceptor copolymers by changing the acceptors: a theoretical study. Theor. Chem. Acc. 129, 257–270.

Wang, H., Zhao, E., Lam, J.W.Y., Zhong Tang, B., 2015. AIE luminogens: emission brightened by aggregation. Mater. Today 18, 365–377.

Wang, J., Lv, F., Liu, L., Ma, Y., Wang, S., 2018a. Strategies to design conjugated polymer based materials for biological sensing and imaging. Coord. Chem. Rev. 354, 135–154.

Wang, L., Chen, X., Xia, Q., Liu, R., Qu, J., 2018b. Deep-red AIE-active fluorophore for hypochlorite detection and bioimaging in live cells. Ind. Eng. Chem. Res. 57, 7735–7741.

Wang, K.-N., Zhu, Y., Xing, M., Cao, D., Guan, R., Zhao, S., et al., 2019a. Two-photon fluorescence probes for mitochondria imaging and detection of sulfite/bisulfite in living cells. Sens. Actuators B Chem. 295, 215–222.

Wang, S., Li, T., Zhang, X., Ma, L., Li, C., Yao, X., et al., 2019b. Stimuli-responsive copolymer and uniform polymeric nanoparticles with photochromism and switchable emission. ChemPhotoChem 3, 1–8.

Wang, S., Liu, J., Feng, G., Guan Ng, L., Liu, B., 2019c. NIR-II excitable conjugated polymer dots with bright NIR-I emission for deep in vivo two-photon brain imaging through intact skull. Adv. Funct. Mater. 29, 1808365.

Wang, X., Geng, Z., Cong, H., Shen, Y., Yu, B., 2019d. Organic semiconductors for photothermal therapy and photoacoustic imaging. ChemBioChem 20, 1–10.

Weber, J., Beard, P.C., Bohndiek, S.E., 2016. Contrast agents for molecular photoacoustic imaging. Nat. Methods 13, 639–650.

Weissleder, R., Mahmood, U., 2001. Molecular imaging. Radiology 219, 316–333.

Wu, D., Huang, L., Jiang, M.S., Jiang, H., 2014. Contrast agents for photoacoustic and thermoacoustic imaging: a review. Int. J. Mol. Sci. 15, 23616–23639.

Wu, I.-C., Yu, J., Ye, F., Rong, Y., Elena Gallina, M., Fujimoto, B.S., et al., 2015. Squaraine-based polymer dots with narrow, bright near-infrared fluorescence for biological applications. J. Am. Chem. Soc. 137, 173–178.

Wu, W., Yang, Y.-Q., Yang, Y., Yang, Y.-M., Wang, H., Zhang, K.-Y., et al., 2019. An organic NIR-II nanofluorophore with aggregation-induced emission characteristics for in vivo fluorescence imaging. Int. J. Nanomed. 14, 3571–3582.

Xia, Y., Zhang, H., Zhu, X., Fang, M., Yang, M., Zhang, Q., et al., 2019. Fluorescent probes for detecting glutathione: bio-imaging and two reaction mechanisms. Dye. Pigm 163, 441–446.

Xiang, J., Cai, X., Lou, X., Feng, G., Min, X., Luo, W., et al., 2015. Biocompatible green and red fluorescent organic dots with remarkably large two-photon action cross sections for targeted cellular imaging and real-time intravital blood vascular visualization. ACS Appl. Mater. Interfaces 7, 14965–14974.

Xu, M., Wang, L.V., 2006. Photoacoustic imaging in biomedicine. Rev. Sci. Instrum. 77, 041101.

Xu, M., Wang, X., Wang, Q., Hu, Q., Huang, K., Lou, X., et al., 2019. Analyte-responsive fluorescent probes with AIE characteristic based on the change of covalent bond. Sci. China Mater. 62, 1236–1250.

Yao, S., Belfield, K.D., 2012. Two-photon fluorescent probes for bioimaging. Eur. J. Org. Chem. 3199–3217.

Yao, J., Yang, M., Duan, Y., 2014. Chemistry, biology, and medicine of fluorescent nanomaterials and related systems: new insights into biosensing, bioimaging, genomics, diagnostics, and therapy. Chem. Rev. 114, 6130–6178.

Yildiz, I., Deniz, E., Raymo, F.M., 2009. Fluorescence modulation with photochromic switches in nanostructured constructs. Chem. Soc. Rev. 38, 1859–1867.

Yoo, S.W., Jung, D., Min, J.-J., Kim, H., Lee, C., 2018. Biodegradable contrast agents for photoacoustic imaging. Appl. Sci. 8, 1567.

Yu, J., Rong, Y., Kuo, C.-T., Zhou, X.-H., Chiu, D.T., 2017. Recent advances in the development of highly luminescent semiconducting polymer dots and nanoparticles for biological imaging and medicine. Anal. Chem. 89, 42–56.

Yu, G., Zhao, X., Zhou, J., Mao, Z., Huang, X., Wang, Z., et al., 2018. Supramolecular polymer-based nanomedicine: high therapeutic performance and negligible long-term immunotoxicity. J. Am. Chem. Soc. 140, 8005–8019.

Yuan, W.Z., Lu, P., Chen, S., Lam, J.W., Wang, Z., Liu, Y., et al., 2010. Changing the behavior of chromophores from aggregation-caused quenching to aggregation-induced emission: development of highly efficient light emitters in the solid state. Adv. Mater. 22, 2159–2163.

Yue, X., Zhang, Q., Dai, Z., 2017. Near-infrared light-activatable polymeric nanoformulations for combined therapy and imaging of cancer. Adv. Drug Deliv. Rev. 115, 155–170.

Zhang, X., Zhang, X., Yang, B., Hui, J., Liu, M., Liu, W., et al., 2014. PEGylation and cell imaging applications of AIE based fluorescent organic nanoparticles via ring-opening reaction. Polym. Chem. 5, 689–693.

Zhang, X., Kurimoto, A., Frank, N.L., Harbron, E.J., 2018. Controlling photoswitching via pcFRET in conjugated polymer nanoparticles. J. Phys. Chem. C 122, 22728–22737.

Zhang, D., Hu, M., Yuan, X., Wu, Y., Hu, X., Xu, S., et al., 2019a. Engineering self-calibrating nanoprobes with two-photon activated fluorescence resonance energy transfer for ratiometric imaging of biological selenocysteine. ACS Appl. Mater. Interfaces 11, 17722–17729.

Zhang, Q., Qu, D.-H., Tian, H., 2019b. Photo-regulated supramolecular polymers: shining beyond disassembly and reassembly. Adv. Opt. Mater. 7, 1900033.

Zhao, M., Li, B., Wang, P., Lu, L., Zhang, Z., Liu, L., et al., 2018. Supramolecularly engineered NIR-II and upconversion nanoparticles in vivo assembly and disassembly to improve bioimaging. Adv. Mater. 30, 1804982.

Zhao, Y., Ma, Y., Lin, W., 2019. A near-infrared and two-photon ratiometric fluorescent probe with a large Stokes shift for sulfur dioxide derivatives detection and its applications in vitro and in vivo. Sens. Actuators B Chem. 288, 519–526.

Zhu, C., Liu, L., Yang, Q., Lv, F., Wang, S., 2012. Water-soluble conjugated polymers for imaging, diagnosis, and therapy. Chem. Rev. 112, 4687–4735.

Zhu, H., Li, J., Qi, X., Chen, P., Pu, K., 2018a. Oxygenic hybrid semiconducting nanoparticles for enhanced photodynamic therapy. Nano Lett. 18, 586–594.

Zhu, S., Hu, Z., Tian, R., Yung, B.C., Yang, Q., Zhao, S., et al., 2018b. Repurposing cyanine NIR-I dyes accelerates clinical translation of near-infrared-II (NIR-II) bioimaging. Adv. Mater. 30, 1802546.

Zhu, X.-Y., Yao, H.-W., Fu, Y.-J., Guo, X.-F., Wang, H., 2019. Effect of substituents on Stokes shift of BODIPY and its application in designing bioimaging probes. Anal. Chim. Acta 1048, 194–203.

Zhuang, W., Yang, L., Ma, B., Kong, Q., Li, G., Wang, Y., et al., 2019. Multifunctional two-photon AIE luminogens for highly mitochondria-specific bioimaging and efficient photodynamic therapy. ACS Appl. Mater. Interfaces 11, 20715–20724.
Zou, J., Lu, H., Zhao, X., Li, W., Guan, Y., Zheng, Y., et al., 2018. A multi-functional fluorescent probe with aggregation-induced emission characteristics: mitochondrial imaging, photodynamic therapy and visualizing therapeutic process in zebrafish model. Dye. Pigm 151, 45–53.

CHAPTER

Polymeric nanoparticles used in tissue engineering

7

Najam ul Hassan, Iqra Chaudhery, Asim. ur.Rehman and Naveed Ahmed
Department of Pharmacy, Quaid-i-Azam University, Islamabad, Pakistan

7.1 Introduction

Tissue engineering (TE) is a discipline that includes biotechnology, bioengineering, and medicinal aspects that involves production of various tissues and cells substituents. It includes various ranges of different materials including polymeric, metallic, and carbon-based structures. These types of substances have power to generate new tissues, repair previous ones, and maintain normal physiological functions of respective tissue and organs (Bakhshandeh et al., 2017). Different kinds of scaffold with various types of cells, along with biological growth factors (GFs) are utilized in TE (Howard et al., 2008). Selection of scaffolds is one of the most important steps in TE along with particular mechanical, physical along with biological properties. A scaffold acts as a time limited architectural, functional, and foreign entity to natural environment. Scaffold disappears once that function has been fulfilled, leaving behind a viable purely normal biological system. Consequently, many materials used in TE are biodegradable, biocompatible and are intended for performing specific objectives (Chen and Liu, 2016; Gurtner et al., 2007). Two basic mechanisms for TE are directly seeding of cells and GFs in scaffold matrix, which is layed down as base for cell culturing and expansion (Fig. 7.1). Furthermore, in second method the Scaffolds themselves behave as GFs, which are implanted in cells throughout tissues matrix (Chen and Liu, 2016).

The human body has a restricted capability to auto regenerate its organs and tissues to retain integrity in most important medical disorders, including tissue dysfunction or devastating deficits (Gurtner et al., 2007, 2008). There is an ever-increasing problem of trauma, degenerative diseases, and congenital abnormalities. Therefore, to develop new biological therapeutics for diverse range of currently intractable diseases, can be regenerative medicine and applied TE as a promising tool. There is a need of research practice to assist and accelerate regenerative procedure by initiating inherited healing potential of patient or alternatively replacing the deteriorated tissues, biological damaged, and lost body fragments (Mao and Mooney, 2015). Such therapeutic strategies adjust physiological conditions in a spatial and temporal manner by mimicking normal mechanisms of tissue repair and regeneration in different parts of the human body (Varner and Nelson, 2014). Even

Advances in Polymeric Nanomaterials for Biomedical Applications. DOI: https://doi.org/10.1016/B978-0-12-814657-6.00005-7

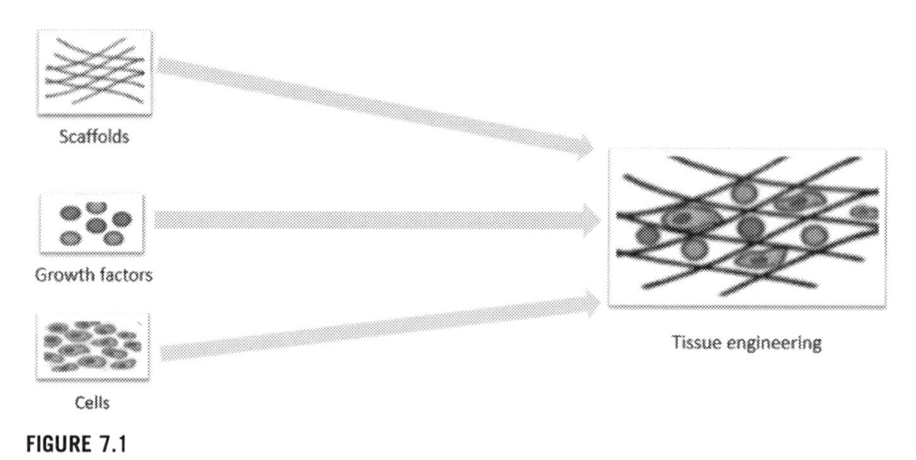

FIGURE 7.1

Components of tissue engineering.

though creating tissue constructs that could serve as an integral part of clinical toolbox, bold steps have been taken but still several of these engineered tissues are not able to completely complement the functional properties of their congenital counterparts. The poor quantitative considerations of adaptive responsive process that change architectural engineered tissues involved in vivo transplantation are responsible for failure to completely match the functional properties (Urciuolo et al., 2013). Living tissues are made up of several repeating units, which are hierarchically assembled across various length scales and retain well-defined three-dimensional (3D) micro architectural characteristics and tissue definite functional properties (Fig. 7.2). Nano-sized and micron tissue modules have got much attention due to their rapidly growing field of interest, and subsequently, this ongoing technological boom can be used in TE (Urciuolo et al., 2013; Rubbens et al., 2008). Alongside with living materials (fillers), such modules are applied to assist as building blocks for generation of large tissue grafts or whole organ implants through "bottom up" approach or can repair wounded tissues at sites of injury (Liu and Gartner, 2012). Considering these applications, it is crucial to summarize not only the structural organization but also the molecular and cellular composition of inborn tissue to increase biological performance. Therefore the total therapeutic outcomes of such engineered tissues build up upon in vivo transplantation (Rubbens et al., 2008). These modular tissues could also be valuable when utilized at sites of injury as injectable living micro tissues repair (Urciuolo et al., 2013).

Even though biotechnology is not yet available that can produce complex organs de novo (Soto Gutierrez et al., 2012), rising evidence recommended that the body's innate strength of regeneration may be augmented by replacing sections of tissue and increasing regenerative cascade (Lee et al., 2010; Feinberg, 2012). Current approach for TE usually involves ex vivo enlargement of multi potential cell populations, for example, mesenchymal stem cells (MSCs), involves

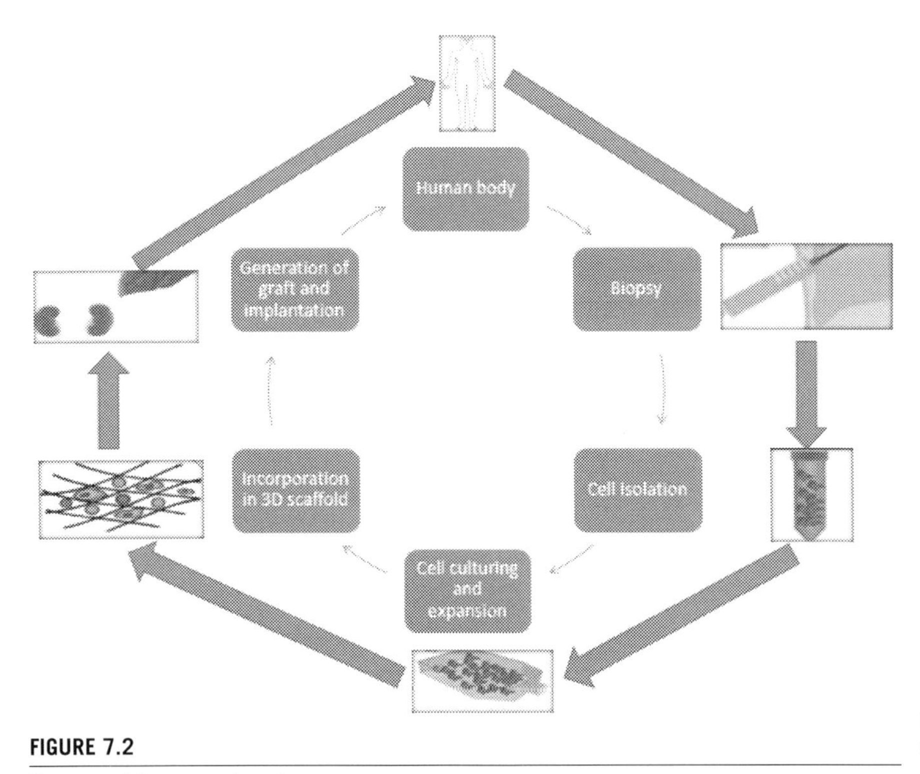

FIGURE 7.2

Process of tissue engineering.

their transplantation into damaged areas (Griffith and Naughton, 2002). Because of their distinctive regenerative potential and immunomodulatory characteristics, MSCs grip great ability in TE and reconstructive therapies. They are not only directly involved in regeneration and wound healing but also have modulating immunogenic reaction to transplants by host foreign body (Hanson et al., 2014). Based on a biodegradable 3D matrix that provides requisite extracellular environment, such cells are usually transplanted within a biomaterial cell construct. For cell-driven tissue development and regeneration, it involves chemical and physical cues (Griffith and Naughton, 2002; Dawson and Oreffo, 2008; Fisher and Mauck, 2013). Further, numerous biological (e.g., a poor knowledge of underlying mechanisms), regulatory (e.g., cost and safety), and technical (e.g., large-scale expansion of stem cells) hurdles linking the use of engineered constructs for human therapeutics and exogenously manipulated stem cells are yet to be controlled (Li et al., 2017; Williams, 2014). Similarly, in cascade of wound healing events, blood clot serving as a natural polymeric scaffold, this kind of matrices must have a desirable shape that provides functionality and supports tissue regrowth until adequate new tissue is formed (Mir et al., 2018). Recently, progress of regenerative biomaterials has promptly evolved to permit sequestration and limited release of GFs that work in concert with materials to achieve tailored biological properties and improved functionalities, which, in a precise and near physiological fashion, can control stem cell fate under niche mimicking, recognizable conditions both in vitro and in vivo (Laurencin et al., 2014). Clinical benefits of bioengineering technologies, based to some extent on the use of biomaterials, in an increasing number of patients place exponentially growing demands on scaffolding materials. Search for an "excellent" TE template has remained a research hotspot as rapidly growing multidisciplinary area of TE continues to advance, along with its intertwined field of "regenerative medicine" (Marino et al., 2015). Although structural, mechanical, and biochemical information coded within natural extracellular matrix (ECM) directs design of new kinds of TE templates. Unfortunately, the network architecture and biological properties of currently existing porous synthetic scaffolds fail to achieve the standards for formation of a complex human tissue (Fong et al., 2012). To facilitate their translation into clinical settings, regenerative biomaterials must be not only effective but also cost operative to support larger number of patients (Holzapfel et al., 2013; Fisher and Mauck, 2013). Focusing on TE, we utilized our wasted freely available building blocks, such as natively derived bio macromolecules to make biomaterials, perfect synthetic tissue template for this purpose (Renth and Detamore, 2012). Some therapeutic biomaterials may be developed from human blood and are used in clinical situations require great fibrinogen content, platelet rich formulations because they contain multiple platelets-derived GFs as natural building blocks (Burnouf et al., 2013). Also, through regulation of cell proliferation, migration, gene expression, and regulation of functional homeostasis such properties have a great influence on cell fate (Holzapfel et al., 2013; Mogoşanu and Grumezescu, 2014).

In TE, one of the most proficient parts is the ability to produce numbers of cells and capability of those cells to maintain, correct phenotype, perform specific biological functions, and differentiate. For instance, in correct organization (a protein based matrix such as collagen in bone), cells necessarily produce an ECM, release cytokines and further signaling molecules, and interact with neighboring cells/tissues (Fitzpatrick and McDevitt, 2015). Primary cells are mature cells of a specific tissue form that are collected from explants material eliminated by surgical method. Primary cells are extremely needed with respect to immunological compatibility but usually they are distinguished as post mitotic cells. It means their proliferation potential is low and no longer has the ability to divide. This may be compounded by ability of some cell types to distinguish in ex vivo cultivation and express an incorrect phenotype, for example, particular chondrocytes in culture often produce fibro cartilage as opposed to hyaline cartilage. This has motivated studies to find and develop substitute cell sources for TE approaches, and limitations of primary cells obtained from explanted tissues stem cells may represent an answer (Meeson et al., 2019). Stem cells are indistinguishable cells that can multiply and have capacity to both self renovate and differentiate to one or more kinds of specialized cells. It should be made wider and applicable to a biological function that could be tempted in a range of cell kinds, involving differentiated cells, rather than a single unit. Stem cells potentially can provide a virtually inexhaustible cell source for TE. Recent research is focused on stimulating stem cell differentiation to needed-lineages and cleansing of consequent cells. It is confirmed that there is no remaining carcinogenic potential in cell population and implantation in a procedure that will substitute or augment function of injured and diseased tissues. First step is choosing most suitable stem cell to form the needed tissue (Sada and Tumbar, 2013). Everyone carries adult stem cells around their own source of stem cells that is found in several tissue niches with liver, bone marrow, brain, skin, and also in circulation. For some stem cell kinds, difficulties with accessibility (e.g., not easy or desirable to tap stem cells in brain), low frequency (e.g., in bone marrow, there is roughly 1 stem cell per 100,000 cells and this might also be affected by age and disease), poor growth, and restricted diversity potential may bound their applicability to TE (Vats et al., 2005). Embryonic stem cells can be evolved from human blastocysts, their capability for multiline age differentiation may be exploited like any tissue, or cell type could be produced on demand in laboratory for cell-based therapies. Human eosinophils stem cells were eventually evolved, providing an incredible enhancement for TE (Place et al., 2009).

Incredible potential of living tissues for auto regeneration might be diminished by innately low regenerative capacity of certain tissues, by an age-related decline in quality and number of host stem cell/progenitor populations, or by negative influence of inflammation on wound repair (Place et al., 2009). Determination to compensate for this reduced healing capacity, TE has been recognized as a potential therapeutic option to reconstruct several of biological methods that occur in tissue development and in natural wound healing cascade in microcosms (Shepherd et al., 2008; Feinberg, 2012). For this reason a harmonious combination of a scaffold/supporting materials, adequate target cells, and growth stimulating bioactive factors is used to promote regeneration of damaged tissues or to replace failing or malfunctioning organs (Harrison et al., 2014). Therefore tissue-engineered constructs have to mimic a certain degree of native complexity of a tissue to assist in restoration of full structure and functionality of tissue. This approach is the first medical therapy wherein engineered tissues can potentially become fully integrated into patient, thus conferring a permanent cure for a diverse range of diseases that are not curable today (Kaur et al., 2019).

Main role of biomaterials in TE is because of their inert, biocompatible, and biodegradable nature. Transitory mechanical provision is provided and mass transport to boost cell adhesion, differentiation, and proliferation to govern shape and size of regenerated tissue (Khan and Tanaka, 2018). Furthermore, biomaterials, typically termed as scaffolds with spatiotemporal accuracy, might present chemical and physical signals in modulation of cell performance and function. They created correct tissue regeneration, as an ECM involves intrinsic signals essential to control and communicate basic cells in TE (Kratochvil et al., 2019). Inert structures working to concept new innovative template for TE, and integrated sense of a structure, actively involved in development of engineered regenerated tissues (Gu et al., 2014). Therefore biomaterial templates in TE should be properly replaced with natively deposited ECM to form new tissues. Newly designed tissue of interest, in the host environment, should be capable to improve manipulate new cells, function, and behavior of desired tissue formation (Aamodt and Grainger, 2016). Any case of TE scaffolds pursue to imitate natural ECM, at least partially, and to form a favorable nano environment to assist and prompt tissue formation (Atala et al., 2012).

7.2 Properties of polymer suitable for tissue engineering

Polymer selected should have compatibility with the body, interacting surfaces and should be safe in usage. Biocompatibility is vital, although it is important to note that "biocompatibility" is not an intrinsic property of a material, but depends on biologic environment that exists with respect to tissue reaction (Berthing et al., 2011). Polymer is designed into material to stimulate response of cell at molecular level. They must have particular type of interactions with cell and initiate cell to undergo adhesion, multiplication, growth along with structuring and processing of ECM (Basu et al., 2016). For biocompatible scaffolds formation, it is reported that single polymer cannot meet all specifications of required systems, thus multi-polymer system has been constructed for optimal biomedical scaffolds. Polymers are cheap in nature and mainly synthetic polymers due to specific properties impart to their structure are relatively higher in cost as compared with the natural polymers. Inertness makes them useful entity for TE along with safety (Koo and Yamada, 2016). Polymers has been classified into natural and synthetic polymers as discussed below while the differences among both classes are discussed in Table 7.1.

7.2.1 Natural polymer

Natural polymer materials function as intrinsic templates for cell attachment and growth, and at same time, they could initiate an immune response. Natural polymers consist of highly organized structures containing extracellular substance called lignin, which is capable of binding to cellular receptors. Although they are considered biocompatible yet they have few disadvantages like deficiency in bulk quantity, expansive, and difficulties in processability for scaffold in clinical applications. Additionally, natural polymer's degradation rate may vary as it depends upon enzyme that varies from patient to patient. Different materials used for TE have two main classes; proteins (collagen, albumin, fibrin, keratin, elastin, gelatin, and silk) and polysaccharides [chitosan, alginic acid, cellulose, chondroitin sulfate (CS), and hyaluronic acid (HA)]. Some of these are discussed below.

7.2.1.1 Collagen

Collagen is mostly applied for tissue regeneration of soft tissues (Chu et al., 2017) due to distinctive physicochemical, mechanical, and biological properties

Table 7.1 Differences of natural and synthetic polymers.

	Natural polymers	Synthetic polymers
Definitions	Natural polymers are ones that derived from natural source. It has several advantages and disadvantages. On basis of these we select whether to use natural polymer or not (Berthing et al., 2011; Basu et al., 2016; Koo and Yamada, 2016).	Synthetic polymers are those, which synthesize from monomers with or without use of copolymer by Polymerization or condensation process (Berthing et al., 2011; Basu et al., 2016; Koo and Yamada, 2016).
Advantages	1. They have property of biological recognition, which helps in cell attachment to carry its mechanism (Koo and Yamada, 2016). 2. They are biocompatible 3. Their surfaces are hydrophilic.	1. They have excellent mechanical properties (Koo and Yamada, 2016). 2. They are cheap in cost. 3. Their form and degradation rate can be easily changed accordingly
Disadvantages	1. They have poor mechanical properties (Basu et al., 2016). 2. They are costly in nature 3. They are limited in supply	1. They have less proper cell recognition (Basu et al., 2016). 2. Their surfaces are hydrophobic 3. They are limited in supply
Examples	Proteins, polysaccharides	Poly(alpha esters)

studied in diverse applications. It can be processed in sheet, tubes sponge's foams, nano fibrous powders, fleeces, injectable viscous solution, and dispersions. By various treatments, degradation rate can be altered. For the treatment of exuding diabetic and ulcer wounds, oxidized cellulose in new spongy collagen matrix has been recently introduced in the United States and European market (Law et al., 2017). For accelerated tissue reproduction, degradable collagen sponges have been widely studied as scaffold material due to their outstanding biocompatibility and permeability. As a biodegradable synthetic bone graft replacement, composite of collagen, hydroxyapatite, and tri calcium phosphate (TCP) is used. It is researched as scaffold for musculoskeletal and nervous TE. Drawbacks of collagen include high cost, variable physicochemical properties, easily degradation, risk of infection, and difficult handling process (Baldwin et al., 2018).

7.2.1.2 Albumin

Albumin protein is found abundantly in blood plasma comprising 50% of total plasma mass. Albumin protein is soluble in water and can be degraded in body (Bertholf, 2014). In healthy human, albumin are half of total protein content (3.5–5 g/dL) of plasma. As supporting substance in lungs TE, albumin is inserted on decellularized scaffold for cell tissue interaction and for easy attachment, growth, and differentiation in different type of cells when seeded (Aiyelabegan et al., 2016). Long-term osteogenic differentiation of MSCs can be furnished by albumin tissue scaffold. Albumin has good material properties and compatibility with cell (Li et al., 2014).

7.2.1.3 Fibrin

Fibrin, a compound derived from fibrinogen and thrombin protein and made up of three pairs of peptide chains, is mostly used in scaffold materials (Lai et al., 2012). Extreme biocompatibility, improved cell attachment, and controlled degradation have been shown by fibrin. Fibrin in situ has been utilized to produce injectable scaffolds to restore damaged cardiac and cartilage tissue. To protect cells from forces during application and cell delivery processes, fibrin gel as a cell carrier has been used by increasing cell viability and tissue regeneration (Soleimannejad et al., 2018). Due to fibrin's bioactivity, biocompatibility, biodegradability, and facile processability, it is used for wound healing. It behaves explicitly in skin TE strategies due to its striking skin repair ability: essential healing properties, adjustable to biomaterial design from its fibrinogen, thrombin precursors, and adaptive physicochemical features (Rodrigues et al., 2013).

7.2.1.4 Polysaccharides

When macromolecules monosaccharide units joined by glycosidic linkages, they produce polysaccharides. Distinctive property of cell signals to immune system is possessed by polysaccharides, and mostly, these are synthesized oligosaccharide moieties. They are significant and extensively studied biomaterials due to their biodegradability and ability to produce appropriate structures (Miao et al., 2018).

7.2.1.5 Hyaluronic acid

HA is glycosaminoglycan family member, linear polysaccharide consisting of alternating units of N-acetyl-D-glucosamine and glucuronic acid, found in almost every invertebrate. By promoting mesenchymal and epithelial cell migration, differentiation and enhancing collagen deposition and angiogenesis HA's immunoneutrality and tissue repair can be used (Peter et al., 2010). Due to chemical structure, it is a hydrophilic polymer and its degradation is fast. HA-based scaffolds on basis of increased biocompatibility, biodegradability, and chemical modification can be appropriate for TE and can be prepared in different forms according to preparation techniques such as hydrogels, sponges, cryogels, and injectable hydrogels (Setayeshmehr et al., 2019).

7.2.1.6 Chondroitin sulfate

CS scaffold with chitosan scaffold is implemented for cartilage TE. CS is a biopolymer with a crucial advantage of being biodegradable, biologically compatible, accessible, and versatile (Kwon and Han, 2016). Cartilage specific gene expression is up regulated by CS-based materials in chondrocytes and MSCs, and it assists osteogenic differentiation by enhancing efficacy of bone anabolic GFs.

CS-based material stimulate wound healing process and regeneration of skin defects. CS can be used in construction of high toughness gels by acquiring a double-network structure. For affluent replacement and restoration of impaired cartilage, bone, skin, and nerve tissues, CS-based materials would be beneficial (Cheung et al., 2015).

7.2.1.7 Chitosan

The word chitosan is originated from chitin. Chitosan is a cationic one-dimensional polysaccharide that comprises D-glucosamine linked B (1, 4) with randomly positioned N-acetyl-glucosamine groups as per the degree of deacetylation of polymer. It is highly biocompatible in vivo. Currently, investigation is being held to estimate potential of utilizing injectables in accordance with chitosan and its derivative products as a scaffold material for variety of TE that includes bones, skin, and cartilage. Permeability of chitosan scaffold can be monitored that may affect mechanical properties (Szekalska et al., 2016).

7.2.1.8 Alginic acid

Alginic acid, a synthetic polysaccharide linear copolymer with homopolymeric blocks of (1–4)-linked-β-D-mannuronate (M) and its C-5 epimer α-L-guluronate (G) residues, respectively, covalently linked together in different sequences or blocks. It is a biocompatible material due to high functionality of alginic acid. For wound dressing and grow new tissues, it is applied as cell transplantation vehicles. Advantages of natural polymer are abundantly available, harmless, biocompatible, biodegradable/bioreabsorbable, and synergic with bioactive components (Sabir et al., 2009) as mentioned in Table 7.1.

7.2.2 Synthetic polymers

7.2.2.1 Poly alpha esters

Saturated aliphatic polyesters are oldest and used often in the field of bone TE. This family includes poly(lactic acid) (PLA), poly(glycolic acid) (PGA), poly (lactic-*co*-glycolate) (PLGA), and other copolymers. PLA, PGA, and PLGA are generally used substances for bone scaffold application. PLA has three forms D PLA, L PLA (PLLA), and blend of D, L PLA (PDLLA). The basic chemical structure of all aliphatic polyester materials is same but difference in pendent groups discussed in Table 7.2, which contributed differences in molecular weight, crystallinity, and directly affecting degradation kinetics. Thus ratio of PLA and PGA present in the compounds decides degradation rate of PLA and PGA copolymer (Ojeda, 2013).

7.2.2.2 Poly(glycolic acid)

PGA is a hard thermoplastic material, with 45%–55% crystallinity, high-melting point, high glass transition temperature, and high degree of crystallization.

Table 7.2 Properties of polymers.

Polymers	Thermal and mechanical properties			Degradation properties		Processing and applications	
	M T[a] (°C)	T_g[b] (°C)	T M[c] (GPa)	Time (months)	Products	Solvent	Applications
Poly(lactic acid) (PLA)	173–178	60–65	1.5–2.7	12–18	Lactic acid	Chloroform Dioxane Acetone DCM[d] Ethyl acetate	Fracture fixation, suture anchors Meniscus repairs Interference screws (Snyder et al., 2015)
Poly glycolic acid (PGA)	225–230	35–40	5–7	3–4	Glycolic acid	Acetone DCM Chloroform Hexafluoroisopropanol	Suture anchors Meniscus repairs Medical devices Drug delivery (Chafran et al., 2019)
Poly (caprolactone) PCL	58–63	~60	0.4 0.6	>24	Caproic acid	DCM Chloroform Hexafluoroisopropanol Toluene	Suture coating Dental and orthopedic implants (Valderrama et al., 2019)
Poly(lactic-*co*-glycolic) PLGA (50/50)	Amorphous	50 55	1.4 2.8	3 6	D, L Lactic Acid and Glycolic acid	DCM Chloroform Ethyl acetate Hexafluoroisopropanol	Suture, drug delivery (Valderrama et al., 2019; Patel et al., 2011)
PLGA (85/15)	Amorphous	50 55	1.4 2.8	3 6	D, L Lactic Acid and Glycolic acid	THF[e] Acetone DCM Chloroform Ethyl acetate	suture anchors Interference screws ACL[f] reconstruction (Patel et al., 2011)

PLGA (90/10)	Amorphous	50 55		<3	D, L Lactic Acid and Glycolic acid	THF Acetone DCM Chloroform Ethyl acetate	Artificial skin Wound healing Suture (Valderrama et al., 2019)
Poly(propylene fumarate) PPF	30–50	~60	2 3	>24	Fumaric Acid, propylene glycol	THF Acetone Ethanol	Orthopedic implants Dental Foam coatings Drug delivery (Valderrama et al., 2019)

[a] *Melting point.*
[b] *Glass transition temperature.*
[c] *Tensile modulus.*
[d] *Dichloromethane.*
[e] *Tetrahydrofuran.*
[f] *Acyl-homoserine lactone.*

Comparison with PLA, it is acidic and more hydrophilic. PGA can modify to foam and porous scaffolds. The type of processing techniques can affect deterioration properties, and in case of PGA, careful control of processing conditions is required as it is very sensitive to degradation. To fabricate PGA-based porous scaffolds, methods like solvent casting, leaching, and compression molding are used as referred in Table 7.2 (Ojeda, 2013). Fiber of PGA is used in sutures due to intense strength and modulus of PGA. Copolymerization in some monomers reduces stiffness in fibers. Degradation products are natural metabolites that are used in bone TE and medical application. Glycolic acid, which is degradation product, is absorbable at high concentration and will cause tissue damage by increased concentration of localized acid. Research is also conducted on development of bone fixation device (Valderrama et al., 2019).

7.2.2.3 Poly(lactic acid)

PLA is synthesized by cyclic dimer of lactic acid existing in two optical isomer forms: Naturally occurring isomers D and L lactate and synthetically DL lactide that is mixture of D lactide and L lactide. Homopolymer L lactide is a semicrystalline polymer. It can be used in load-bearing applications such as sutures and orthopedic fixation due to high tensile strength, elongation, and modulus (Chafran et al., 2019). For 3D scaffolds creation by solution casting, gel casting, solvent casting and particulate leaching, high pressure gas foaming, particulate, and electrospinning, PLA and their derivatives can be used. Copolymerization of aliphatic polyesters can intensify mechanical and physical properties. Lactic acid and glycolic acid copolymers have been explored since several years. Amount of each comonomer decides its degradation rate (Patel and Atala, 2011).

7.2.2.4 Polyanhydrides

Polyanhydrides that are aromatic, aliphatic, or a mixture of both components with evident biocompatibility and excellent characteristics such as controlled release characteristics are used in TE. However, these are hydrolytically unstable. Polyanhydrides are not widely used in orthopedic implantation. Injectable photo-crosslinked polyanhydrides due to low bearing and mechanical properties but can be used in renovation of irregularly shaped bone imperfection or soft tissue repairs. Advantages of scaffolds are nonpoisonous, injectability, low degradation, and high compatibility, and various properties can be modified during manufacturing of scaffolds (Snyder et al., 2015).

7.2.2.5 Polyorthoesters

Being amorphous, hydrophobic, and biodegradable polymers, polyorthoesters have many specific features like surface wearing down mechanism (removal of upper surface gradually deposing new surfaces by deformation) and pH sensitive degeneration rate (Lyu and Untereker, 2009). They are hydrophobic and easily dissolved in organic solvents like chloroform, methylene chloride, and dioxane. Through surface erosion, these polymers perform heterogeneous degradation. Variation in mechanical properties of poly(orthoesters) can be done by selecting starting materials with different compositions and molecular weights as mentioned in Table 7.2 (Sander et al., 2004).

7.2.2.6 Polyphosphazene

Phosphazene polymer constitutes a great diversity of performance materials possessing a backbone of alternating nitrogen and phosphorous atoms (Zhang et al., 2017). Polyphosphazene is mainly studied as a substance for blood connecting devices due to its high blood compatibility. Its metabolites are natural and harmless (Guo and Ma, 2014). All members of this class were homopolymer comprising all phosphorous atoms in polymer chain with same kind of organic substituents. For TE applications and for drug delivery, polyphosphazene is more suitable. Biodegradable polyphosphazene has likely to be used for bone TE, and their amino acid ester group are brilliant biodegradable materials with amino acids as decomposition products (Deng et al., 2010).

There are also some other synthetic polymers, poly(ethylene glycol), poly (propylene fumarate), polyphosphoesters, poly(ester amides), etc.

7.3 Method of preparation of polymers for tissue engineering

Three production methods are commonly used for producing polymeric nanofibers for TE which are: phase separation, electrospinning, and self-assembly. Every technique has inherent benefits and drawbacks regarded to TE.

7.3.1 Electrospinning

Electrospinning is one of the simple and economical techniques as compared with other available practices. Equipment involved is of high-voltage source along with collector and syringe pump. Polymer fibers obtained from this technique are greater than 3 nm, and some also exceeds 5 nm (Wang et al., 2019). The polymer solution is placed under the needle tip dipped in solution. Electric field is applied with help of a source of high voltage, which induces charge at polymer causing charge repulsion into solution. These repulsive forces overcome surface tension and cause the start of jet. As soon as this jet moves across solvent, it will get evaporated and polymer fiber would be collected. This method is used to prepare many natural and synthetic polymers into fibers of greater length. It produces stable scaffolds utilized within TE (Ifegwu and Anyakora, 2018). Reneker and Chun explained stable electrospinning jet as actually made up of four parts: collection, base, jet, and splay. In lower region, from needle jet appears to form a cone called Taylor cone (Reneker et al., 2007). Shape of base depends upon force of electric field and surface tension of liquid; if electric field is durable enough jets might be evicted from surfaces, which are necessarily flat. They are being more conducive to jet formation with solutions of higher conductivity, jet charging take place at the base. Polymer jet is accelerated and stretched by electric forces, which cause diameter to lessen as its length upsurges. Furthermore, with high vapor pressure solvents might start to evaporate, which cause decreased jet diameter and velocity (Shin et al., 2001).

7.3.2 Self-assembly

Self assembly is spontaneous arrangement of nanomaterials definite structures depending upon shape and composition of nanomaterials. This is done under specific heat and kinetic movements which allow localized and definite interactions like hydrogen bonding inter molecular forces, lipophilic interactions, and pie to pie interactions. These interactions decrease energy of molecules and make them stable structure. It is one of most important technique because of cheap and higher scale production. Both native and synthetic polymers utilized for grounding with nanomaterials (Berbezier and Maurizio, 2015). To nanofibers fabrication, self-assembly is a bottom up technique that depends on weak noncovalent interactions to construct nanofibers from trivial molecules, peptides, nucleic acids, and proteins (Sun et al., 2017). This approach can be utilized for assembling nanofibers in vivo for tissue repair to build an injectable scaffold. Although this technique generates nanofibers of least scale (5–8 nm), fabrication procedure is a challenging approach, restricted to a limited polymers, and could only make tiny fibers with lengths of one to several mm (Sun et al., 2017). A common building block for self assembled nanofibers is peptide amphiphilic (PAs) and utilized for over a decade. PAs involves a hydrophobic aliphatic tail connected by an amide bond to a hydrophilic peptide arrangement of four or more amino acids. Stimulation of PA assembly could be controlled by changing ion content of PA solution that results in a gel-like structure (Castelletto et al., 2009). When electrostatic repulsion among molecules is counter-balanced, peptides will suddenly, with hydrophobic tails clustered in center, arranged into cylindrical, micelle-like structures (Qiu et al., 2018).

7.3.3 Phase inversion

Phase inversion is a technique used for preparation of nanomaterials by fabrication of artificial membrane. This preparation is done by entrapment of different nanomaterials within a membrane matrix. The phase inversion works on principal of phase transition due to change of concentration of surfactant with respect to the surroundings. Common technique used for phase inversion is based on different affinities of polymer/surfactants with temperature. As there is a positive charge on nonionic surfactant and it has property of hydrophilic at lower temperature, it can lead to oil in water emulsion. Water in oil emulsion can be obtained, as there is a negative charge on nonionic surfactant and property of hydrophobic nature at higher temperature. At moderate temperature, charge become zero and homogeneous micro emulsion is obtained (Esfahani et al., 2018).

Phase separation is a procedure to make porous polymer membranes and scaffolds by persuading parting of a polymer solution into a polymer poor phase and a polymer rich phase. Currently, technique has been used to generate polymeric nano fibrous constructs from aliphatic polyesters. Matrices appear to have up to 98.5% porosity and fiber diameters extending from 50 to 500 nm. To generate matrices, a polymer, for example PLLA, is dissolved in a solvent, like tetrahydrofuran, and quickly cooled to persuade phase separation. Subsequently, solvent is replaced with water, and construct is freeze-dried (Berro et al., 2015). Nanofibers could be attained by selecting suitable gelling temperature. Higher gelling temperatures appear to cause microfiber formation, nevertheless with decreased gelling temperatures diameter eliminated to nanofibers dimensions. Variations of this approach may be utilized with controlled and carefully designed macro porous architectures to generate nano fibrous constructs. Initially, approach was established with PLLA or PLGA, but more newly, practice has been completed with polyhydroxyalkanoate, chitosan, gelatin, and gelatin/apatite composites. Benefits of this technique are that it does not need specialized equipment, and there is some disparity among batches. Furthermore, constructs can be formed in a mold to attain a definite geometry (Yang et al., 2017).

7.4 Polymer scaffolds used in tissue engineering

7.4.1 Natural and synthetic polymers for scaffolds

Polymers for TE scaffolds has been selected on the basis of their hydrophilicity/hydrophobicity, solubility, shape material chemistry, molecular weight and structure, water absorption, degradation, lubricity, surface energy, and erosion mechanism. Due to qualities such as high surface to volume ratio, very small pore size, biodegradability, and mechanical property with advantages of biocompatibility, versatility, and biological properties in TE and organ substitution (Chopade et al., 2019). Scaffold materials can be divided into synthetic, biologic, degradable, and nondegradable depending on properties such as composition, structure, and arrangement of their macromolecules. It can be categorized into ceramics, glasses, polymers, etc. as biomaterials can be applied naturally occurring polymers and synthetic biodegradable polymers (Rodríguez Vázquez et al., 2015). Naturally occurring polymers have bioactive properties that lead to better interactions with cells and enhance performance of cells in biological system (Porzionato et al., 2018). Classification of natural polymers can be done as proteins (silk, fibrinogen, elastin, keratin, actin, and myosin), polysaccharides (cellulose, amylase, dextran, chitin, and glycosaminoglycan) (Dhandayuthapani et al., 2011). Synthetic biomaterial provides facilities of restoration of structure and function of damaged tissues. They have been extensively used in biomedical field yet to be paid through their ideal porosity, degradation time; mechanical features, and cheap production methods with long shelf time. Their physicochemical and mechanical properties can be comparable to biological tissues owing to appropriate tensile strength, elastic modulus, and degradation rate (Chopade et al., 2019). They are used in TE as PLA and PGA.

7.4.2 Three-dimensional polymeric scaffolds

These can be used to provide mechanical strength, interconnected porosity, varying surface chemistry, and unique geometries to be used in tissue regeneration, which is essential to act as a 3D template for tissue ingrowths (Malliaras et al., 2013). Designs of scaffold have includes meshes, fibers, sponges, foams, etc. chosen because of their uniform cell distribution, diffusion of nutrients, and growth of organized cell communities. Fabrication techniques involve use of heat and/or pressure to polymer or dissolving it in an organic solvent to get desired shape, which depends upon bulk surface properties of material and proposed function of scaffold. 3D scaffolds must be designed, fabricated, and utilized to regenerate tissue similar to original tissue or organ to be replaced in order to repair and regenerate damaged tissue and organs (Nooeaid et al., 2012).

7.4.3 Porous scaffold

Polymeric porous scaffolds have higher porosity having interconnected pore network. Their porous network simulates ECM formation, for example, sponge or foam porous scaffold have been used especially for growth of bone or organ vascularization (Neto and Ferreira, 2018). Foam polymeric scaffold provides a physical surface that inhibits growth of adherent contact cells, improves nutrient transport, and limit cluster to pore size of foam clearing clusters that can develop a necrotic center (Chen and Liu, 2016). Foams can be made to form either random or oriented pore architectures, which depends on choice of solvent and phase separating conditions improvement in porous scaffold properties like increase in interconnected pore network is required for development of artificial blood vessels or peripheral nerve growth in bodies. Pore sizes vary for different cells and tissues. Porous controlled release systems have pores, large enough to enable good diffusion of drug. As porous scaffolding materials PLLA, PGA, PLGA, poly(caprolactone) (PCL), PDLLA, and PEE based on PEO and PBT are used (Ayala Caminero et al., 2017). Latest development in this field includes creating porous scaffolds composed of nano and microscale biodegradable fibers by electrospinning (Kamaly et al., 2016).

7.4.4 Hydrogel scaffold

Hydrogels have been playing an ever-increasing role in the field of TE as scaffolds to guide growth of new tissues and in biomedical field for controlled drug delivery (Mantha et al., 2019). They have advantages of biocompatibility, cell controlled degradability, and intrinsic cellular interaction but may exhibit batch variations with narrow limited range of mechanical properties. They have structural similarity to macromolecular-based components in body so they are considered biocompatible. It is commonly believed that degradation rates of tissue scaffolds must be matched at rate of various cellular processes in order to optimize tissue regeneration (Dhandayuthapani et al., 2011). Therefore degradation behavior of all biodegradable hydrogels should be well defined, reproducible, and tunable via hydrogel chemistry or structure. Biocompatible hydrogels are currently used in cartilage wound healing, bone regeneration, wound dressings, as carriers for drug delivery. Hydrogel with GF can act directly to support development and diversity of cells in newly formed tissues (Zhu and Marchant, 2011). Hydrogels are mostly good for enhancing cell migration, angiogenesis, high water content, and rapid nutrient diffusion. Collagens are examples of hydrogel forming polymers of natural origin, gelatin, fibrin, HA, alginate, and chitosan. Synthetic polymers are PLA, poly (propylene fumarate)-derived copolymers, polyethylene glycol (PEG) derivatives, and PVA (Lev and Seliktar, 2018).

7.4.5 Fibrous scaffold

Development of nanofibers has improved scope for fabricating scaffolds that can potentially mimic architecture of natural human tissue at nanometer scale. Electrospinning is most extensively studied approach, also appears to display most promising outcomes for TE applications. Nanofibers manufactured by self-assembly and phase separation have had comparatively limited studies that discovered their application as scaffolds for TE. High surface area to volume ratio of nanofibers combined with their microporous structure favors cell adhesion, proliferation, migration, and differentiation, all of which are highly desired properties for TE applications. Nanofibers used as scaffolds for musculoskeletal TE including bone, cartilage, ligament, skeletal muscle, skin, vascular, neural TE, and as vehicle for controlled delivery of drugs including proteins and DNA (Liu et al., 2013). Natural polymers and synthetic polymers discovered for fabrication of nanofibers, for example, collagen, gelatin, chitosan, HA, silk fibroin, PLA, poly(urethane), PCL, PLGA, poly(ethyl vinyl acetate), and PLLA are fibrous scaffold in biomedical application. Blending (or mixing) approach is a common choice for nanofibers functionalization. Though, most of polymer nanofibers do not possess any specific functional groups, and they must be specifically functionalized for successful applications (Dhandayuthapani et al., 2011).

7.4.6 Microsphere scaffold

Microsphere grounded TE scaffold designs, in recent years, have gained substantial attention. Microsphere scaffolds have longitudinal extension and time-based duration control that provides rigid gradients for interfacial TE. Impact of nanotechnology on scaffold design and possibility of continued discharge formulations of GFs through microspheres are presentation of promising progresses (Gupta et al., 2017). Particle aggregation methodology is recommended in bilayered scaffolds formation for osteochondral TE in order to attain an enhanced integrative bone and cartilage alignment. PLGA microsphere as porous scaffolds matrix of trabecular bone array have represented potential for bone TE. Sintered microsphere matrix was given assurance to bone regeneration scaffold. The benefit of sintered microsphere structure is its pore interconnectivity and desirable 3D pore size. Gel microsphere matrix and sintered microsphere matrix prepared using random packing of PLGA microspheres to make 3D porous structures for bone regeneration. For bone applications, fabrication of polymer ceramic matrices composite microspheres is utilized. Chitosan microsphere scaffolds generated for osteochondral and cartilage TE (Dhandayuthapani et al., 2011).

7.4.7 Polymer bioceramic composite scaffold

Their mechanical and physiological needs of host tissue by governing volume fraction, morphology, and arrangement of reinforcing phase is significant for creation of complex material, which is suited for TE (Chen and Liu, 2016). Ceramics in fabricating implants can be categorized as nonabsorbable (relatively inert), biodegradable or resorbable (inert), and bioactive or surface reactive (semi inert). The inert bio ceramics are alumina, zirconia, silicone nitrides, and carbons. Certain glass ceramics and dense hydroxyapatite (HAP) are semiinert (bio reactive) and resorbable ceramics. Examples are aluminum calcium phosphate, coralline, plaster of Paris, HAP, and TCP. Ceramics are recognized for their good compatibility, corrosion resistance, and high compression resistance. Shortcomings of ceramics involve brittleness, low fracture strength, difficulty to fabricate, low mechanical reliability, lack of resilience, and high density. Blending of polymers and inorganic phases form composite materials with enhanced mechanical properties due to inherent higher rigidity and power of inorganic material (Masuelli, 2013). Then, addition of bioactive phases to bio resorbable polymers can change polymer deprivation behavior of scaffolds (Baino et al., 2015). Due to its excellent mechanical properties and osteoconductivity highly porous polymer/ceramic, composite scaffolding appears to be a capable substrate for bone TE. PLGA/HAP composite scaffold has excellent biocompatibility with hard tissues, high osteoconductivity, and bioactivity. Most important inorganic component of natural bone is bio ceramics, including CP, HAP, and TCP are composite with PLLA, collagen, gelatin, and chitosan are extensively utilized as scaffolding materials for bone repair (Thavornyutikarn et al., 2014).

7.4.8 Cellular scaffold

Cellular tissue matrices could be made by forming artificial scaffolds or by eliminating cellular components from tissues by mechanical and chemical management to yield collagen rich matrices. Such matrices gradually damage implantation and are usually substituted by ECM proteins released by growing in cells (Patel and Atala, 2011). Decellularized biological scaffold was introduced to gain a physiological matrix scaffold that look like of native blood vessels. Cellular bladder matrix has assisted as a scaffold for ingrowths of host bladder walled modules in rats. Since structures of proteins (e.g., collagen and elastin) in cellular matrices are well preserved and normally arranged, mechanical properties of cellular matrices are not considerably diverse from those of natural bladder submucosa. Matrix was made through mechanically and chemically eliminating all cellular components from bladder tissue (Serrano Aroca et al., 2018). The decellularisation process assists similar biomechanical characteristics as similar to native tissues that are essential for long-term functionality of grafts (Edgar et al., 2016). Certainly, derived materials and cellular tissue matrices have potential advantage of biological recognition. TE that has been familiarized is the use of biological/polymeric complex materials as starter matrices. These hybrids can be complex structures, for example, heart valves, invented from decellularized porcine aortic valves, and dip covered with a biodegradable polymer (He and Lu, 2016).

7.5 Applications

7.5.1 Cardiomyocytes tissue engineering

Cardiovascular TE is one of the beneficial use of nanomaterials in last few years. Any part of muscles of heart or myocardium does not receive enough quantity of blood for their proper functioning is said to be myocardial infarction. This deprived condition cause destruction of cardiomyocytes results into condition called arrhythmia, ventricular reconstruction leading to heart failure (Grenadyorov et al., 2020). Previously, heart transplants were the best treatment for patients with last stage of heart failure. It was limited due to limitations of donor hearts and risks associated with hemolytic clot formation. Alternative methods of TE for cardiomyocytes were advancing in this regard. This technique is used to enhance contractility of muscle tissue of heart for efficient working (Grenadyorov et al., 2020). The properties required for nanomaterials in TE of heart are nanoscale fabrication higher surface area to volume ratio and increase in surface roughness, which in turn increases electromechanical properties. Scaffolds used for TE should be having proper mass transfer highly biodegradable at specific rates mediate cell attachment, cell division, electromechanical properties similar to body tissues and can be transformed into different forms. The cardiac TE field has been evolved from last 20 years but more work and effort is required as cardiovascular diseases cannot be treated easily (Kitsara et al., 2017).

Scaffolds used are

1. Synthetic material (PEG and PGA)
2. Natural materials (collagen, gelatin)
3. Nanotubes and nanoparticles (carbon nanotubes)
4. Electrospun scaffolds (poly glycerol sebecate)

Patches are one of other processes for TE of heart. These patches are mostly made up of biodegradable polymers and nonbiodegradable polymers. They make cell to works as single component due to their low level of conductivity Examples are carbon nanofiber-reinforced patch and gold nanofiber-reinforced patch. Injectable scaffolds are used due to the easy procedure and substitute of surgery as they can be administered via catheter or syringe. They are used for anesthetic purposes also for vaccinations, for example, injectable scaffold (Amezcua et al., 2016).

7.5.2 Bone tissue engineering

Bone tissue transplants are one of the most common transplants worldwide. It is done by using cell or tissue from same individual. Various problems related to this procedure are present such as different resorptions, an increases in failures, less blood supply, and donor site issues. These troubles can be solved through use of synthetic biomaterials but these materials cannot be used due to hyper sensitivity and auto immune response (Wang and Yeung, 2017). Bone is composing of 30% organic collagen fibrils and 70% inorganic CaP crystals. It also contains various ions (calcium, zinc, and magnesium) and other molecules. Bone grafting is a process that is started with movement of bone forming cell to area and then it divides into multiple cells along with differentiation into osteoblasts with formation of matrix and remodeling of bone (Neto and Ferreira, 2018) (Fig. 7.3).

Four elements are essential in bone TE

1. Signal from which process starts
2. Host which responds to signal
3. Carrier that can pass on signal as well as act as scaffolds
4. Well-connected host bed (Sundelacruz and Kaplan, 2009).

Substances accustomed bone TE must have high electromechanical characteristics and structural components necessary for reformation of stem cells. Such graphene coatings or fabrication increase scaffolds aspects (differentiations of stem cells, cell adhesion, and multiplication of osteoblasts) (Chocholata et al., 2019). Carbon allotropes are utilized in bone TE. To enhance quality of polymers involves graphene, single-walled nanotubes, multiwalled carbon nanotubes, and ultrashort carbon nanotubes derivatives. Number of inorganic materials is in use innovative kind of TE as tungsten disulfide nanotubes and molybdenum nano platelets. To increases quality of epoxy composites, electro spin fibers, and biodegradable polymers, reinforcing agent is used (Tozzi et al., 2016).

Synthetic polymeric scaffolds are near to eradicate the need of bone grafts for TE applications. This is also a step toward regeneration of bone by nanostructure materials, because they have capability to generate reactions at cellular level (Stratton et al., 2016). For bone regeneration, hydroxyapatite is one of most prominent scaffold materials, because resemblance in structure β-TCP and bioactive glass. Inorganic materials largely comprise squeezing force and osteoconductivity

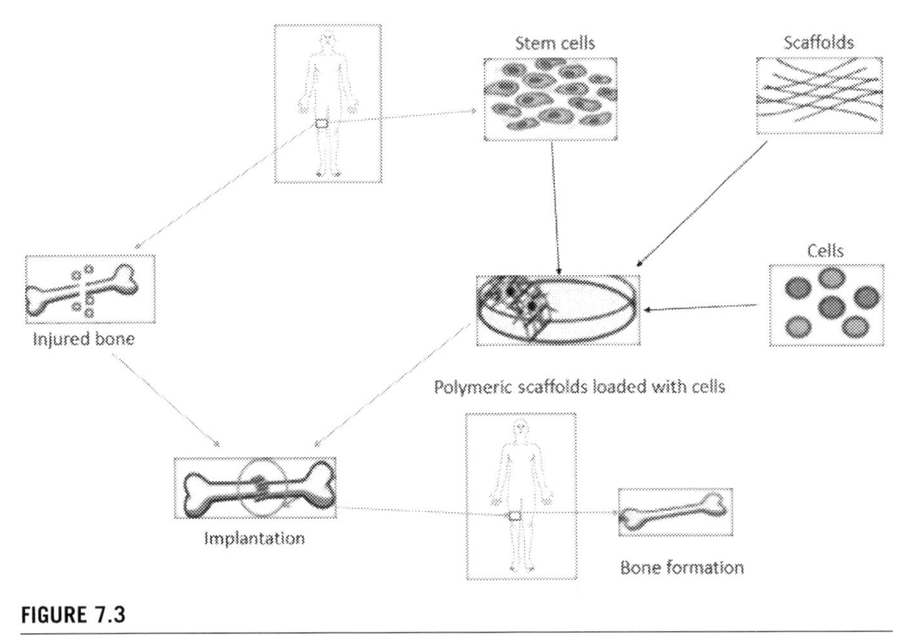

FIGURE 7.3

Bone tissue engineering.

potential. Such materials sometimes mixed with further biodegradable polymers for considerable bioactivity. Inventing new kind of nano hydroxyapatite/PCL spiral structured scaffolds (1:4 ratio), manufactured by an improved salt leaching technique implanted with human fetal osteoblasts (hFOBs), and mineralized by an ECM (Jeong et al., 2019). Bone mineralization markers were assessed by utilizing reverse transcriptase polymerase chain reaction analysis and these markers are lining up as bone sialoprotein, osteonectin (ON), osteocalcin (OC), and type I collagen. For bone regeneration, grain size is often major aspect of scaffold in TE. Grain size involves size of every individual speck of substance or "grain." With respect to cellular attachment, proliferation and differentiation of most osteogenic lineages smaller grain sizes seems as more suitable (Jeong et al., 2019). Nevertheless, fabrication processes often carryout to produce compact grain sizes because of observed cell attachment account. By utilizing hydroxyapatite scaffolds, grain size indicates to be relied upon sintering temperature. In order to reach an ideal, little grain size without accommodating porosity, was ground in perfect sintering temperature (1325°C). These findings are substantial step forward for researchers who want a standardized method for sintering such biomaterials. Exception of grain size, mechanical power is another important factor for bone regeneration that imitates native tissue. For this purpose, in case of bone TE applications, polymeric materials having great mechanical power are sometimes utilized as scaffolds, for example, silk protein, chitosan, chitosan nanofibers, PLLA, and bioactive glass materials. Due to their high compressive power, porosity, and fatigue resistance, metallic scaffolds are famous, for example, those of titanium (Stratton et al., 2016). Bone TE applications also for vascularization potential mechanical strength of scaffolds are currently available. For bone TE, vascularization is critical, although numerous potential solutions established in current years. Within scaffold inadequate vascularization can create a strong deficiency of important nutrients for survival of cell and give rise to unpredicted and hazardous irregularities in differentiation (Maisani et al., 2017). One method to initiate vascularization is to present specific GFs within scaffold. GFs, for example, vascular endothelial growth factor (VEGF) significantly upsurge blood vessel density, besides to carry osteoprogenitor cells to faulty sites in vivo in mice models, vascularization was described over a 28 day period using intravital microscopy. Remarkably accumulation of VEGF was revealed a responsible factor for vascularization, inadequate concentrations, and as inhabitant of deformed vasculature. GFs can similarly be united in a scaffold to assist numerous functions (García and García, 2016). An amalgamation of BMP 2 (for regeneration of bone, burdened in PLGA microspheres) and VEGF (for vascularization laden in gelatin hydrogel) GFs rooted into polypropylene scaffold to permit both improved bone formation and boosted vascularization. Fascinatingly enough, a combination of BMP 2 and VEGF was found to upsurge bone formation above 56 day period itself greater than BMP2, regardless of conventional role of VEGF includes frequently vascularization. This validates that a mixture of GFs is looked for in most cases. To accomplish both mechanical strength plus offer an environment favorable for vascularization, for bone TE, PLGA scaffolds have specifically been believed. They are feasible contenders, particularly when mixed with additional bioactive materials for superior cell attachment (De Witte et al., 2018). For bone TE, new PLGA/silk hybrid scaffold applications were united with hydrophilic silk polymer, hydroxyapatite nanoparticles to advance their biocompatibility and effectiveness. Adjustable pressure field discharge perusing electron microscopy high-resolution, variable-pressure, field-emission, scanning electron microscope (VP FE SEM) is utilized to prove porous kind of scaffold and approach angle dimensions established that silk component add extra hydrophilicity to scaffold (Sheikh et al., 2016). These results are vital step in indicating how PLGA scaffolds may be improved or blended for larger cell infiltration and complete bioactivity. The osteoblasts refined for 14 days period on scaffold and by examining with MTT, displayed cell attachment and proliferation throughout culture. Furthermore, when rooted within rat calvarial defect over a period of 4 weeks, and when exposed to Haemotoxylin and Eosin (H&E) staining, bone formation were seen. Therefore notions such as grain size, mechanical strength, and vascularization last to pursue dilemmas in regeneration bone field, with a constant research to enhance these parameters (Stratton et al., 2016).

7.5.3 Nerve regeneration

Central nervous system (CNS) and peripheral nervous system (PNS) are two divisions of nervous system. It is essential to differentiate among the two, in that, CNS comprises brain, spinal cord, ganglia, and nervous tissue, and outside of

CNS, are parts of PNS. Conventionally, in TE, nerve regeneration applications involve both systems. There have been varieties of challenges that are still to be addressed, and they do not hold up well in vivo models as in mice nerve axons are slighter and tinier than those in humans, and to achieve functional recovery is difficult by atrophy in target tissues (Stratton et al., 2016). On vast animal models parallel to humans, further *in vivo* testing is essential in order to tie gap between what is hypothesized and what is verified. In PNS regeneration applications, Schwann cells are at front of examination, as they play a role in myelination of axons and provide structural support. Therefore 3D scaffolds promote myelination; outgrowth and structural support for axons via Schwann cells for nerve regeneration applications must be bioactive. Nanofibers seem to play a significant part in nerve regeneration, aimed to guide axonal outgrowth of neuritis in above mentioned 3D structures. Nerve guidance conduits (NGCs) have multiple uses, such as to direct growth of axons from one proximal nerve end, aiding in regeneration of tissue secrete GFs, and in elimination of inhibitory scar tissue at injury site (Stratton et al., 2016). From visual analysis, it might be observed that NGC is intended to tie nerve gap among two broken ends and permit for outgrowth of nerve. Recently, this manages recovery of nerve from injuries. NGCs are commonly subjected to innovative customization in laboratory setting. New combination of both united and arbitrarily orientated electrospun PCL nanofibers in a double layer is valuable in guiding outgrowth of neuritis in vitro when preseeded with Schwann cells and permitted for moderate functional recovery in a 14 mm rat sciatic nerve injury model in vivo (Grinsell and Keating, 2014). This unique combination of bilayered NGCs, made up of aligned nanofibers in the inside layer and randomly orientated nanofibers on outside layer, may also be witnessed during surgical techniques. They are strongly tear resistant when compared with the conventional NGCs made exclusively of traditional, aligned nanofibers. Such scaffolds that are far more robust and tear resistant in vivo validate their real world competence. Stimulatingly enough, although nanofibers still remain highly popular for NGCs, it was just revealed that significant amount of neuritis extension, as well as Schwann cell area growth in vitro demonstrated by protein films contains blended silk fibroin and coated human tropo-elastin protein (Xie et al., 2014). Comparing with the standard poly- D-lysine film coating this new biodegradable scaffold acquired both a robust resembling biomaterial constituent from silk and enhanced 2–4 fold rise in neuritis extension capabilities from tropo-elastin protein. NGCs sometimes functionalized with proteins, for example, collagen or laminin, which further initiate outgrowth of nerve axons and increase nerve functional recovery. For regeneration of nervous system in TE, hydrogels have also been working as scaffold, as Schwann cell-based axonal recovery systems supported by this type. Proliferating and differentiating neuro progenitors in chitosan-based hydrogels (1.5 kPa stiffness) can be injected in vivo for central nervous system regeneration by using Zebrafish injury model (White et al., 2015). Uniqueness of this study originates from a point that this is one of the rare occasions in which a self-healing hydrogel, in next year's, has been presented to be operative in vivo for regeneration of nerve applications. Silk fibroin-based hydrogels are woefully yet hardly used regeneration of nerve applications, beyond the fact when utilized with Schwann cell cultures in vitro. They have displayed slight to no cytotoxicity and permit for significant regeneration of nerves. It has stated that culturing neural stem cells on softer hydrogels permits variation in atrocities and neurons, whereas stiffer hydrogels tends to permit differentiation into oligodendrocytes (Stratton et al., 2016).

7.5.4 Cell labeling and gene delivery

In labeling of cell from inside or outside along with nanoparticles, number of nanomaterials were used and locating in artificial tissues or increasing electromechanical structures of polymer scaffold like carbon nanotubes. It is hard to find such type of a tube having ability for loading bio macromolecules with material detecting, and it must be biocompatible with body (Boer et al., 2016). For delivery of drugs into cell in sustained manner, Halloysite nanotubes are ideal. Halloysite has the capability to get deposited around nucleus or to move inside cell. Because of these characteristics it can easily be utilized for visualization purpose as labeling agent. Frequently to perform confocal visualization, materials are placed with fluorescent agent. As Halloysites might easily move inside cell illustrates that it has the ability of acting as drug delivery agent. Drugs like curcumin and brilliant green are delivered by Halloysites (Jeevanandam et al., 2018).

7.5.5 Orthopedic implants

Orthopedic implants are utilized in defected bone or joint to provide strength to a broken bone. To give strength and for artificial cartilage, it is mainly comprised titanium alloys and stainless steel, plastic coatings may also be used. Orthopedic implants have limits of infection relevant to site and bone tissue integration. Composition and surface morphology of materials are major factors effecting properties of implants. Bone modeling and inhibition of bacterial infections are completed by coating. Implants surfaces along with various polymeric coatings can resolve problems related implants. New forms of coatings are chitosan, graphene, and oxide hydroxyapatite are used (Navarro et al., 2008).

7.5.6 Skin tissue engineering

Skin is the first line of barrier in human body and it is major organ of the body. It mainly performs functions like protection of body from external environment and maintains temperature of body. It comprises outer epidermis and then inner epidermis, each layer has specific functions like production of Vitamin D, to inhibit dehydration, inhibit microbes to enter into body and to stop trauma. Epidermis mainly made of Keratinocytes, and it has additional power of regeneration due to the presence of large number of stem cells, which is significant for wound healing. Many cell types, that is, Xenogeneic, allogenic, and autogenic are there for TE beside scaffolds to use for skin regeneration (Fig. 7.4). For tissue regeneration, fibrous scaffolds, hydrogel scaffolds, porous scaffolds, composite scaffolds, and cellular scaffolds, microsphere scaffolds are available (Boer et al., 2016).

Skin is being subjected to genetic, metabolic, and inflammatory diseases. Decline in human skin function is resulted with aging such as sensory perception, immune response, barrier efficacy, sensory perception, wound healing, and DNA repair is due to senescent cells. Deviations in collagen formation, flattening of basement membrane, a reduction in blood supply to skin, flattening of basement membrane, and a slower inflammatory response reduce the ability to achieve skin repair (Farage et al., 2008). Cutaneous wound healing is a coordinative biological process that includes integrated interaction of various cytokines, GFs, and cell types, such as inflammatory cells, Keratinocytes, enzymes, endothelial cell and fibroblasts. Including an initial inflammatory response, a proliferative phase, and a final remodeling phase, tissue repair is achieved by tightly regulated processes that overlay in space and time (Gainza et al., 2015). Chronic wounds do not have the ability to proceed through those sequential phases, afterwards resulting in postponed or incomplete healing. Many factors take part in poor wound healing. Between them, a key role has been accredited to an abnormal and constant inflammatory response, a trademark of nonhealing skin wounds, leads to an extreme proteolysis activity because of protease inhibitor degradation, and eventually to inflammation arbitrated tissue damage (Trengove et al., 1999). A reduced vascular supply is usual the cause of ulcer formation. Additionally, wound repair is affected by a reduction in quantity of existing and biologically active GFs in wound environment. Infection is one of the most usual complications of chronic

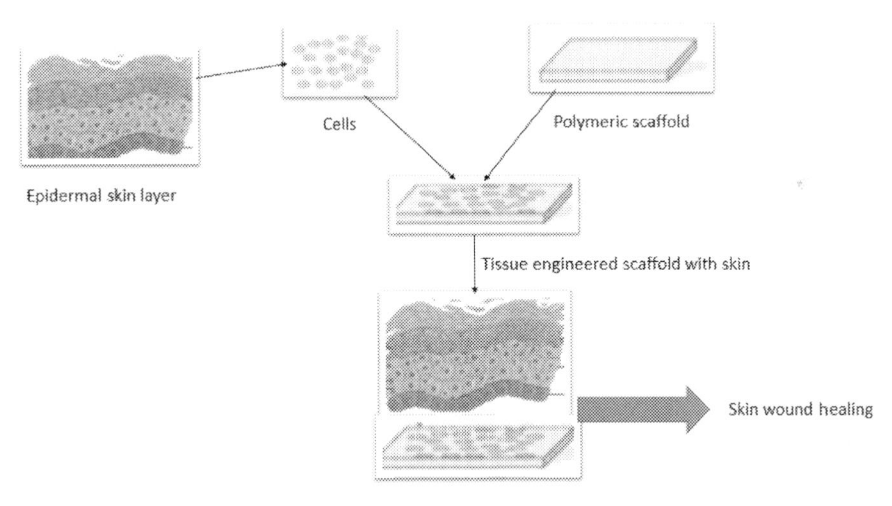

FIGURE 7.4

Utilization of tissue engineering in skin wound healing.

wounds. Intact skin is disrupted in open wounds. Higher levels of bacterial content commonly present on open wounds and can initiate a pro-inflammatory environment. Hereafter, process of wound healing can be diminished partially because of the elongation in an inflammatory phase, which suppresses regenerative phases (Trengove et al., 1999). Bacteria not only contend for inadequate oxygen and nutrients existing in wound, also discharge toxins and induce an amplified production of enzymes that promote cellular failure. Chronic wounds contain vascular (venous or arterial), pressure, and diabetic foot ulcers (DFUs). A pressure ulcer was a localized skin underlying tissue damage resulted owed to bony distinction with pressure and shear (George Broughton et al., 2006). Vascular ulcers commonly contained on lower limbs and caused by a circulation disorder that leads to decrease in arterial blood flow or a diminished venous blood return. Vascular ulcers involve a group of lesions of specific relevance because of their high prevalence. These ulcers are a primary cause of morbidity between patients of peripheral vascular disease (Gainza et al., 2015). Lastly, DFU is a key complication of diabetes due to high level of concerns created on patients' quality of life. A number of contributing factors cause DFUs, for example mechanical alterations in bony architecture of foot, peripheral vascular disease (blocked arteries), peripheral neuropathy (damaged nerves), all of which occur in diabetic population with greater frequency and intensity (Gainza et al., 2015). Nontraumatic lower extremity amputations are highly linked with DFUs within the industrialized world. Major skin burns occurred by chemicals, heat, electricity, radiation or electricity believed as chronic wounds. Skin integrity effected by major burn cause fluid loss and creates way for bacterial infection. Severity of a burn depends on location, depth, and affected body surface area.

7.5.7 Muscle tissue regeneration

Scaffolds should have both structural integrity and at the same time have the ability to bring both force regeneration and strong contraction. There are three types of muscles named as cardiac, smooth, and skeletal. Cardiac muscle tissue is situated at walls of heart, smooth muscle tissue is present mostly in walls of some other organs, and skeletal muscle fibers are attached to skeleton. Furthermore, cardiac muscle regeneration is of specific significance, due to cardiac muscle tissue commonly has very limited natural regenerative ability in most mammals (Stratton et al., 2016). Cardiomyocytes are at forefront of cardiac muscle regeneration, which are capable of differentiating to form most simple structures for cardiac tissues. Cardiomyocytes are often implanted onto PGA, collagen scaffolds, gelatin, and alginate, even though it is suggested that layering cell sheets in a 3D structure devoid of an artificial scaffold may cause better bioactivity. Peptides such as RGD attachment to scaffold improve cellular functionality (Zimmermann, 2009). Neonatal rat, greater cellular adhesion, and accelerated cardiac tissue regeneration in vitro on heart patches than unmodified alginate scaffolds promoted by cardiac cells seeded onto RGD. Western staining verified expression of proteins necessary for cellular vitality likes N cadherin, actinin and connexin 43. Furthermore, in contrast to the control group, cellular apoptosis lessened considerably in RGD immobilized macro porous alginate scaffolds (Shachar et al., 2011). Like those of PCL and collagen nanofibers are presented as useful particular for smooth muscle TE scaffolds, by orientating cells to maintain a classic phenotype shape (Shachar et al., 2011). Without external intervention skeletal muscle has a great, already made in ability for regeneration. If severe injury occurs, this regenerative capacity may be limited or completely lost. Throughout repair and regeneration phase, satellite cells play a very significant role in migrating to defect site, proliferating, and differentiating to preserve functional properties (Ibsirlioglu et al., 2020). Satellite cells for skeletal muscle TE applications have ability to create over one hundred myofibers in vivo by seeding only seven of these cells into irradiated mice muscle tissue. Common biomaterials as scaffolds for implantation of stem cells to stimulate skeletal muscle tissue are fibrous meshes, hydrogels and patterned substrates. Electrical stimulation is presented as a unique catalyst on 3D scaffolds in vitro having potential for expansion of several myogenic progenitor cells, which might be a significant future technique for expansion of other kinds of cell such as satellite cells (Stratton et al., 2016). Whereas electrical stimulation did not influence cellular viability, a satellite cell activator, NO(x), improved with a 65% greater emission rate. Further myogenic markers, for example desmin, also amplified according to control group that could be utilized in regeneration of all tissue type (Flaibani et al., 2009).

7.5.8 Tendon/ligament regeneration

After injury, tendons do not naturally regenerate completely and even slight injuries may create challenges in overall healing process. Due to these reasons, 3D scaffolds are of importance for tendon regeneration. Conventional methods, such as grafts, stimulate cellular proliferation and are unsuccessful to bring back structural mechanical properties of original tendon, and various solutions have been suggested from years to this dilemma. ECM of tendon is frequently made of collagen type I and displayed itself in an interwoven, complex structure forming a 3D, biomimetic environment relatively hard to replicate (Pedde et al., 2017). One main hurdle in regeneration of Achilles tendon (AT), owed in huge part to continuous mechanical load placed onto it. Tendon regeneration applications, polymeric materials having exceptionally powerful mechanical properties may also use as scaffolds, for example silk and PLGA. It is stated that PLGA/silk fibrous scaffolds are utilized as devices to yield bFGF, initiating mesenchymal progenitor cell distinction and attachment in vitro. PLGA fibers were used to release and encapsulate bFGF, whereas microfibrous silk was utilized as reinforcement (Wongpanit et al., 2012). Fallouts showed an upsurge in gene expression of ECM proteins in typical ligament, tendon, and higher collagen production. Immuno histochemically analysis discovered that collagen type I and collagen type III were highly expressed, showing a reconstruction of native ECM environment. Ligaments, in a dense matrix composed mainly of fibroblasts encircled by collagen types I and III, due to critical role that anterior cruciate ligament (ACL) plays in knee stabilization have increased attention within field of TE. Polymeric scaffolds such as PLLA and silk fibers which have been used to deliver GFs and mimic mechanical properties of native tissue environment can be used in place of ACL, because of its poor healing abilities and less mechanical stability. Recently, a novel scaffold for ACL regeneration has been reported, composed of mechanically strong extruded PLLA nanofibers combined with a flexible shell of electrospun PCL nanofibers, allowing for integration of bFGF and platelet-derived GF in a controlled release manner, as well as proliferation of hMSCs in vitro. Both PLLA and PCL fibers were fabricated via electrospinning. Gene expression appears as an up regulation of vital ligament markers necessary for cellular viability, for example collagen type I, collagen type III, tenascin C, and scleraxis over a 21 day period. AT and ACL appeared to be the two largest hurdles to overcome for tendon and ligament regeneration due to their complex nature (Yu, 2016).

7.6 Future perspective

Nanotechnology gives opportunity to improve in vivo effectiveness of GFs, avoiding proteolysis degradation and prolonging emission at abrasion. A wide variety of nanoscale delivery systems have been designed to support wound healing, mainly polymeric, lipid, and nano fibrous structures. Biocompatible polymeric devices have currently turned into a proficient substitute for controlled emission of active compounds, involving GFs. Such nanometric colloidal systems can be engaged in different diseases, administration routes, and dosage ranges. Nanospheres could be made utilizing natural or synthetic biomaterials, also other polymer combinations. As in many drug delivery systems, synthetic PLGA is one of the most extensively utilized polymers to make nanosphere. This advanced way of rhEGF burdened (recombinant human epidermal growth factor) PLGA NPs utilize to improve double emulsion process and evaluated their efficiency afterward topical administration in full thickness wounds produced on diabetic rats. Recent advancement in drug delivery includes mixture of various technological methodologies that might enhance dressing integration. Generally, such conclusions that fibrin based scaffolds comprising GF loaded NPs are an interesting strategy for sustained release of VEGF and bFGF, because they acted as a double DDS for GF delivery. Therefore initial burst release of GFs and leak out of particles from wound site after topical administration might be eliminated, if a more sustained release of GFs was utilized.

References

Aamodt, J.M., Grainger, D.W., 2016. Extracellular matrix based biomaterial scaffolds and host response. Biomaterials 86, 68–82.

Aiyelabegan, H.T., et al., 2016. Albumin based biomaterial for lung tissue engineering applications. Int. J. Polymeric Mater. Polymeric Biomater. 65 (16), 853–861.

Amezcua, R., et al., 2016. Nanomaterials for cardiac myocyte tissue engineering. Nanomaterials 6 (7), 133.

Atala, A., Kasper, F., Mikos, A., 2012. Engineering complex tissues. Sci. Transl. Med. 4 (160), 160. 112.

Ayala Caminero, R., et al., 2017. Polymeric scaffolds for three dimensional culture of nerve cells: a model of peripheral nerve regeneration. MRS Commun. 7 (3), 391–415.

Baino, F., Novajra, G., Vitale Brovarone, C., 2015. Bioceramics and scaffolds: a winning combination for tissue engineering. Front. Bioeng. Biotechnol. 3, 202.

Bakhshandeh, B., et al., 2017. Tissue engineering; strategies, tissues, and biomaterials. Biotechnol. Genet. Eng. Rev. 33 (2), 144–172.

Baldwin, M., et al., 2018. Augmenting endogenous repair of soft tissues with nanofibre scaffolds. J. R. Soc. Interface 15 (141), 20180019.

Basu, A., et al., 2016. Poly (α hydroxy acid) s and poly (α hydroxy acid co α amino acid) s derived from amino acid. Adv. drug. delivery Rev. 107, 82–96.

Berbezier, I., Maurizio, D.C., 2015. Self-assembly nanostructures nanomaterials. J. Nanotechnol. 1397–1398.

Berro, S., et al., 2015. From plastic to silicone: novelties in porous polymer fabrications. J. Nanomater. 16 (1), 123.

Berthing, T., et al., 2011. Intact mammalian cell function on semiconductor nanowire arrays: new perspectives for cell-based biosensing. Small 7 (5), 640–647.

Bertholf, R.L., 2014. Proteins and albumin. Laboratory Med. 45 (1), e25–e41.

Boer, M., et al., 2016. Structural and biophysical characteristics of human skin in maintaining proper epidermal barrier function. Adv. Dermatol. Allergol./Postępy Dermatologii i Alergologii 33 (1), 1.

Burnouf, T., et al., 2013. Blood derived biomaterials and platelet growth factors in regenerative medicine. Blood Rev. 27 (2), 77–89.

Castelletto, V., et al., 2009. Helical-ribbon formation by a β-amino acid modified amyloid β-peptide fragment. Angew. Chem. Int. Ed. 48 (13), 2317–2320.

Chafran, L.S., et al., 2019. Preparation of PLA blends by polycondensation of D, L lactic acid using supported 12 tungstophosphoric acid as a heterogeneous catalyst. Heliyon 5 (5), e01810.

Chen, F.M., Liu, X., 2016. Advancing biomaterials of human origin for tissue engineering. Prog. Polym. Sci. 53, 86–168.

Cheung, R.C.F., et al., 2015. Chitosan: an update on potential biomedical and pharmaceutical applications. Mar. Drugs 13 (8), 5156–5186.

Chocholata, P., Kulda, V., Babuska, V., 2019. Fabrication of scaffolds for bone tissue regeneration. Materials 12 (4), 568.

Chopade, S.S., Nangare, K., Bagal, V., 2019. Bionanocomposite: a novel approach for drug delivery system. Int. J. Pharm. Res. Sci. 10 (7), 1000–1007.

Chu, C., et al., 2017. Collagen membrane and immune response in guided bone regeneration: recent progress and perspectives. Tissue Eng. Part. B: Rev. 23 (5), 421–435.

Dawson, J.I., Oreffo, R.O., 2008. Bridging regeneration gap: stem cells, biomaterials and clinical translation in bone tissue engineering. Arch. Biochem. Biophysics 473 (2), 124–131.
De Witte, T.M., et al., 2018. Bone tissue engineering via growth factor delivery: from scaffolds to complex matrices. Regenerative Biomater. 5 (4), 197–211.
Deng, M., et al., 2010. Polyphosphazene polymers for tissue engineering: an analysis of material synthesis, characterization and applications. Soft Matter 6 (14), 3119–3132.
Dhandayuthapani, B., et al., 2011. Polymeric scaffolds in tissue engineering application: a review. Int. J. Polym. Sci. 2011.
Edgar, L., et al., 2016. Heterogeneity of scaffold biomaterials in tissue engineering. Materials 9 (5), 332.
Esfahani, M.R., et al., 2018. Nanocomposite membranes for water separation and purification: fabrication, modification, and applications. Sep. Purif. Technol. .
Farage, M., et al., 2008. Intrinsic and extrinsic factors in skin ageing: a review. Int. J. Cosmetic Sci. 30 (2), 87–95.
Feinberg, A.W., 2012. Engineered tissue grafts: opportunities and challenges in regenerative medicine. Wiley Interdiscip. Reviews: Syst. Biol. Med. 4 (2), 207–220.
Fisher, M.B., Mauck, R.L., 2013. Tissue engineering and regenerative medicine: recent innovations and transition to translation. Tissue Eng. Part. B: Rev. 19 (1), 1–13.
Fitzpatrick, L.E., McDevitt, T.C., 2015. Cell derived matrices for tissue engineering and regenerative medicine applications. Biomater. Sci. 3 (1), 12–24.
Flaibani, M., et al., 2009. Muscle differentiation and myotubes alignment is influenced by micropatterned surfaces and exogenous electrical stimulation. Tissue Eng. Part. A 15 (9), 2447–2457.
Fong, E.L., et al., 2012. Building bridges: leveraging interdisciplinary collaborations in development of biomaterials to meet clinical needs. Adv. Mater. 24 (36), 4995–5013.
Gainza, G., et al., 2015. Advances in drug delivery systems (DDSs) to release growth factors for wound healing and skin regeneration. Nanomed.: Nanotechnol., Biol. Med. 11 (6), 1551–1573.
García, J.R., García, A.J., 2016. Biomaterial mediated strategies targeting vascularization for bone repair. Drug. Delivery Transl. Res. 6 (2), 77–95.
George Broughton, I., Janis, J.E., Attinger, C.E., 2006. Wound healing: an overview. Plastic Reconstructive Surg. 117 (7S), 1e S–32e S.
Grenadyorov, A.S., et al., 2020. Modifying the surface of a titanium alloy with an electron beam and aC: H: SiOx coating deposition to reduce hemolysis in cardiac assist devices. Surf. Coat. Technol. 381, 125. 113.
Griffith, L.G., Naughton, G., 2002. Tissue engineering current challenges and expanding opportunities. Science 295 (5557), 1009–1014.
Grinsell, D., Keating, C., 2014. Peripheral nerve reconstruction after injury: a review of clinical and experimental therapies. BioMed. Res. Int. .
Gu, X., Ding, F., Williams, D.F., 2014. Neural tissue engineering options for peripheral nerve regeneration. Biomaterials 35 (24), 6143–6156.
Guo, B., Ma, P.X., 2014. Synthetic biodegradable functional polymers for tissue engineering: a brief review. Sci. China Chem. 57 (4), 490–500.
Gupta, V., et al., 2017. Microsphere based scaffolds in regenerative engineering. Annu. Rev. Biomed. Eng. 19, 135–161.
Gurtner, G.C., Callaghan, M.J., Longaker, M.T., 2007. Progress and potential for regenerative medicine. Annu. Rev. Med. 58, 299–312.

Gurtner, G.C., et al., 2008. Wound repair and regeneration. Nature 453 (7193), 314.

Hanson, S., D'Souza, R.N., Hematti, P., 2014. Biomaterial–mesenchymal stem cell constructs for immunomodulation in composite tissue engineering. Tissue Eng. Part. A 20 (15 16), 2162–2168.

Harrison, R.H., Pierre St., J.P., Stevens, M.M., 2014. Tissue engineering and regenerative medicine: a year in review. Tissue Eng. Part. B: Rev. 20 (1), 1–16.

He, Y., Lu, F., 2016. Development of synthetic and natural materials for tissue engineering applications using adipose stem cells. Stem Cell Int. 4 (11), 43.

Holzapfel, B.M., et al., 2013. How smart do biomaterials need to be? A translational science and clinical point of view. Adv. Drug. Delivery Rev. 65 (4), 581–603.

Howard, D., et al., 2008. Tissue engineering: strategies, stem cells and scaffolds. J. Anat. 213 (1), 66–72.

Ibsirlioglu, T., Elçin, A.E., Elçin, Y.M., 2020. Decellularized biological scaffold and stem cells from autologous human adipose tissue for cartilage tissue engineering. Methods 171, 97–107.

Ifegwu, O.C., Anyakora, C., 2018. Place of electrospinning in separation science and biomedical engineering. Electrospinning Method Used to Create Functional Nanocomposites Films. IntechOpen, p. 17.

Jeevanandam, J., et al., 2018. Review on nanoparticles and nanostructured materials: history, sources, toxicity and regulations. Beilstein J. Nanotechnol. 9 (1), 1050–1074.

Jeong, J., et al., 2019. Bioactive calcium phosphate materials and applications in bone regeneration. Biomater. Res. 23 (1), 4.

Kamaly, N., et al., 2016. Degradable controlled release polymers and polymeric nanoparticles: mechanisms of controlling drug release. Chem. Rev. 116 (4), 2602–2663.

Kaur, A., et al., 2019. Functional skin grafts: where biomaterials meet stem cells. Stem Cell Int. 20, 44.

Khan, F., Tanaka, M., 2018. Designing smart biomaterials for tissue engineering. Int. J. Mol. Sci. 19 (1), 17.

Kitsara, M., et al., 2017. Fibers for hearts: a critical review on electrospinning for cardiac tissue engineering. Acta Biomater. 48, 20–40.

Koo, H., Yamada, K.M., 2016. Dynamic cell–matrix interactions modulate microbial biofilm and tissue 3D microenvironments. Curr. Opin. Cell Biol. 42, 102–112.

Kratochvil, M.J., et al., 2019. Engineered materials for organoid systems. Nat. Rev. Mater. 4 (9), 606–622.

Kwon, H.J., Han, Y., 2016. Chondroitin sulfate based biomaterials for tissue engineering. Turkish J. Biol. 40 (2), 290–299.

Lai, V.K., et al., 2012. Microstructural and mechanical differences between digested collagen–fibrin co gels and pure collagen and fibrin gels. Acta Biomater. 8 (11), 4031–4042.

Laurencin, C.T., et al., 2014. Delivery of small molecules for bone regenerative engineering: preclinical studies and potential clinical applications. Drug. Discovery Today 19 (6), 794–800.

Law, J.X., et al., 2017. Electrospun collagen nanofibers and their applications in skin tissue engineering. Tissue Eng. Regen. Med. 14 (6), 699–718.

Lee, K., Silva, E.A., Mooney, D.J., 2010. Growth factor delivery based tissue engineering: general approaches and a review of recent developments. J. R. Soc. Interface 8 (55), 153–170.

Lev, R., Seliktar, D., 2018. Hydrogel biomaterials and their therapeutic potential for muscle injuries and muscular dystrophies. J. R. Soc. Interface 15 (138), 20170380.

Li, P.S., et al., 2014. A novel albumin based tissue scaffold for autogenic tissue engineering applications. Sci. Rep. 4, 5600.

Li, X., et al., 2017. Administration of signaling molecules dictates stem cell homing for in situ regeneration. J. Cell. Mol. Med. 21 (12), 3162–3177.

Liu, J.S., Gartner, Z.J., 2012. Directing assembly of spatially organized multicomponent tissues from bottom up. Trends Cell Biol. 22 (12), 683–691.

Liu, H., et al., 2013. Electrospinning of nanofibers for tissue engineering applications. J. Nanomater. 2013, 3.

Lyu, S., Untereker, D., 2009. Degradability of polymers for implantable biomedical devices. Int. J. Mol. Sci. 10 (9), 4033–4065.

Maisani, M., et al., 2017. Cellularizing hydrogel based scaffolds to repair bone tissue: how to create a physiologically relevant micro environment? J. Tissue Eng. 8, 2041731417712073.

Malliaras, K., et al., 2013. Cardiomyocyte proliferation and progenitor cell recruitment underlie therapeutic regeneration after myocardial infarction in adult mouse heart. EMBO Mol. Med. 5 (2), 191–209.

Mantha, S., et al., 2019. Smart hydrogels in tissue engineering and regenerative medicine. Materials 12 (20), 3323.

Mao, A.S., Mooney, D.J., 2015. Regenerative medicine: current therapies and future directions. Proc. Natl Acad. Sci. 112 (47), 14452–14459.

Marino, A., et al., 2015. Biomimicry at nanoscale: current research and perspectives of two photon polymerization. Nanoscale 7 (7), 2841–2850.

Masuelli, M.A., 2013. Introduction of fiber reinforced polymers–polymers and composites: concepts, properties and processes. Fiber Reinforced Polymers Technology Applied for Concrete Repair. IntechOpen.

Meeson, R.L., et al., 2019. In vitro behavior of canine osteoblasts derived from different bone types. BMC Veterinary Res. 15 (1), 114.

Miao, T., et al., 2018. Polysaccharide-based controlled release systems for therapeutics delivery and tissue engineering: from bench to bedside. Adv. Sci. 5 (4), 1700513.

Mir, M., et al., 2018. Synthetic polymeric biomaterials for wound healing: a review. Prog. Biomater. 7 (1), 1–21.

Mogoşanu, G.D., Grumezescu, A.M., 2014. Natural and synthetic polymers for wounds and burns dressing. Int. J. Pharm. 463 (2), 127–136.

Navarro, M., et al., 2008. Biomaterials in orthopaedics. J. R. Soc. Interface 5 (27), 1137–1158.

Neto, A.S., Ferreira, J.M., 2018. Synthetic and marine derived porous scaffolds for bone tissue engineering. Materials 11 (9), 1702.

Nooeaid, P., et al., 2012. Osteochondral tissue engineering: scaffolds, stem cells and applications. J. Cell. Mol. Med. 16 (10), 2247–2270.

Ojeda, T., 2013. Polymers and environment. Polym. Sci. 23.

Patel, M.N., Atala, A., 2011. Tissue engineering of penis. Sci. World J. 11, 2567–2578.

Patel, H., Bonde, M., Srinivasan, G., 2011. Biodegradable polymer scaffold for tissue engineering. Trends Biomater. Artif. Organs 25 (1), 20–29.

Pedde, R.D., et al., 2017. Emerging biofabrication strategies for engineering complex tissue constructs. Adv. Mater. 29 (19).

Peter, M., et al., 2010. Novel biodegradable chitosan–gelatin/nano bioactive glass ceramic composite scaffolds for alveolar bone tissue engineering. Chem. Eng. J. 158 (2), 353–361.

Place, E.S., Evans, N.D., Stevens, M.M., 2009. Complexity in biomaterials for tissue engineering. Nat. Mater. 8 (6), 457.

Porzionato, A., et al., 2018. Tissue engineered grafts from human decellularized extracellular matrices: a systematic review and future perspectives. Int. J. Mol. Sci. 19 (12), 4117.

Qiu, F., et al., 2018. Amphiphilic peptides as novel nanomaterials: design, self assembly and application. Int. J. Nanomed. 13, 5003.

Reneker, D., et al., 2007. Electrospinning of nanofibers from polymer solutions and melts. Adv. Appl. Mech. 41, 43–346.

Renth, A.N., Detamore, M.S., 2012. Leveraging "raw materials" as building blocks and bioactive signals in regenerative medicine. Tissue Eng. Part. B: Rev. 18 (5), 341–362.

Rodrigues, M.T., Reis, R.L., Gomes, M.E., 2013. Engineering tendon and ligament tissues: present developments towards successful clinical products. J. Tissue Eng. Regen. Med. 7 (9), 673–686.

Rodríguez Vázquez, M., et al., 2015. Chitosan and its potential use as a scaffold for tissue engineering in regenerative medicine. BioMed. Res. Int. 3 (2), 33–38.

Rubbens, M.P., et al., 2008. Intermittent straining accelerates development of tissue properties in engineered heart valve tissue. Tissue Eng. Part. A 15 (5), 999–1008.

Sabir, M.I., Xu, X., Li, L., 2009. A review on biodegradable polymeric materials for bone tissue engineering applications. J. Mater. Sci. 44 (21), 5713–5724.

Sada, A., Tumbar, T., 2013. New insights into mechanisms of stem cell daughter fate determination in regenerative tissues. Int. Rev. Cell Mol. Biol. 1–50. Elsevier.

Sander, E.A., et al., 2004. Solvent effects on microstructure and properties of 75/25 poly (d, l-lactide-co-glycolide) tissue scaffolds. J. Biomed. Mater. Res. Part. A 70 (3), 506–513.

Serrano Aroca, Á., Vera Donoso, C.D., Moreno Manzano, V., 2018. Bioengineering approaches for bladder regeneration. Int. J. Mol. Sci. 19 (6), 1796.

Setayeshmehr, M., et al., 2019. Hybrid and composite scaffolds based on extracellular matrices for cartilage tissue engineering. Tissue Eng. Part. B: Rev. 25 (3), 202–224.

Shachar, M., et al., 2011. Effect of immobilized RGD peptide in alginate scaffolds on cardiac tissue engineering. Acta Biomater. 7 (1), 152–162.

Sheikh, F.A., et al., 2016. Hybrid scaffolds based on PLGA and silk for bone tissue engineering. J. Tissue Eng. Regen. Med. 10 (3), 209–221.

Shepherd, B.R., et al., 2008. Human aortic smooth muscle cells promote arteriole formation by coengrafted endothelial cells. Tissue Eng. Part. A 15 (1), 165–173.

Shin, Y., et al., 2001. Experimental characterization of electrospinning: electrically forced jet and instabilities. Polymer 42 (25), 09955–09967.

Snyder, S.S., Anastasiou, T.J., Uhrich, K.E., 2015. In vitro degradation of an aromatic polyanhydride with enhanced thermal properties. Polym. Degrad. Stab. 115, 70–76.

Soleimannejad, M., et al., 2018. Fibrin gel as a scaffold for photoreceptor cells differentiation from conjunctiva mesenchymal stem cells in retina tissue engineering. Artif. Cells, Nanomed., Biotechnol. 46 (4), 805–814.

Soto Gutierrez, A., et al., 2012. Perspectives on whole organ assembly: moving toward transplantation on demand. J. Clin. Investigation 122 (11), 3817–3823.

Stratton, S., et al., 2016. Bioactive polymeric scaffolds for tissue engineering. Bioact. Mater. 1 (2), 93–108.

Sun, L., Zheng, C., Webster, T.J., 2017. Self assembled peptide nanomaterials for biomedical applications: promises and pitfalls. Int. J. Nanomed. 12, 73.

Sundelacruz, S., Kaplan, D.L., 2009. Stem cell and scaffold based tissue engineering approaches to osteochondral regenerative medicine. Seminars in Cell & Developmental Biology. Elsevier.

Szekalska, M., et al., 2016. Alginate: current use and future perspectives in pharmaceutical and biomedical applications. Int. J. Polym. Sci. 2016.

Thavornyutikarn, B., et al., 2014. Bone tissue engineering scaffolding: computer aided scaffolding techniques. Prog. Biomater. 3 (2 4), 61−102.

Tozzi, G., et al., 2016. Composite hydrogels for bone regeneration. Materials 9 (4), 267.

Trengove, N.J., et al., 1999. Analysis of acute and chronic wound environments: role of proteases and their inhibitors. Wound Repair. Regen. 7 (6), 442−452.

Urciuolo, F., et al., 2013. Building a tissue in vitro from bottom up: implications in regenerative medicine. Methodist DeBakey Cardiovascular J. 9 (4), 213.

Valderrama, M.A.M., van Putten, R.J., Gruter, G.J.M., 2019. Potential of oxalic and glycolic acid based polyesters (review). Towards CO2 as a feedstock (carbon capture and utilization CCU). Eur. Polym. J. .

Varner, V.D., Nelson, C.M., 2014. Toward directed self-assembly of engineered tissues. Annu. Rev. Chem. Biomol. Eng. 5, 507−526.

Vats, A., et al., 2005. Stem cells and tissue engineering. Stem Cell Repair and Regeneration. World Scientific, pp. 81−98.

Wang, W., Yeung, K.W., 2017. Bone grafts and biomaterials substitutes for bone defect repair: a review. Bioact. Mater. 2 (4), 224−247.

Wang, C., et al., 2019. Fabrication of electrospun polymer nanofibers with diverse morphologies. Molecules 24 (5), 834.

White, J.D., et al., 2015. Silk−tropoelastin protein films for nerve guidance. Acta Biomater. 14, 1−10.

Williams, D.F., 2014. Biomaterials conundrum in tissue engineering. Tissue Eng. Part. A 20 (7-8), 1129−1131.

Wongpanit, P., Pornsunthorntawee, O., Rujiravanit, R., 2012. Silk fibre composites. Natural Polymers: Composites. Royal Society of Chemistry, Cambridge, pp. 219−222.

Xie, J., et al., 2014. Nerve guidance conduits based on double layered scaffolds of electrospun nanofibers for repairing peripheral nervous system. ACS Appl. Mater. Interfaces 6 (12), 9472−9480.

Yang, G.Z., et al., 2017. Influence of working temperature on formation of electrospun polymer nanofibers. Nanoscale Res. Lett. 12 (1), 55.

Yu, Q., 2016. Applications of Human Bone Materials and Synthesized Biomaterials for Bone related Tissue Engineering. University of Akron.

Zhang, J., et al., 2017. Synthetic biodegradable polymers for bone tissue engineering. Handb. Compos. Renew. Mater. 355−375.

Zhu, J., Marchant, R.E., 2011. Design properties of hydrogel tissue engineering scaffolds. Expert. Rev. Med. Devices 8 (5), 607−626.

Zimmermann, W.H., 2009. Remuscularizing failing hearts with tissue engineered myocardium. Antioxid. Redox Signal. 11 (8), 2011−2023.

CHAPTER

Polymeric nanomaterials as broad-spectrum antimicrobial compounds

8

Abhilasha Mishra[1], Rekha Goswami[2] and Neha Bhatt[1]

[1]*Department of Chemistry, Graphic Era Deemed to be University, Dehradun, India*

[2]*Department of Environmental Science, Graphic Era Hill University, Dehradun, India*

8.1 Introduction

Nowadays, bacterial contamination frequently increases, and its resistance toward antibiotics is also growing highly, resulting in a higher demand for the development of new-generation antibiotics to combat the chronic health problems. Antibiotics are commonly used to kill or inhibit the growth of bacteria for many years. But the antimicrobial resistance is becoming more serious as the worldwide use of antibiotics is increasing day by day due to improper use of antibiotics in general medical practice and also in animals for increasing meat production (Kumarasamy et al., 2010; Jansen et al., 2018). The US Centers for Disease Control and Prevention (CDC) reported that approximately 2 million people get contaminated with antibiotic-resistant bacteria, resulting in increased mortality rate annually (Talbot et al., 2006). Recently, many of the new infectious pathogens such as extensively antibiotic-resistant tuberculosis, Ebola virus, and avian influenza A (H5N1) (Burman, 2010; Christian et al., 2013) were recorded. Fig. 8.1 shows pathogens that are resistant to the most commonly used antimicrobial agents in clinical treatment. Development of efficient, long-lasting, and broad-spectrum antimicrobial agents is required to combat these resistant microorganisms.

Compared to conventional antimicrobial agents, antimicrobial polymeric materials provide better antimicrobial effectiveness with reduced toxicity (Ilker et al., 2004) An antimicrobial polymer possesses more chemical stability and hence shows antimicrobial activity for long term (Majumdar et al., 2009). Over the last few years, polymeric nanoparticles (NPs) obtained high attention in the biomedical field due to their unique properties such as nanosize (Parveen and Sahoo, 2008). In biomedical applications, various NPs act as nanocarriers such as solid lipid NPs (Nassimi et al., 2010), micelles (Mao et al., 2016), nanosized lipid carriers (Chakraborty et al., 2017), polymeric NPs (Masood, 2016), dendrimers (Caminade and Turrin, 2014), carbon nanotubes (Zhang et al., 2011), and liposomes (Daraee et al., 2016). Among them, liposomes and polymeric NPs are the most dominant nanocarriers for drug delivery (Kumari et al., 2019). Development

Advances in Polymeric Nanomaterials for Biomedical Applications. DOI: https://doi.org/10.1016/B978-0-12-814657-6.00008-2

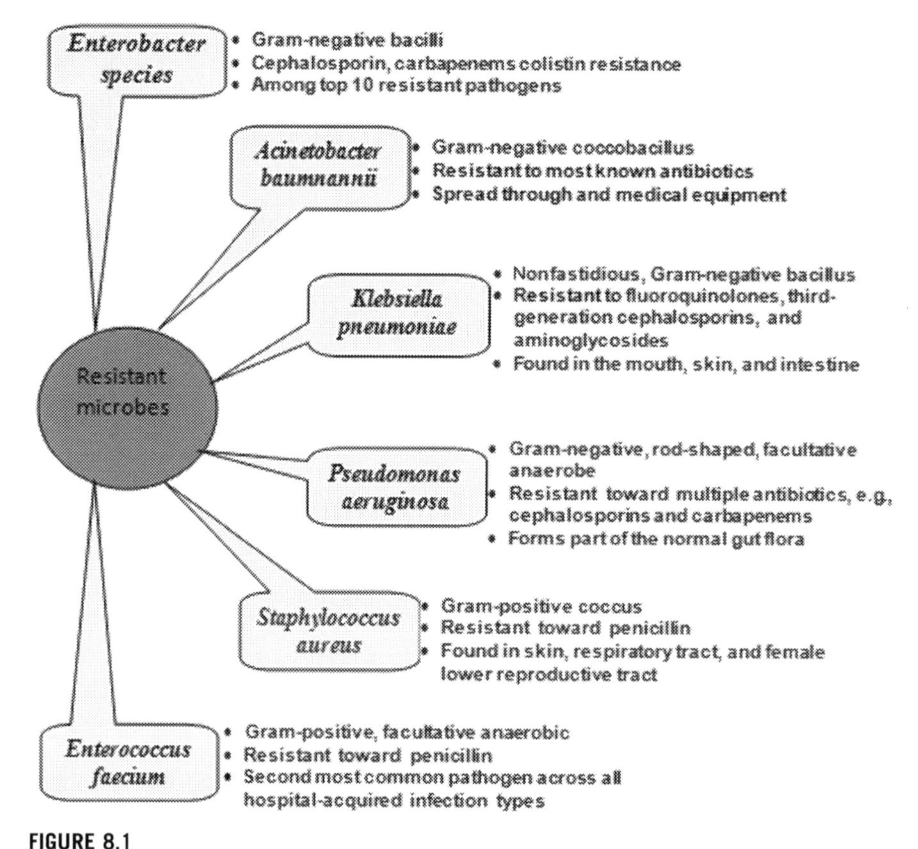

FIGURE 8.1

Pathogens resistant to most commonly used antimicrobial agents in clinical treatment.

of nanotechnology in biomedical field enhances the effectiveness of the drug within the body. For proper drug delivery system, many NPs have been approved in the past few years (Uddin et al., 2017; Badwaik et al., 2018). Due to antimicrobial property and its nanosize structure, polymeric nanoparticles (PNPs) attain immense attention in the field of biomedical application as well as in other areas such as food, environment, and water.

Polymeric nanomaterials (PNMs) with antimicrobial property show a tendency to hinder the growth of microbes on the surface and in nearby areas. PNMs either have antimicrobial activity itself or can act as controlled release carrier for antimicrobial agents. In 1965 researchers introduced antimicrobial polymers by preparing polymers and copolymers from 2-methacryloxytroponones that destroy bacterial growth (Cornell and Donaruma, 1965). In the 1970s many researchers prepared salicylic acid and quaternary ammonium groups–based polymeric structures that showed antimicrobial activity (Vogl and Tirrell, 1979; Panarin et al., 1971). It was found that antimicrobial characteristics of PNMs depend on several

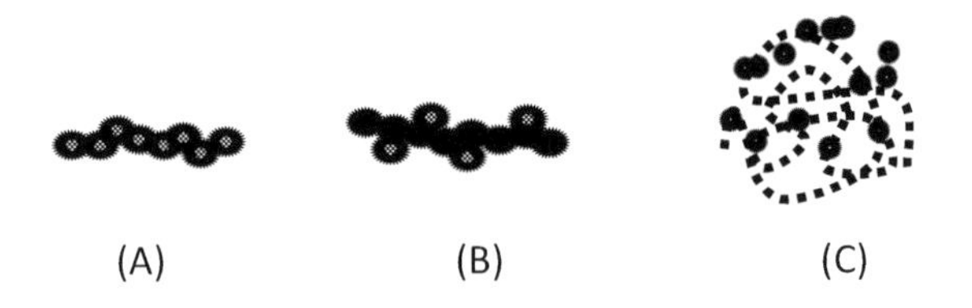

FIGURE 8.2

An illustration of (A) antimicrobial polymer, (B) polymer modified for antimicrobial activity, and (C) polymeric carrier for antimicrobial agent.

features such as molecular weight, distribution of charge, and type and degree of alkylation (Timofeeva and Kleshcheva, 2011). NMs can complement and support traditional antibiotics "as a good carrier" (Zhang et al., 2010).

Some PNPs made up of polymers such as compounds with quaternary nitrogen, chitosan, halamines, and poly-ε-lysine have a natural tendency to show antimicrobial property, and some are incorporated with others to display their activity (Jain et al., 2014). Since 2013, as per the Google Patent Search database, around 27,845 patents have been filed for antimicrobial polymers (Siedenbiedel and Tiller, 2012). PNPs are polymeric carriers in the size range of 1–1000 nm, prepared by various natural or synthetic polymers, in which the antimicrobial agent can be immobilized in solid or solution form or are adsorbed on the surface physically or by chemical linkages (Tosi et al., 2008). Antimicrobial NMs can be broadly classified into three types: (1) NMs prepared from antibacterial polymers, (2) PNMs modified to show antimicrobial activity, and (3) NMs as carrier for antimicrobial agents. A schematic illustration of these three types is shown in Fig. 8.2.

8.2 Nanomaterials prepared from antimicrobial polymers

Polymers having covalently linked biologically active repeating units having antimicrobial activity are known as antimicrobial polymers or polymeric biocides (Francolini et al., 2015). These types of polymers have the ability to kill microbes. These can be directly used for antimicrobial applications or can be used in combination with other antimicrobial agents. Antimicrobial activity of responsible functional group may increase or decrease during and after the polymerization reaction (Huang et al., 2016).

8.2.1 Cationic polymers

Cationic polymers attract the negatively charged phosphatidylethanolamine which is present in bacterial cell as a key constituent. Micro/nanosized polymeric particles and gels having positive charge are popularly utilized as effective antimicrobial agent. Strong interaction between cationic DNA and polymer colloids, ability to swell in acid, and the ability to form oriented bonds with proteins make them suitable for antimicrobial activity. Destructive interaction with cytoplasmic membranes and/or the cell wall is responsible for bactericidal action of the polycationic biocides (Kenawy et al., 2007). Particle sizes and presence of functional groups on these polymers have a high impact on pharmacokinetics and biodistribution. It was found that positively charged NPs show higher removal velocity as compared to negatively charged NPs. Mononuclear phagocyte system quickly removed the protected particles in a size range of 100 and 200 nm (Zhang et al., 2008). Some cationic monomers used for preparing antibacterial polymers are given in Table 8.1.

Table 8.1 Cationic monomers used for the preparation of polymers with antimicrobial activity.

Class	Monomer name	Structure
Vinylpyridines and their quaternary ammonium salts	2-VP	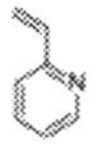
	4-VP	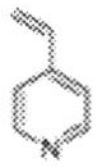
	MVPC MVPI	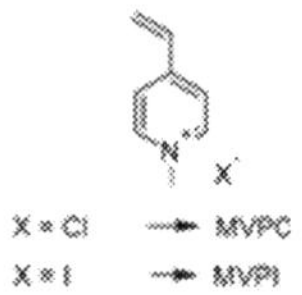 X = Cl → MVPC X = I → MVPI
	DMVP	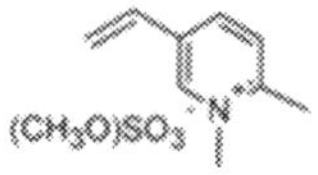 $(CH_3O)SO_3^-$
	EMVPB	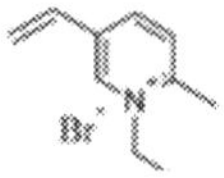 Br^-
(Dialkylamino)ethyl methacrylates	DMAEMA DEAEMA	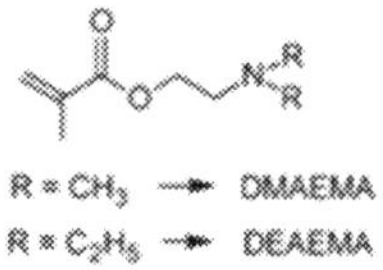 R = CH_3 → DMAEMA R = C_2H_5 → DEAEMA
QACMs	VBTMAC	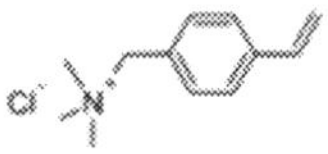 Cl^-

(Continued)

Table 8.1 Cationic monomers used for the preparation of polymers with antimicrobial activity. *Continued*

Class	Monomer name	Structure
	MATMAC MATMAI	X = Cl → MATMAC X = I → MATMAI
	MAPTMAC	
	DADMAC	
	DMBEMAB	
DMBMAPAB		
Primary amino-functionalized monomers	VBAH	
	AMEH	
Other cationic monomers	VBIC	
	VBH	

2-VP, *2-Vinylpyridine;* 4-VP, *4-vinylpyridine;* AMEH, *aminoethyl methacrylate hycrochloride;* DADMAC, *diallyldimethyl ammonium chloride;* DEAEMA, *2-(diethylamino)ethyl methacrylate;* DMAEMA, *2-(dimethylamino)ethyl methacrylate;* DMBEMAB, *N,N-dimethyl-N-butyl-N-ethyl methacrylate ammonium bromide;* DMBMAPAB, *N,N-dimethyl-N-butyl-N-methacrylamidino propyl ammonium bromide;* DMVP, *1,2-dimethyl-5-vinylpyridinium methyl sulfate;* EMVPB, *1-ethyl-2-methyl-5-vinylpyridinium bromide;* MAPTMAC, *[3-(methacryloyl-amino) propyl] trimethylammonium chloride;* MATMAC, *[2-(methacryloyloxy)ethyl] trimethylammonium chloride;* MATMAI, *[2-(methacryloyloxy) ethyl] trimethylammonium iodine;* MVPC, *1-methyl-4-vinylpyridinium chloride;* MVPI, *1-methyl-4-vinylpyridinium iodide;* QACMs, *quaternary ammonium cationic monomers;* VBAH, *vinylbenzylamine hydrochloride;* VBH, *4-vinylbenzyl hydrazine;* VBIC, *vinylbenzyl isothiouronium chloride;* VBTMAC, *vinylbenzyl trimethylammonium chloride.*

Reproduced with permission from Ramos, J., Forcada, J., Hidalgo-Alvarez, R., 2013. Cationic polymer nanoparticles and nanogels: from synthesis to biotechnological applications. Chem. Rev. 114 (1), 367–428 (Ramos et al., 2013).

8.2.1.1 Polymers containing nitrogen/phosphorous in polymeric backbone

These types of polymers show antimicrobial properties due to the presence of biocidal quaternary ammonium salt (QAS) and quaternary phosphonium salt (QPS) in the main chain (Tosi et al., 2008; Fidkowski et al., 2005; Tamami et al., 2012; Rodič et al., 2013). Polymers containing QAS groups are commonly used as polymeric biocides.

Researchers developed antimicrobial surfaces by using releasable NPs having covalently linked QAS/QPS (Shi et al., 2004). Li et al. fabricated antimicrobial thin film having two different functional layers—the top layer was made up of NPs immobilized [3-(trimethoxysilyl) propyl] octadecyl-dimethylammonium chloride and below this a silver-ion reservoir was present. The coating was found to be bifunctional and showed antibacterial activity by releasing biocide and contact-killing surface. Due to this bifunctional nature, the prepared coating showed a better bactericidal effect even after the exhaustion of silver ions (Li et al., 2016).

8.2.1.2 Cationic quaternary polyelectrolytes

Acrylic/methacrylic derivatives are cationic quaternary polyelectrolytes that are widely used as antimicrobial polymers. Mostly, these antibacterial polymers are prepared by using 2-(dimethylamino)ethyl methacrylate, which is a methacrylic monomer. Antimicrobial properties of these polymers can be improved by alteration during preparation in composition, charge, molecular weight, hydrophobicity, etc. Gottenbos et al. (2001) prepared trimethylaminoethyl methacrylate chloride and antimicrobial activity against *Staphylococcus epidermidis*, *Staphylococcus aureus*, *Escherichia coli*, and *Pseudomonas aeruginosa* were evaluated. Researchers found that the antimicrobial nature of cationic quaternary polyelectrolytes is majorly dependent upon the property of amine side chains and hydrophobic nature. It was further observed that the reversible protonation of amine group is required to achieve toxic-free antimicrobial polymers. Methacrylamide copolymers that contain few polar ester groups required much high content of hydrophobic comonomer to stimulate hemolysis (Palermo and Kuroda, 2010). Cationic-conjugated polyelectroytes are also having antimicrobial activity but are less studied due to difficult preparation methods.

8.2.1.3 Polyoxazolines

Polyoxazolines having quaternary ammonium end groups show appreciable antibacterial properties. They are also known as pseudopeptides (Hoogenboom, 2009). Flexible nature and low toxicity of polyoxazolines makes them excellent end-functionalized antibacterial polymers. Waschinski and coworkers used QAS for the end functionalization of polyoxazolines and prepared a series of antibacterial polymers. They found that the antimicrobial activity is largely affected by polymeric backbone. They also found aggregation of polyoxazolines which results in the formation of unimolecular micelles that leads to an improved antimicrobial activity (Waschinski and Tiller, 2005).

8.2.2 Polymers containing aromatic or heterocyclic structures

Some cationic polymers that contain aromatic/heterocyclic skeleton structures are known to have antibacterial activity. Polymers obtained from vinylpyridine (VP) and polystyrene (PS) which contain quaternary ammonium moieties are having great antimicrobial potential. Reactive pyridine moieties in poly(vinylpyridine) (PVP) are responsible for their antimicrobial activity. Antimicrobial activity quaternized PVP depends on the alkyl chain length. Researchers prepared an antibacterial thin film with covalently attached alkylated pyridinium polymers which was able to kill bacteria on contact to coated glass slide (Siedenbiedel and Tiller, 2012). Quaternized PVP with alkyl bromides can kill drug-resistant bacteria such as *P. aeruginosa*, *S. epidermidis*, and *E. coli*. It works more efficiently with *N*-hexylated PVP. It was also found that block and random copolymer having quaternized PVP and PS also shows appreciable antimicrobial activity (Park et al., 2004a,b).

Imidazole derivatives are excellent examples of antimicrobial polymers having aromatic/heterocyclic structures (Anderson and Long, 2010). Imidazole derivatives are compatible with living tissues and biodegradable. The imidazole ring shows resistance to hydrogenation process and provides excellent chemical consistency. By aromatic substitution reactions the imidazoles form various functional derivatives that are antimicrobial in nature. Due to this reason, many researchers developed vinyl- and acryl-substituted imidazole derivatives for antimicrobial applications. It was found that imidazolium salt prepared by quaternization of neutral imidazole acts as polycationic biocide (Soykan et al., 2005).

Phenols are antibacterial agents active in the bacterial membrane. These phenolic derivatives degenerate the bacterial cell membrane that results in liberation of intracellular material and hence cell death. Park et al. developed antimicrobial polymer by using vinyl monomers having benzoic acid a phenol pendant group. They evaluated antimicrobial activity of polymer against *Aspergillus fumigates*, *Penicillium pinophilum* fungi and *S. aureus*, *P. aeruginosa* bacteria. They reported that the polymerization reaction reduces the bactericidal action of the monomers (Park et al., 2001). Many derivatives of benzaldehyde are also extensively used as safe broad-spectrum bactericide, algaecide, and fungicide. Subramanyam et al. copolymerized *p*-acryloyloxybenzaldehyde with methyl methacrylate (MMA) to prepare antifouling polymer. They evaluated antibacterial efficiency of copolymer against *P. aeruginosa* and *Bacillus macroides* by paper disk method and found considerable antibacterial activity (Subramanyam et al., 2009).

8.2.3 Hyperbranched and dendritic polymers

Dendrimers are sphere like, hyperbranched, nanosized, symmetric molecules having well-defined, monodisperse structure with tree-like arms (Sampathkumar and Yarema, 2007). Hyperbranched polyethyleneimine (PEI) shows great antimicrobial potential. Hydrophobic substituent in hyperbranched PEI improves its antimicrobial activity. Quaternization helps in not only conserving water solubility of

PEI but also increasing the ability to absorb in bacterial membrane. PEI is generally prepared by tertiary amination reactions (Gao et al., 2007).

Andreas et al. prepared a series of nanocomposite films by solvent-casting technique in which as a base polymer, they used poly(vinyl alcohol) (PVA), and in place of active material, they used a multiwalled carbon nanotube that was functionalized with quaternized hyperbranched PEI. Due to hydrophilic nature the prepared carbon-based functionalized dendritic polymer showed appreciable water solubility. The prepared films were transparent with better mechanical properties and excellent antibacterial activity (Sapalidis et al., 2018).

Researchers prepared branched PEI with quaternary ammonium–functionalized primary amine groups having alkyl chains of different length, allylic, and benzylic groups. Due to this grafting strategy the hydrophobic/hydrophilic balance, molecular weight of the functional branched PEIs, the length of the hydrophobic groups can be easily tuned. Antimicrobial activity of this polymer was evaluated against *Bacillus subtilis* and *E. coli* and found appreciable antimicrobial activity (Pasquier et al., 2008). Abid et al. prepared various generation of poly(ethylene glycol)diacrylate-based dendrimers, which was quaternized with hydrochloric acid. The antibacterial activity of this dendritic copolymer was tested against *S. aureus* and *E. coli*. They reported that the antibacterial activity mainly depends on the surface porosity and the concentration of quaternary ammonium group. It was also found that the mechanical strength decreases as the generation of the dendrimer increases (Abid et al., 2010).

8.2.4 Polymers mimic natural peptides

Polymers mimicking natural peptides are generally based on norbornene (Michl et al., 2014), polyguanidines, polybiguanidines, and β-lactams (Gabriel et al., 2008), they are also prepared by guanylation reaction with 1*H*-pyrazole-1-carboxamidine hydrochloride (Bernatowicz et al., 1992; Michl et al., 2014). Polyguanidines and polybiguanides received high attention as antimicrobial polymeric compound due to good antibacterial efficiency, broad-spectrum antimicrobial activity, high water solubility, and nontoxic nature (Ganewatta and Tang, 2015). Polyguanidines inhibit bacterial growth by adhesion and subsequent disruption of Ca^{2+} salt bridges which results in cell death (Jain et al., 2014). Preparation of guanidine-containing polymers is generally done by the reaction of cyanamide/dicyanamide (polybiguanides) and chlorcyan with a diamine or by polycondensation of a diamine with a guanidinium salt (Zhang et al., 1999). Researchers worked on some guanidine-based oligomers and evaluated the minimum average molecular weight of the oligomers to maintain the antibacterial activity and the influence of the diamine and guanidinium salt on it. They evaluated antimicrobial activities against *B. subtilis*, *S. aureus*, *E. coli*, and *Saccharomyces cerevisiae* and found good antimicrobial activity (Feiertag et al., 2003; Albert et al., 2003).

8.2.5 Halogen polymers

Polymers containing halogen molecule in its structure show broad-spectrum antimicrobial activity. These polymers show hydrophobic and oleophobic characters due to firm electronegativity and low polarizability. Surface activity and high hydrophobic character are responsible for its antimicrobial activity. Moon et al. synthesized a polymer having quinolone moieties bearing a fluorine atom. They analyzed the antimicrobial action against *Micrococcus luteus*, *E. coli*, *S. aureus*, and *B. subtilis* by shake flask method and found appreciable antimicrobial activity (Moon et al., 2003). Guittard and his coworkers prepared various surfactants, called Quaterfluo, in which perfluoroalkyl chains were inserted in the gemini structure. They evaluated antimicrobial activity against *S. aureus*, *P. aeruginosa*, bacteria, *Aspergillus niger* fungus, and *Candida albicans* and found no count of bacteria detected after 1 h of contact (Guittard and Geribaldi, 2001).

2,4,4-Trichloro-2′-hydroxydiphenylether, triclosan having antifungal and antibacterial properties and also have acrylate functionality, was copolymerized to develop terpolymers with varying composition of hydroxyethyl acrylate and butyl acrylate. Antimicrobial activity was evaluated against *E. coli* and *S. epidermidis* bacteria as well as against two other marine-fouling microorganisms. They reported that an increase in amount of triclosan moieties enhances the antimicrobial activity (Kugel et al., 2009). Patel and his coworkers have developed 4-chloro-3-methylphenol and 2,4-dichloro-based acrylic monomers and copolymerized them with vinyl acetate (VA), MMA, methyl acrylate, or 8-quinolinyl methacrylate in different studies. Prepared polymers were examined against *B. subtilis*, *Staphylococcus citreus*, *E. coli* bacteria; *Candida utilis*, *S. cerevisiae*, *Pichia stipitis* yeasts; and *A. niger*, *Trichoderma lignorum*, *Sporotrichum pulverulentum* fungi. They reported that the presence of chlorine groups in these polymers enhances the antimicrobial activity, and the antimicrobial property decreases with the decreased amount of chlorine (Kugel et al., 2009; Patel et al., 2003, 2005, 2006, 2009).

8.3 Modified nanomaterials for antimicrobial activity

For adding antimicrobial activity into polymers, different methods were adopted by the researchers. Following are some common approaches used for chemical modification of the polymer to achieve antimicrobial property:

- covalent attachment of polymers with small molecules having antimicrobial characteristics;
- antimicrobial peptides (AMPs) set on an inactive polymer; and
- grafting of antimicrobial polymer on an inactive polymer.

8.3.1 Covalent attachment of polymers with small antimicrobial molecules

Sun and his coworkers added cyclic halamine precursors with high-performances fibers, such as polybenzimidazole/poly(*p*-phenylene terephthalamide), poly(aromatic imide-amide), and poly(*m*-phenylene isophthalamide) blend (Sun and Sun, 2001). They also inserted these cyclic halamines into polypropylene by reaction extrusion. Antibacterial properties of the modified polymers were tested against *E. coli*. All of them showed high potent activity. The best activity was shown by 2,4-diamino-6-diallylamino-1,3,4–5-triazine derivative. Park et al. modified copolymer of ethylene and VA with three antimicrobial salicylic acid, 4-aminobenzoic acid, and 4-hydroxy benzoic acid. The antimicrobial effectiveness was tested against *P. aeruginosa* and *S. aureus* by shake flask method. They reported that the copolymer that was modified with salicylic acid (SA) had higher antimicrobial activity as compared to other (Park et al., 2004a,b).

8.3.2 Coupling of antimicrobial peptides

AMPs represent a group of short, cationic, gene-encoded peptide antibiotics which is virtually present in every organism. AMPs have been regarded as a promising solution to combat multidrug-resistant bacteria (Melo et al., 2009). However, limited success in clinical trials was found for AMP due to salt sensitivity, poor in vivo stability, and high toxicity to mammalian cells (Dann and Hontela, 2011; Chu et al., 2013; Xie et al., 2017). Researchers have been conjugated AMPs by coupling or polymerization with some functional polymers to solve these problems (Costa et al., 2015; Siriwardena et al., 2017; Zhou et al., 2013). NPs from AMP polymer conjugates show better antibacterial activity compared to AMPs and their linear analogs (Lam et al., 2016; Hou et al., 2017). It was found that poly(ethylene glycol) (PEG) can protect the positive charges on AMPs, which shield them from the attack of immune system and provide prolong circulation time in blood (Hamley, 2014). Liu et al. prepared conjugate of N-termini of monomeric peptides RWRW-NH2 and RRWW-NH2 with polymaleic anhydride. They protected all side chains to avoid cross-linking and observed enhanced antimicrobial activity against Gram-negative *E. coli* and Gram-positive *B. subtilis* (Liu et al., 2006). Becker et al. prepared a micellar assembly by an AMP (tritrpticin) conjugated with amphiphilic block copolymer i.e. poly(acrylic acid) and polystyrene (PAA-*b*-PS). They found that the PS segment was forming the core and AMP was distributed on the surface with a hydrodynamic diameter of 51 ± 5 nm. They determined the antibacterial activity of micelle against *S. aureus* and *E. coli* and found minimum inhibition concentration (MIC) was 13 μg/mL for both microorganisms, whereas MIC of the tritrpticin alone for *S. aureus* and *E. coli* were 16 and 32 μg/mL, respectively (Becker et al., 2005).

8.3.3 Grafting other antimicrobial polymers

Grafting method is largely used for the surface modification for creating antibacterial surfaces such as fabric, packaging materials, and other polymeric surfaces. Cen et al. were grafted polyethylene terephthalate (PET) films with 4-VP followed by quaternization with hexyl bromide to get pyridinium groups. They evaluated a modified surface against *E. coli* and found that the killing efficiency was greatly affected by pyridinium concentration on the surface. They reported that the modified surface was highly effective when pyridinium concentration on surface was larger than $1.5 \times 10-4\ \text{mol/m}^2$. Natural polymers were also grafted to synthetic polymers for creating antimicrobial properties (Cen et al., 2003). Yang et al. grafted nonwoven polypropylene fabric with acrylic acid (AA) and immobilized it with chitosan (poly-β(1−4)-D-glucosamine). The antimicrobial activity was evaluated against *P. aeruginosa* and it was found that the antibacterial activity increased with the increase in AA grafting. An increase in antimicrobial activity was noticed upon incorporation of chitosan due to its antimicrobial nature (Yang et al., 2003).

8.4 Polymeric nanomaterial as carrier for antimicrobial agent

PNMs are promising candidates for controlled release of antimicrobial agents. Polymeric nanocarriers increase the effectiveness of drug (Kalhapure et al., 2015). They provide many benefits as a carrier for antimicrobial agent such as good biocompatibility, low toxicity, improved bioavailability, and enhanced drug solubility (Yang and Pierstorff, 2012). Polymeric nanocarriers such as micelles, nanocapsules, nanospheres, nanogels, liposomes, etc. have attracted much more attention for the controlled delivery of antimicrobial agent to target site. Polymers that are used for the preparation of nanosized carriers range from natural to synthetic. A schematic illustration of some widely used polymeric nanocarriers is shown in Fig. 8.3.

Polymeric nanocarriers can be prepared from different polymers, from natural to synthetic. Polymers that are broadly used for the preparation of nanocarriers for antimicrobial agents are summarized in Table 8.2.

8.5 Mechanisms for antimicrobial activity

NMs as antimicrobial agents are complementary to conventional antimicrobial agents that are highly potential and gaining popularity among researchers as they may decrease the harmful side effects and limitations of simple antimicrobial agents. This includes fight against biofilms, multidrug failure, and mutants

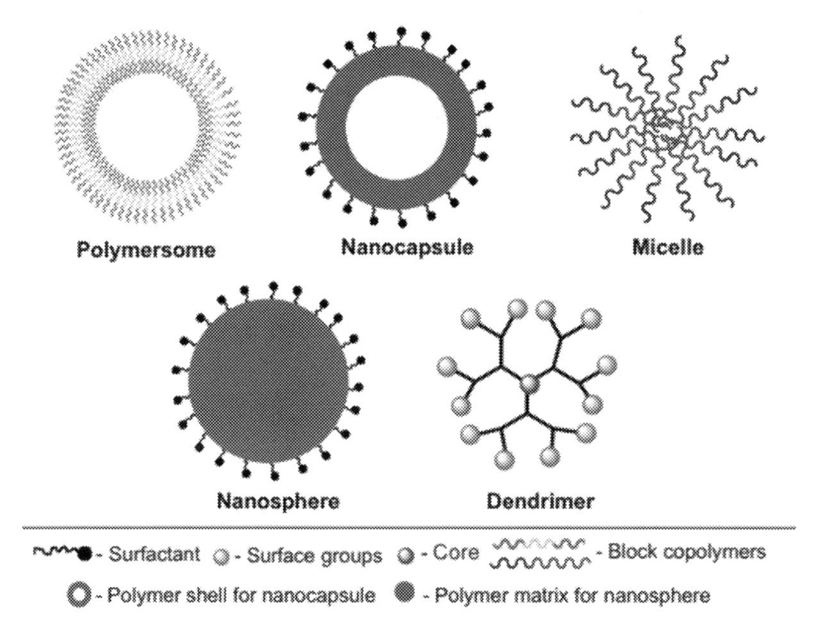

FIGURE 8.3

Schematic illustration of various polymeric nanocarriers.

Reproduced with permission from Iyisan, B, Landfester, K., 2019. Polymeric nanocarriers. In: Gehr, P., Zellner, R. (Eds.), Biological Responses to Nanoscale Particles, Nanoscience and Technology. Springer, Cham, pp. 53–84 (Iyisan and Landfester, 2019).

(Zhang et al., 2010; Pelgrift and Friedman, 2013). Polymeric antimicrobial NMs show a variety of intrinsic properties due to altered chemical compositions; hence, they have various modes of action. The planktonic or sessile states of the microbe, growth rate of biofilm, and type of microbes greatly influence the activity of NMs against microbes (Baek and An, 2011; Nath and Banerjee, 2013).

Active agent–loaded polymeric NPs release the antimicrobial agents at a controlled rate to kill microorganisms or polymeric surfaces with quaternary ammonium compounds, alkyl pyridiniums, or quaternary phosphonium kill microorganisms by contact killing. Researchers proposed several mechanisms of action for disruption of bacterial cell wall by cationic groups. Overall, the mechanism of antimicrobial activity of antibacterial PNMs can be categorized as passive or active mechanisms. A schematic diagram of active and passive mechanisms is shown in Fig. 8.4.

8.5.1 Passive mechanism

In passive mechanism the polymers have the ability to prevent adhesion of bacteria and also repel bacteria. In this mechanism the polymer does not interact

Table 8.2 Nanocarriers prepared from different types of polymers.

Type of polymer	Name	Type of nanomaterial	Antimicrobial active component	Reference
Natural	CS	Nanocapsule	Encapsulated gold	Belbekhouche et al. (2019)
		Nanocapsule	Antibacterial polypeptide and as a carrier for anticancer and antiepilectic drug	Zhou et al. (2013)
		Nanoparticle	Antimicrobial activities against phytopathogens	Oh et al. (2019)
		Nanocapsule	CD sulfate nanocapsule as drug carrier	Gnanadhas et al. (2013)
		Nanofilm	Drug triclosan	Chen et al. (2018)
		CS–fatty acid nanomicelles	Ciprofloxacin	Farhangi et al. (2018)
	Alginate	Nanocapsule	Encapsulated gold	Belbekhouche et al. (2019)
		Nanocomposite	Sodium alginate film containing functional Au-TiO_2 nanocomposites	Tang et al. (2018)
		Nanobiocomposite	AL/AgNP biocomposites	Nam et al. (2016)
	Starch	Nanoparticles	Starch stabilized silver	Kumar et al. (2018)
		Nanoparticle	Antibiotic	Ismail and Gopinath (2017)
		Nanoparticle	CS–starch–silver nanoparticle	Jung et al. (2018)
	Dextran	Nanogel	Silver nanoparticle	Ferrer et al. (2014)
		Nanofibers	Moxifloxacin antibiotic	Shawki et al. (2010)
		Nanogel	Polysaccharide nanogels, loaded with zinc ions	Malzahn et al. (2014)
	Lysozyme	Nanogel	Silver nanoparticle	Ferrer et al. (2014)
	Cellulose	Nanofiber	Zinc oxide (ZnO) nanoparticle	Panaitescu et al. (2018)
	Albumin	Nanomicelles	Doxorubicine	Xu et al. (2011)
Biosynthesized polymer	Poly(3-hydroxybutyrate) (PHB)	Bionanocomposites	ZnO nanoparticles	Pascual and Vicente (2014)
		Nanofibers	Zinc oxide (ZnO) nanoparticle	Panaitescu et al. (2018)
	PHBV	Nanoparticles	Eugenol-containing nanoparticles	Rodriguez et al. (2019)
		Nanocomposites	Silver	Castro-Mayorga et al. (2016)
Chemically synthesized polymer	Poly(lactic acid)	Nanocomposites	ZnO nanoparticle, polyvinyl alcohol	Restrepoa et al. (2018)
		Nanofiller	CS-coated with nanosilver as a filler	Nootsuwan et al. (2018)
	Polylactic-*co*-glycolic acid (PLGA)	Nanofibers	Silver nanoparticles	Almajhdi et al. (2014)

AL/AgNP, *Alginate/silver;* CD, *chitosan–dextran;* CS, *chitosan;* PHBV, *poly(3-hydroxybutyrate-co-3-hydroxyvalerate);* PLA, *poly(lactic acid).*

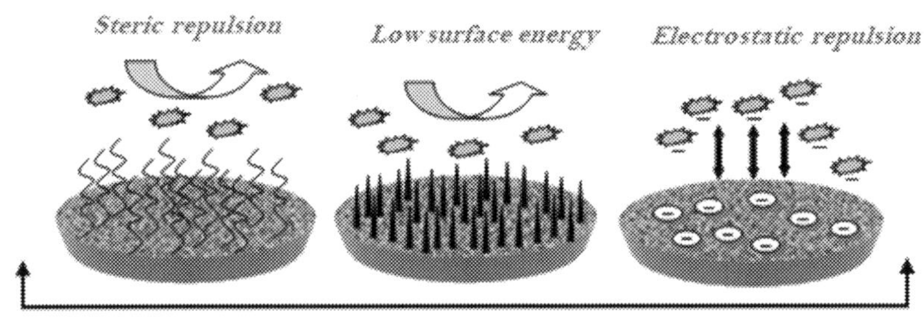

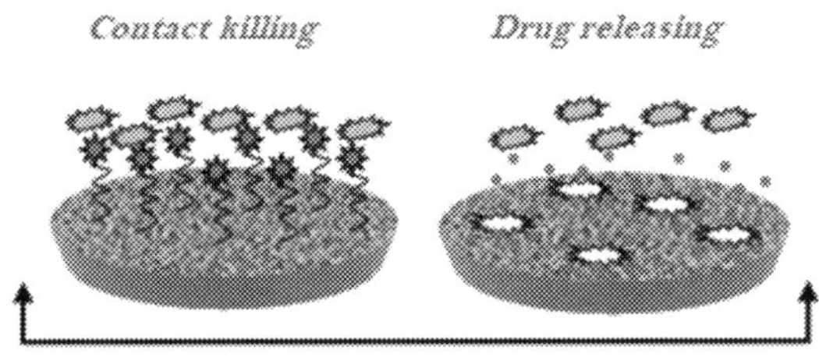

FIGURE 8.4

Schematic diagram of active and passive mechanisms.

actively to kill microbes. Because of hydrophilic nature and negatively charge of teichoic acids present in microbes, passive mechanism is shown by the polymers that are either positively charged or having hydrophobic surface with low surface free energy (Francolini et al., 2015; Zhang and Chiao, 2015).

Typical passive polymers include the following:

1. polymers with hydrophobic, porous surface, self-healing properties such as poly(dimethyl siloxane);
2. poly(*N*-vinylpyrrolidone) (PNVP), PEG, poly(2-methyl-2-oxazoline), and poly (dimethyl acrylamide) which are neutral polymers; and
3. polyampholytic polymers and polymers having zwitterionic structures, for example, phospholipid-, phosphobetaine-, sulfobetaine-based polymers (Liu et al., 2014; Ye and Zhou, 2015).

PEG has been studied broadly and found to have good antimicrobial effects. PEG reduces the adsorption of protein that results in decreased bacterial adhesion. PEG acts as a passive antimicrobial polymeric material due to large exclusion volume, high chain mobility, and steric hindrance by extensively hydrated layer (Zhang and Chiao, 2015; Liu et al., 2014; Ye and Zhou, 2015; Yu et al., 2014). Some passive polymers and their biomedical applications are given in Table 8.3.

Table 8.3 Passive polymers and their biomedical applications.

Passive polymer	Biomedical application	References
PEG, OEG	Used in antifouling or protein resistant coatings	Lee and Voros (2005), Zhang et al. (2001)
PCBMA	Protein adsorption	Ladd et al. (2008)
PC	Grafted PC helps in improving antithrombotic properties	Yu et al. (2014)
Zwitterionic BCMs	BCM films are used for its antiadhesive property	Hippius et al. (2014)
Protein-based bioplastics (albumin, soy, and whey)	Antimicrobial property	Jones et al. (2015)
Polyphenols (PPh)	Showing antimicrobial tendency toward periodontitis, a chronic infectious disease	Shahzad et al. (2015)

BCMs, *Block copolymer micelles;* OEG, *oligo ethylene glycol;* PC, *phosphorylcholine;* PCBMA, *poly (carboxybetaine methyl acrylate);* PEG, *poly(ethylene glycol).*

8.5.2 Active mechanism

Active polymers kill microbes that come in contact with polymeric surfaces. Polymers showing active killing of microbes are usually functionalized with some active antimicrobial substances, namely, AMPs, cationic antimicrobial agents, or antibiotics. The mechanism of active killing entirely depends on the nature of antimicrobial agents that are used for functionalization. Polymers functionalized with QAS are the most commonly used active antimicrobial polymer. Quaternary ammonium–functionalized polymers destroy the cytoplasmic membrane by interacting with the cell wall and results in the cell rupture that results in cell death (Xue et al., 2015).

Polyethylenimine, *N*-halamine, and polyguanidine are some of the common active polymeric antimicrobial agents. Polyethylenimine electrostatically interacts with cell membrane to rupture it and cause cell death. Oxidative halogens that are present at amino or thio groups of cell receptors are attacked by *N*-halamine and cause cell death. Polyguanidine interrupts the function of calcium salt bridges which results microbial cell death (Jain et al., 2014).

In active killing the PNMs act by two major destructive pathways: (1) interfere in membrane potential and disturbing the microbial cell integrity; (2) formation of reactive oxygen species (ROS)/oxygen-free radicals that catalyze the killing mechanism. These two pathways are complementary to each other and usually occur simultaneously (Pelgrift and Friedman, 2013; Huh and Kwon, 2011; Blecher et al., 2011). Electrostatic binding of NMs with microbial cell wall and membrane alters the membrane potential due to which depolarization occurs and microbial cell loses its integrity that results in cell lysis and finally cell death

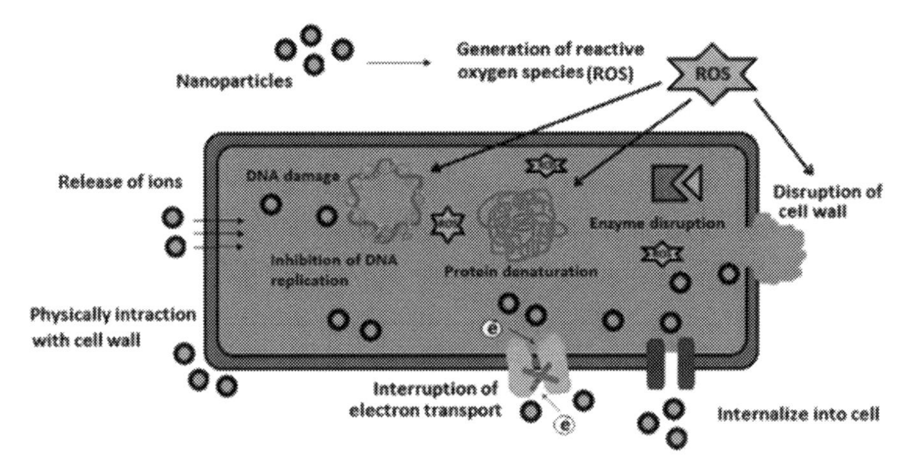

FIGURE 8.5

Various active mechanisms of antimicrobial activity by the nanoparticles.

Reproduced with permission from Chiriac, V., Stratulat, D.N., Calin, G., Nichitus, S., Burlui, V., Stadoleanu, C., et al., 2016. Antimicrobial property of zinc based nanoparticles. IOP Conf. Ser. Mater. Sci. Eng. 133 (1), 012055 (Chiriac et al., 2016).

(Pelgrift and Friedman, 2013). Various active mechanisms of antimicrobial activity by the NPs are depicted in Fig. 8.5.

Production of ROS is considered as the most efficient way for cytotoxicity of NMs (Nathan and Cunningham-Bussel, 2013). Sudden release of ROS due to severe oxidative stress leads to alteration of protein structures, inhibition of enzymes, lipid peroxidation, and nucleic acid damage. High concentrations of the ROS cause cell death, and low concentration leads to mutations and DNA damage (Pan et al., 2010; Wang et al., 2011). The toxicity of NM can be photocatalyzed by inducing production of ROS with visible or UV light (Matejka and Tokarsky, 2014). For example, Maness et al. (1999) studied bactericidal activity of photocatalytic TiO_2 and found that TiO_2 NPs induce lipid peroxidation under UV light that results respiratory disturbance in *E. coli* cells and leads to cell death. Some polymers showing active mechanisms and their biomedical applications are given in Table 8.4.

8.6 Factors influencing antimicrobial activity

Antimicrobial activity of the polymers depends on many factors such as spacer length (alkyl chain length), molecular weight, and types of counterion (Ikeda et al., 1984). These factors play a very important role during antimicrobial action and its mechanism. The ratio between the microbial population and the amount of NM is a very critical factor for toxic effect exerted by NM against microbe (Huh and Kwon, 2011). Environmental factors such as temperature, pH, and aeration also play an important parameter and greatly influence the toxicity of NM for

Table 8.4 Polymers showing active mechanisms and their biomedical applications.

Active polymers	Biomedical application	Reference
Nisin peptides	Helps in preventing bacterial biofilm formation and maintain surface hygiene	Duday et al. (2013)
Carbamate containing QAS with polyurethane	QASs used as active agent, combined with polyurethane by cross-linking with terpene-based polyol and polyisocyanate This combination is used as antimicrobial coating	Liu et al. (2015)
Cationic polymers containing tertiary amine	By means of polymerization novel dual-function amphiphilic random copolymers produced Helps in preventing biofilm infections also reduces the risk of emergence of drug-resistant bacteria	Taresco et al. (2015)
Fluorosilicone copolymers having poly(2(dimethylamino) ethyl methacrylate) and poly (hexafluorobutyl methacrylate)	Used for antimicrobial coating	Zhou et al. (2015)
QAC	Helps in preventing the transmission of pathogens in medical wards	Yuen et al. (2015)

QAC, Quaternary ammonium chloride; QAS, quaternary ammonium salt.

microbes. Shape, size, chemical architect, composition, solvent used, and combination of different NPs in various ratios also affect the antibacterial activity (Gatoo et al., 2014). Some main factors that greatly influence antimicrobial activity of polymeric NMs are discussed in the following subsections.

8.6.1 Molecular weight

Molecular structures of various PNM highly influence the antimicrobial properties; hence, many researchers have evaluated the dependency of molecular weight on toxic effects of PNMs (Tashiro, 2001; Kenawy et al., 2007). Polymers containing quaternary and alkyl structures such as *N*-hexyl-poly vinyl pyrrolidine required minimum a molecular weight of 160 and 25 kDa, respectively, to show efficient antibacterial effects on various microbial species (Klibanov, 2007). Huang and coworker prepared poly(2-(dimethylamino) ethyl methacrylate) (PDMAEMA)-coated PP surface by grafting method. The tertiary amine group presents in PDMAEMA converted into quaternary ammonium that was the limiting factor for the antibacterial activity of the coated surface. They observed that the antibacterial action of the coated surface was directly proportional to the quantity of the grafted polymers. The results showed that polymer containing high molecular weight (> 10,000 g/mol) exhibits high killing efficiency up to 100%; on the other hand, low MW (1500 g/mol) grafted polymers observed less efficient (Huang et al., 2007). Timofeeva et al. prepared aqueous solutions of the secondary and tertiary polydiallylamines cationic polymers, and their antimicrobial activities were evaluated against Gram-positive and Gram-negative bacteria. They found that antibacterial activity of the polymers was directly dependent on molecular weight. They observed that 100% killing of bacteria decreases at MW a range 24–60 kDa (Timofeeva et al., 2009).

The bacterial cell surface is negatively charged due to the presence of teichoic acids. Therefore polycationic polymers adsorbed negatively charged bacterial population to a great extent as compared to monomeric cations. Hence, it can be concluded that antimicrobial activity is more for polymers as compared to their monomers. Ikeda et al. prepared polycationic–polymeric antibacterials having pendent phosphonium salts, and a comparative evaluation of antibacterial activity for prepared polymer and corresponding monomers was done. They found that the antimicrobial activity was enhanced with the increase in molecular weight (Dizman et al., 2004; Kanazawa et al., 1993a,b). Chen et al. prepared poly(propyleneimine) dendrimers and functionalized them with quaternary ammonium. They reported that the antimicrobial activity of the prepared dendrimers showed a parabolic dependence on molecular weight (Chen et al., 2000).

8.6.2 Counterion

Kanazawa et al. studied the antimicrobial effect of [tributyl (4-vinyl benzyl) phosphonium] on *S. aureus* and evaluated counter-anion dependency. They observed that the antimicrobial activity was greatly influenced by the counter anions. Initially, the antimicrobial activity was lower for the counter anions that facilitate the formation of tight ion pair with phosphonium ion, whereas it was higher for those facilitating ionic dissociation to form free ions. The extent of antimicrobial activity was found to be in the order chloride > tetrafluoride > perchlorate > hexafluorophosphate, which was attributed to the solubility products of the polymers (Kanazawa et al., 1993a,b). Chen et al. synthesized quaternary ammonium dendrimers and evaluated their antimicrobial activity and found that the activity was greatly influenced by counterion. They found that dendrimers having bromide anions show a higher activity compared to those having chloride anions (Chen et al., 2000).

Dutta and coworker prepared a range of amino acid–based hydrogelating amphiphiles by varying the counter anion from chloride to carboxylate. They studied the extent of antimicrobial activity and found that the change in counter ion greatly influences antimicrobial properties. They reported that the inclusion of a hydrophobic group in the counterion enhances the antibacterial activity of prepared amphiphiles (Dutta et al., 2011). Dong et al. prepared antimicrobial surface by using poly(1-(2-methacryloyloxyhexyl)-3-methylimidazolium bromide) (PILBr) having counterion-responsive nature. The properties of these PILBr can be shift repeatedly as bacterial killing and release mode. They replaced the counter-anion chains with lithium bis(trifluoromethanesulfonyl)amide and found that the surface becomes hydrophobic from hydrophilic. Counter-anion switching results in a collapsed chain conformation that permits the release of dead microbes. The switching of killing and releasing actions of the surface was maintained up to three cycles (Dong et al., 2016).

8.6.3 Spacer length and alkyl chain

Antimicrobial activity of the polymeric material is highly influenced by the spacer length as it affects the change in conformation and charge density of the polymer. Conformation and charge density affect the interaction between cytoplasmic membrane and polymer; hence, the spacer length is a major factor that affects the antimicrobial activity of PNMs. Tiller et al. (2001) reported that for synthesizing alkylated quaternized PVP polymers the optimum alkyls tail length should be C6 and above this may affect the antimicrobial efficiency of the synthesized polymer. The polymeric microbeads were prepared by using phase inversion techniques in which the poly(4-VP) and poly(vinylidene fluoride) were mixed to use as a substrate. The pyridine group was converted to pyridinium by quaternization with alkyl bromide to impart antibacterial activity. The alkyl bromide has about 4–10 carbon atoms chain, resulting N-alkylated polymeric beads having a capacity to breakdown the bacterial and fungal spores upon contact. It was also concluded during research that as longer the C10 hydrophobic chains found to be highly effective in degrading the fungal wall (Hu et al., 2005).

Sawada et al. (1999) developed end-capped 2-(3-acrylamidopropyldimethylammonio) ethanoate with perfluoro-propyl and perfluoro-oxaalky. The fluorinated polymers were tested for antimicrobial activities against *S. aureus* and *P. aeruginosa*. It was observed that the polymer with oxaalkyl group was more effective than polymer having propyl group that was attributed to the longer chain length. Nonaka et al. prepared copolymers of methacryloylethyl trialkyl phosphonium chlorides/*N*-isopropylacrylamide. They reported that the antimicrobial activity for *E. coli* was increased with the increase in the alkyl chain length in the phosphonium groups of the copolymer (Nonaka et al., 2003).

8.6.4 Branching in polymeric chain

Antimicrobial activity is also affected by branching in structure of PNM. Generally, branching increases the antibacterial activity such as in the case of dendrimers. Branched polymers and some hyperbranched dendrimers act as polyvalent inhibitors which means they fight both bacterial and viral diseases. Chen and Cooper (2002) compared the antimicrobial activity between cationic dendrimers and imperfect dendritic polymers. They found that poly(propyleneimine) dendrimers functionalized with QAS show parabolic dependence of the antimicrobial properties (Chen et al., 2000). Wang and coworkers studied the antimicrobial activity of a set of cationic poly(sulfone amines) (PSAs) by changing the branched structures and their silver nanocomposites (PSA/Ag). They reported that the size of silver NPs (AgNPs) decreases with an increase in branching in polymeric structure. The antimicrobial activity was decreased with the branched structure of PSAs, due to the decreased zeta-potential; whereas an increased antimicrobial activity with increase in branched architecture was found for PSA/Ag nanocomposites (Wang et al., 2012a,b).

8.7 Application of polymeric antimicrobial nanomaterials

In this section, we will discuss some common applications of PNMs based on their antimicrobial activity. Developments in the field of nanotechnology helped in creating new and more efficient antimicrobial agents with improved properties. Some main applications of antimicrobial PNMs are shown in Fig. 8.6.

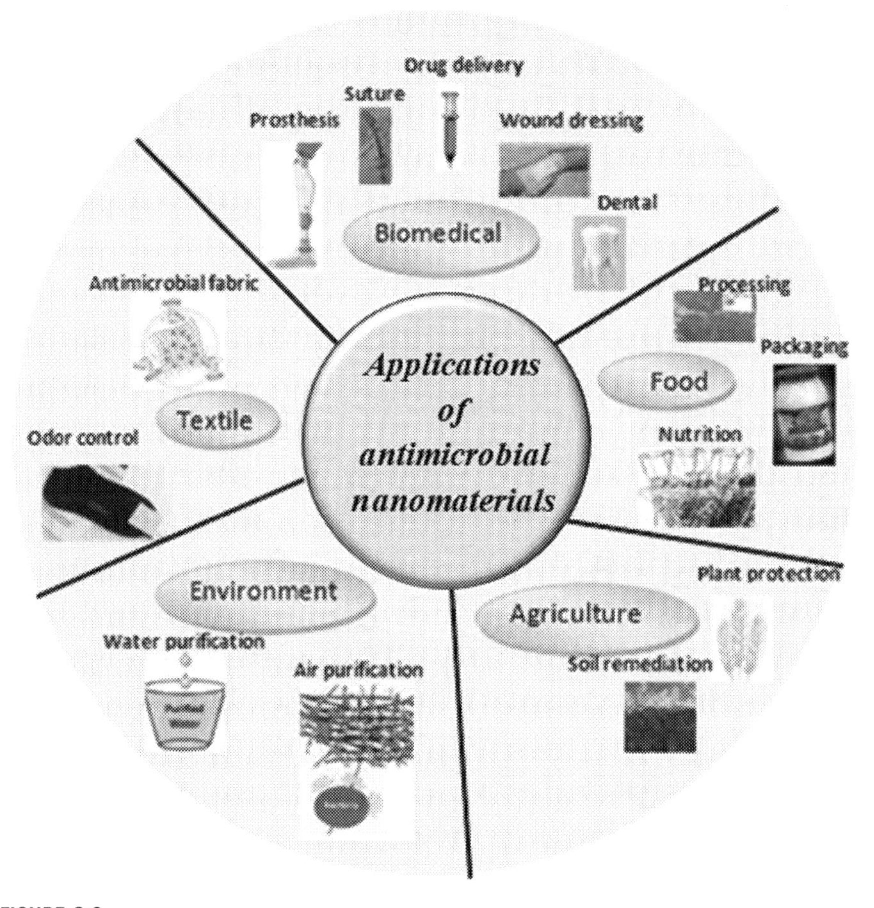

FIGURE 8.6

Main applications of antimicrobial PNMs. *PNM*, Polymeric nanomaterial.

8.7.1 Biomedical applications

The major objectives for developing antimicrobial NMs for biomedical purposes are to avoid biofilm formation and to decrease the risk of spreading the infection among people. As already discussed, resistant microbes are becoming an alarming threat to human health due to improper use of antibiotics; hence, the search for more efficient antimicrobial agent is continuously increasing for biomedical applications.

8.7.1.1 Wound dressing

Wound type, wound healing time, should be considered in the designing of a successful wound dressing. Physical, chemical, and mechanical properties of the dressing are also an important parameter. By using an appropriate wound dressing, it is possible to achieve faster healing rates and better esthetic repair of the wound (Zahedi et al., 2010). Electrospinning is a low-cost, simple, and very commonly used method for manufacturing preparing wound dressings (Agarwal et al., 2013). Chitosan that is having antibacterial activity is extensively used to treat wound and burn infections. Due to its biocompatible, nontoxic, and hemostatic nature, it stimulates wound healing (Dai et al., 2011; Jayakumar et al., 2011). Dutta and his coworkers prepared chitosan-based wound dressing. They blended chitosan with synthetic polymer PNVP and added TiO_2/Ag_2O NPs to enhance antimicrobial property (Archana et al., 2013), a synthetic polymer with good biocompatibility. The prepared polymeric solution was electrospun to fibers to use as wound dressing. Lin et al. (2013) electrospun chitosan with nanocellulose, which has found extensive application in biotechnological areas such as drug delivery, tissue engineering, and wound dressing.

8.7.1.2 Dental applications

NPs with polymers have been found to exhibit good antimicrobial properties in the oral cavity (Saafan et al., 2018). Metal and organic NPs have been applied in many areas of dentistry due to broad-spectrum antibacterial properties (Magalhaes et al., 2016). Pietrokovski and Nisimov combined nanosized calcium phosphate with quaternary ammonium PEI (Pietrokovski et al., 2016) and found appreciable antibacterial activity with long durability. A composite containing quaternary ammonium dimethacrylate and silver NPs was prepared by Cheng and Zhang having a stronger antibacterial activity up to 12 months of water-aging (Cheng et al., 2016). Beyth and his coworkers synthesized (Beyth et al., 2006; Yudovin-Farber et al., 2008) PEI-based cationic NPs by cross-linking and subsequent quaternization and methylation with bromooctane and methyl iodide, respectively. They incorporated 1% NP in commercial dental resin. They reported strong antimicrobial activity of modified dental resin against *Streptococcus mutans*. Also, over 1-month NP–modified dental composite maintained full mechanical property and antimicrobial activity without leaching of NPs. Fik et al. prepared antimicrobial polymers of poly(2-metyloxazoline) with quaternary ammonium end group for dental application. They used this antimicrobial polymer as additive in a commercial dental adhesive. The modified dental adhesive was able to kill *S. mutans* in the tubule of tooth (Fik et al., 2014).

8.7.1.3 Drug delivery

Antibiotics given via conventional routes, that is, oral, ocular, intravenous, and intramuscular are found to have lack of control over release rates; hence, large and multiple doses of active agents are required to attain therapeutic concentrations at the site of infection. Large and multiple doses may result undesirable toxicity and side effects. Polymeric NPs are a promising alternative for controlled release of antibacterial agent and also increase its effectiveness (Kalhapure et al., 2015). These antibiotics loaded polymeric nanocarriers can be rapidly taken up by the microorganisms followed by intracellular release of the active agent. Many synthetic and natural polymers have been used to prepare nanocarriers for the controlled release of antibiotics (Álvarez-Paino et al., 2017). Kumar et al. prepared polylactic co-glycolic acid (PLGA) NPs for the encapsulation of levofloxacin followed a modified emulsion–diffusion–evaporation method in which they used mannitol and sucrose as lyoprotectants (Kumar et al., 2012). The best result was found with mannitol showing higher stability and less aggregation. After a single oral administration of encapsulated levofloxacin in mice, drug release into the blood plasma NPs was sustained up to 4 days in mice after single oral administration. Also, there was no sign of toxicity was found in mice up to 2 weeks of treatment.

A list of some commonly used PNMs used in biomedical applications is given in Table 8.5.

8.7.2 Food applications

8.7.2.1 Food packaging

In the field of food packing, shelf life and better storage are one of the crucial factors to maintain its freshness. Antimicrobial coating plays a vital role during food packing by enhancing its shelf life (Muriel-Galet et al., 2012). Generally, PET, polyethylene, PS, ethylene/VA copolymer, polypropylene (PP), and ethylene-vinyl alcohol copolymer are the various petroleum-based polymeric materials that are used in food packaging in the form of antimicrobial films (Joerger, 2007). Usually, natural polymers are not used because comparatively they are not as strong as synthetic polymers. However, few natural polymers like chitosan have antimicrobial property, due to which it is used in food-packaging process (Hoagland, 1999). Chitosan can also be used to encapsulate other antibacterial agents to enhance antimicrobial activity (Hong et al., 2005; Lee et al., 2003). Polymeric antimicrobial agents can be coated on packaging by lamination (Hoagland, 1999), spraying (nebulization) (Contini et al., 2011), immersion (Vasile et al., 2011; Stoleru et al., 2016), etc.

Table 8.5 Biomedical applications of antibacterial polymeric nanomaterials.

Polymer type	Type		Application	References
Natural	Chitosan	Chitosan/pluronic hydrogels	Show better transfection efficiency and also enhance local transgene expression at the site of injection for gene therapy	Lee et al. (2009)
		Cisplatin-loaded chitosan microspheres	Drug release	Bergisadi (1999)
		Nanocomposite	Helps in promoting cell growth and mineral-rich matrix deposition by osteoblasts cells in culture	Seol et al. (2004)
		Chitosan–TPP nanoparticles	siRNA delivery	Katas and Alpar (2006)
	Alginate	Hydrogel	Cell encapsulation, cell transplantation, and tissue engineering	Rowley et al. (1999), Saxena et al. (1999), Kolambkar et al. (2011), Roman et al. (2009)
	Cellulose	Nanocrystal	Drug delivery	Vinatier et al. (2009)
		Hydrogel	Tissue engineering, controllable delivery system, blood purification, sensor, chromatographic supports	Vinatier et al. (2009), Chang et al. (2010), Ye et al. (2003), Sannino et al. (2007), Xiong et al. (2005)
	Starch	Microsphere	Used as drug delivery carrier produced by emulsion cross-linking method	Malafaya et al. (2006)
Biosynthesized	Poly (ε-caprolactone)	Heparin-conjugated poly(ε-caprolactone) electrospun fiber	Used for the development of vascular grafts to lower the mortality rate due to various vascular diseases	Wang et al. (2012a,b)
	PGS	Microfabricated capillary networks	Helps in tissue-engineered microvascular network scaffold	Fidkowski et al. (2005)
Chemically synthesize PNPs	Polylactic (PLA)	Nanofibers	Helps in controlling biodegradation rate, as well as the hydrophilicity rate during biomedical application	Kim et al. (2003)
	Polyurethane	Grafted films	Blood compatibility	He et al. (2011)
	Polylactic Co-glycolic acid (PLGA)	Nanoparticles	Gene delivery, vaccine delivery system, cancer imaging and cancer therapy, cerebral diseases	Panyam and Labhasetwar (2003), Beaudette et al. (2009), Chittasupho et al. (2009), Edwards (2001)
	PMMA	Nanomaterial scaffolds	Bone-fixation materials, dental materials, artificial crystal	Zhao et al. (2013)

PGS, *Poly(glycerol sebacate)*; PMMA, *polymethyl methacrylate resin*; TPP, *tripoly phosphate*.

Antimicrobial nanocomposite films that are prepared by impregnating the fillers (having at least one dimension in the nanometric range or NPs) into the polymers offer two-way benefit because of their structural integrity and barrier properties (Rhim and Ng, 2007). Variety of antimicrobial agents was used for the formation of antimicrobial nanocomposites used in food packaging such as metal oxide NPs (MgO, TiO_2, MgO), metals NPs (silver, copper), modified nanoclays, chitosan, nisin, and essential oils–laden particles, and synthetic compounds such as QASs, antibiotics, and organic acids (Sung et al., 2013; Azeredo, 2013). Generally, synthetic and natural polymer–based antimicrobial food-packaging films were having a tendency to enter into the food and prevent microbial growth in the food surface by direct contact. The working mechanism mainly depends on the preparation method and the type of the antimicrobial NPs incorporated into the matrix. Some parameters like dispersibility, particle size, interaction between NP, and the polymer are responsible for influencing the antimicrobial activity of the nanocomposites (Huang et al., 2018).

8.7.2.2 Preservation or shelf life

To increase the freshness of the packed food, bioactive components are added, and to prevent it from degradation and inactivation due to unfavorable environment, nanoencapsulation of antimicrobial NM is done. By encapsulating NPs, the shelf life of food products increases by lowering degradation process or it hinders degradation until the product is to be delivered at the designated site area. Variety of food products used nanocoating results in preventing moisture content loss, any gas exchange. It also helps in maintaining the flavors, color, antioxidants, and enzymes and provides long shelf life even after the packed food product is opened (Weiss et al., 2006; Renton, 2006). Moreover, the edible nano-coatings encapsulating the functional components within the droplets often enable a slowdown of chemical degradation processes by engineering the properties of the interfacial layer surrounding them. For example, *Curcuma longa* (curcumin) is known for most active and least stable bioactive component; upon encapsulating, this component shows stability at varying ionic strength to pasteurization process (Sari et al., 2015).

8.7.3 Textile

Textile products such as bedding, pillows, and surgical gowns are potential sources of health care–associated infections in hospital. Almost all clothing and textile materials carry microbes that can readily be colonized. Textile materials provide a good substrate for the growth and colonization of microbes in hospitals. An ideal antimicrobial fabric finishing should be nontoxic, safe, and environment friendly (Corcoran, 1998). Neely and Maley (2000) evaluated the survival lifetimes of staphylococci and enterococci typically found on the surface of textile and other materials commonly found in hospitals and reported around 1–8 weeks for different fabrics. Bozja et al. (2003) developed light-activated antimicrobial fabric in which they were used protoporphyrin IX and zinc protoporphyrin IX to nylon fibers by using grafting method. These fibers were investigated against *S. aureus* and *E. coli* in the presence of light. It was concluded that these fabrics are activated only during availability of suitable light source; in its absence, it shows ineffective nature toward both the strains. Worley and his coworkers (Ren et al., 2009; Cerkez et al., 2013) used halamine compounds such as polypropylene or polyacrylonitrile to enhance the antimicrobial action of synthetics and cotton fabrics. They also observed hydantoin diol–based cotton with TiO_2 NPs combination and concluded that modified fabric has excellent antimicrobial tendency against *S. aureus* and *E. coli*.

Busila et al. prepared Ag:ZnO/chitosan nanocomposite coatings modified by sol–gel method using 3-glycidyloxypropyltrimethoxysilane and tetraethoxysilane as functionalization agents. They applied coating on various fabric blends of cotton/polyester and evaluated its antimicrobial activity. The coated fabric exhibited high antimicrobial and higher thermal stability than that of only chitosan-coated fabric. The best antibacterial effect was found with cotton/polyester (50%/50%) fabric (Busila et al., 2015). Natural fibers contributing to the reduction of environmental pollution as well as the burden of waste disposal have recently received considerable attention and became highly valuable materials. A new type of textile consisting of mulberry fibers uniformly laden with titania nanorods was prepared using sol–gel electrospinning and facile dip-coating methods. The mulberry fiber–TiO_2 composite textile exhibited improved antimicrobial activity compared with pure mulberry textile. Furthermore, the advantages of this unique natural-synthetic composite textile are its antiyellowing and self-cleaning properties, which are due to the scattering effect of UV radiation by titania nanorods (Jang et al., 2015). For fabricating eco-friendly antimicrobial textile material the impregnation of polypropylene (PP) and corona-modified PP nonwoven material with thymol by supercritical solvent impregnation with carbon dioxide as a working fluid was proposed. The thymol impregnation yield was approximately 7% for both PP and corona-modified PP nonwoven fabrics, providing antimicrobial activity against *S. aureus*, *E. coli*, and *C. albicans*. Nevertheless, the higher rate of thymol release from the corona-modified material was due to the higher fiber surface hydrophilicity (Markovic et al., 2015).

8.7.4 Environmental applications

8.7.4.1 Air purification

Contamination in the air majorly occurs due to the bacterial and fungal cells, endospores, and spores that enter the environment through biological and nonbiological routes. Various bacterial and fungal strains such as *Pseudomonas*, *Micrococcus*, *Bacillus*, *Mucor*, *Cladosporium*, *Penicillium*, Phoma, and *Aspergillus* are responsible for infecting the environment. Therefore it is necessary to control such infection in the prone areas like hospitals and food-manufacturing industries (Álvarez-Paino et al., 2017). To cope up with the air-purification issue, antimicrobial polymer shows tremendous growth. Researchers used soybean crops and poly-ethylene-oxide (PEO) for making high bacterial filtration efficiency (BFE) nanofilters that are mainly used against bacterial aerosols consisting of *E. coli*. For the formation of BFE, nanofilter blending of pure soy flour (SF) and PEO in a ratio of 7:3 is done by adopting electrospinning method. Protein derived from the soybean crop is available in three different forms—soy protein isolate, soy protein concentrate, and defatted SF—which hold approximately 90%, 70%, and 52% protein, respectively. Generally, agar diffusion tests are performed to detect the antimicrobial property of the produced nanofibers. In this study the BFE of the nanofiber filter was analyzed by passing the aerosolized *E. coli* through the testing equipment. After that the filtered aerosol again passes through agar gel that results in the deposition of bacteria present in the aerosol. The quantitative measurement of the filter BFE is done by counting bacterial colonies after incubation period. Researchers compared the BFE between nanofiber filters consisting of pure PEO and soy protein nanofiber filter with different mass ranging from 1 to 5 g/m^2.

It was observed that the PEO nanofiber and soy protein nanofiber having a 5 g/m^2 mass show 100% and 81.5% BFE values, respectively. The results also suggested that BFE value becomes high as the protein content in the nanofiber increases. Scanning electron microscopy (SEM) images and the bacterial filtration tests specify that nanofibers containing soy protein effectively entrapped Gram-negative bacteria due to the presence of positive charge on the nanofiber surface. It is also noted that the small quantity, that is, 3 g/m^2 of soy protein–based nanofibers effectively captured 100% of the airborne bacteria present in the environment (Lubasova et al., 2014). Usually, high-efficiency particulate air (HEPA) filter is used within the hospitals units such as oncology, surgical wards, and hematology units (Duce et al., 2000) to remove infectious microorganism from the circulated air. As per the Department of Energy, it is recorded that HEPA efficiently removed about 99.97% of airborne particles having a diameter of 0.3 μm from infectious air. Taylor and coworkers used the bactericidal activity polymer coating over HEPA filter with broad-spectrum polyurethane with quaternary ammonium group and analyzed it against eight bacterial species mainly responsible for nosocomial infection. The results suggested that by increasing the coating solution concentration the bactericidal action of the coated HEPA against infectious airborne particle also increased. The minimum coating concentration of 4 mg/mL is efficient but taking about 2 h to kill all the bacteria in the solution, whereas the maximum concentration of about 8 mg/mL takes 30 min to kill all the bacteria present. The bactericidal activity of the coated filter majorly depends upon its thickness which is measured by using an SEM imaging system. It is noted that the coated HEPA filter showed an improved tendency toward air purification (Taylor et al., 2015).

8.7.4.2 Water purification

Generally, for water purification, chlorine disinfection method is highly used; during purification process, chlorine ions get reacted with organic substance present in wastewater, resulting in the formation of trihalomethane that is carcinogenic in nature. Due to this reason, antimicrobial PNMs are used with high interest; various classes of polymers were used for water purification such as polymeric phosphonium material (Kenawy et al., 2002), polymeric quaternary ammonium compound (Waschinski et al., 2008). Various crosslinked anion exchange resins such as polyiodide resins, quaternary ammonium-type resins, insoluble polyelectrolytes, macroporous, and macroreticular resins are also used for water-disinfection process, they are known as insoluble disinfectants (Abid et al., 2010).

Phenols are known to be one of the highly polluted organic compounds; its discharge into the environment causes obnoxious taste and smell in the drinking water. The major sources are coal-processing plant, pesticides, paper and paint industries, refineries, etc. For the removal of phenol from wastewater researchers synthesized curcumin formaldehyde resin (CFR), a bio-based polymeric adsorbent by using polycondensation method with formaldehyde. Various analytical methods are used such as carbon, hydrogen and nitrogen analyser (CHN), Fourier transform infrared (FTIR), thermogravimetric analysis, differential thermal analysis, differential scanning calorimetry (TGA-DTA-DSC), nuclear magnetic resonance (NMR), Brunauer–Emmett–Teller analysis (BET), SEM for the characterization of CFR. During study, it was observed that CFR has a very high removal rate for phenol. And by means of CFR the phenol removal rate is quite fast and stability sets within 1 h (Alshehri et al., 2014). For the removal of bacterial species from the wastewater, Bonenfant et al. modified the carboxymethylcellulose and β-CD-based polymers by synthesizing with various quaternary ammonium compounds. The recorded results showed that these compounds were positively used for the elimination of *E. coli* from the wastewater (Bonenfant et al., 2011).

8.7.5 Agriculture

Polymeric NPs help the agricultural sector in various ways. By applying polymeric coating, it enhances the capability of the plant to intake nutrients and helps plant tissue to combat with the plant pathogen and various plant diseases, resulting in increased productivity without damaging the soil profile. Use of parasite in agricultural field for high production decreased the soil and land productivity; to overcome these problems, many researchers use natural polymers like alginate or PVA polymeric film to cover the soil which results in keeping the soil moist and also ensures decontamination of the soil. The usage of natural polymer for coating is beneficial due to the reason that they degrade itself after use (Hajji et al., 2016; Russo et al., 2005).

To protect the cultivated field from various pests, pathogens, and weeds, many researchers investigate new formulation by utilizing nanotechnology. An effective modern fungicide TEB—which stands for Tebuconazole—known for its fungicidal activity exhibits triazole components that help in regulating plant growth (Hedden et al., 1989; Child et al., 1993). To improve its efficiency in the agriculture sector, many researchers formulate advanced fungicides by incorporating polymeric NP into TEB. To produce slow-release fungicide formulation, TEB is embedded in the polymer matrix—films and pellets consist of the natural degradable P3HB [poly(3-hydroxybutyrate)]. FTIR spectroscopy, differential scanning calorimetry, X-ray structure analysis are some methods by which formulated fungicide were studied (Volova et al., 2015). Other polymeric particles like poly (methyl methacrylate) and poly(styrene-*co*-maleic anhydride) were also used by some researchers for encapsulating TEB. This formulation helps in controlling wheat rust, Puccinia recondite well-known plant diseases (Asrar et al., 2004).

In the agriculture sector, plastic film is used drastically, which results in poor nutrient availability due to its nondegradable behavior. To overcome these difficulties, many researchers suggest the use of modified biodegradable polymeric NPs. They modified biodegradable p polymer with antimicrobial agent such as silver and chitosan, and bio-based alcohols (glycerol and PEG) are also used. Plasma technique was used to modify polymeric surface by incorporating an efficient antimicrobial agent silver into PLA polymer. Low molecular weighted antimicrobial polymer agents such as chitosan, glycerol, and PEG were used for the bulk modification of PLA. By means of surface modification, polar groups on the surface are generated, which enhance the hydrophilicity of the PLA resulting in high adhesion and colonization; it also enhances the antimicrobial property. Against *E. coli*, *Listeria monocytogenes* and *Salmonella typhimurium* bacteria–modified PLA shows positive growth inhibition factor whereas observed less efficient toward the growth inhibition of *S. aureus* (Turalija et al., 2016).

To prevent the use of chemically hazardous pesticides, many researchers extract the essential oil of various aromatic plants such as lavandin by means of steam distillation process and use it as an alternative for insect repellent. For encapsulation, two high-pressure precipitation methods are used, namely, particles from gas saturated solutions (PGSS) and PGSS-drying. In PGSS process, simply extracted essential oil is encapsulated into PEG polymer, whereas in PGSS-drying, *n*-octenyl succinic–modified starches are used for the encapsulation of extracted oil; before encapsulation, it is necessary to remove all the water by forming oil-in-water emulsion process (Varona et al., 2010).

8.8 Conclusion and future prospects

With the increase in resistant microbes, it is difficult to treat such microbial infections with the conventional antimicrobial agents. Researchers are continuously developing new carriers to target such resistant microbes and increase the bioavailability of antimicrobial agent. Various PNMs are a promising candidate to develop broad-spectrum antimicrobial agents. Polymers with covalently linked biologically active repeating units show excellent antimicrobial activity. Also, antimicrobial activity can be incorporated by covalent attachment, coupling or grafting of antimicrobial polymer on inactive polymer. Various polymeric nanocarriers such as nanocapsule, micelle, nanosphere, and dendrimers are commonly used for broad-spectrum antimicrobial activity. The polymeric nanocarriers show both passive and active mechanism. Molecular weight, counter ion, spacer length, and branching in polymeric chains are the main features influencing the antimicrobial activity of PNMs. Broad-spectrum antimicrobial PNMs are very useful in biomedical agricultural, food processing, textile, and environmental applications in treating microbial infections.

References

Abid, C.Z., Chattopadhyay, S., Mazumdar, N., Singh, H., 2010. Synthesis and characterization of quaternary ammonium PEGDA dendritic copolymer networks for water disinfection. J. Appl. Polym. Sci. 116 (3), 1640–1649.

Agarwal, S., Greiner, A., Wendorff, J.H., 2013. Functional materials by electrospinning of polymers. Prog. Polym. Sci. 38 (6), 963–991.

Albert, M., Feiertag, P., Hayn, G., Saf, R., Honig, H., 2003. Structure activity relationships of oligoguanidines influence of counterion, diamine, and average molecular weight on biocidal activities. Biomacromolecules 4 (6), 1811–1817.

Almajhdi, F.N., Fouad, H., Khalil, K.A., Awad, H.M., Mohamed, S.H., Elsarnagawy, T., et al., 2014. In-vitro anticancer and antimicrobial activities of PLGA/silver nanofiber composites prepared by electrospinning. J. Mater. Sci. Mater. Med. 25 (4), 1045–1053.

Alshehri, S.M., Naushad, M., Ahamad, T., Alothman, Z.A., Aldalbahi, A., 2014. Synthesis, characterization of curcumin based ecofriendly antimicrobial bio-adsorbent for the removal of phenol from aqueous medium. Chem. Eng. J. 254, 181–189.

Álvarez-Paino, M., Muñoz-Bonilla, A., Fernández-García, M., 2017. Antimicrobial polymers in the nano-world. Nanomaterials 7 (2), 48.

Anderson, E.B., Long, T.E., 2010. Imidazole-and imidazolium-containing polymers for biology and material science applications. Polymer 51 (12), 2447–2454.

Archana, D., Singh, B.K., Dutta, J., Dutta, P.K., 2013. In vivo evaluation of chitosan–PVP–titanium dioxide nanocomposite as wound dressing material. Carbohydr. Polym. 95 (1), 530–539.

Asrar, J., Ding, Y., La Monica, R.E., Ness, L.C., 2004. Controlled release of tebuconazole from a polymer matrix microparticle: release kinetics and length of efficacy. J. Agric. Food Chem. 52 (15), 4814–4820.

Azeredo, H.M.C.D., 2013. Antimicrobial nanostructures in food packaging. Trends Food Sci. Technol. 30 (1), 56–69.

Badwaik, H.R., Nakhate, K., Kumari, L., Sakure, K., 2018. Oral delivery of proteins and polypeptides through polysaccharide nanocarriers. Polysaccharide Based Nano-Biocarrier in Drug Delivery. Taylor & Francis, pp. 1–24.

Baek, Y.W., An, Y.J., 2011. Microbial toxicity of metal oxide nanoparticles (CuO, NiO, ZnO, and Sb_2O_3) to *Escherichia coli*, *Bacillus subtilis*, and *Streptococcus aureus*. Sci. Total Environ. 409 (8), 1603–1608.

Beaudette, T.T., Bachelder, E.M., Cohen, J.A., Obermeyer, A.C., Broaders, K.E., Frechet, J.M., et al., 2009. In vivo studies on the effect of co-encapsulation of CpG DNA and antigen in acid degradable microparticle vaccines. Mol. Pharm. 6 (4), 1160–1169.

Becker, M.L., Liu, J., Wooley, K.L., 2005. Functionalized micellar assemblies prepared via block copolymers synthesized by living free radical polymerization upon peptide-loaded resins. Biomacromolecules 6 (1), 220–228.

Belbekhouche, S., Bousserrhine, N., Alphonse, V., Floch, F.L., Mechiche, Y.C., Menidjel, I., et al., 2019. Chitosan based self-assembled nanocapsules as antibacterial agent. Colloids Surf. B Biointerfaces 181, 158–165.

Bergisadi, J.A., 1999. Effect of formulation variables on cis-platin loaded chitosan microsphere properties. J. Microencapsulation 16 (6), 697–703.

Bernatowicz, M.S., Wu, Y., Matsueda, G.R., 1992. 1*H*-Pyrazole-1-carboxamidine hydrochloride an attractive reagent for guanylation of amines and its application to peptide synthesis. J. Org. Chem. 57 (8), 2497–2502.

Beyth, N., Yudovin-Farber, I., Bahir, R., Domb, A.J., Weiss, E.I., 2006. Antibacterial activity of dental composites containing quaternary ammonium polyethylenimine nanoparticles against *Streptococcus mutans*. Biomaterials 27 (21), 3995–4002.

Blecher, K., Nasir, A., Friedman, A., 2011. The growing role of nanotechnology in combating infectious disease. Virulence 2 (5), 395–401.

Bonenfant, D., Bourgeois, F.R., Mimeault, M., Monette, F., Niquette, P., Hausler, R., 2011. Synthesis and structure-activity study of quaternary ammonium functionalized β-cyclodextrin-carboxymethylcellulose polymers. Water Sci. Technol. 63 (12), 2827–2832.

Bozja, J., Sherrill, J., Michielsen, S., Stojiljkovic, I., 2003. Porphyrin-based, light-activated antimicrobial materials. J. Polym. Sci. A Polym. Chem. 41 (15), 2297–2303.

Burman, W.J., 2010. Rip Van Winkle wakes up: development of tuberculosis treatment in the 21st century. Clin. Infect. Dis. 50 (Suppl. 3), S165–S172.

Busila, M., Musat, V., Textorbc, T., Mahltigd, B., 2015. Synthesis and characterization of antimicrobial textile finishing based on Ag:ZnO nanoparticles/chitosan biocomposites. RSC Adv. 5 (28), 21562–21571.

Caminade, A.M., Turrin, C.O., 2014. Dendrimers for drug delivery. J. Mater. Chem. B 2 (26), 4055–4066.

Castro-Mayorga, J.L., Fabra, M.J., Lagaron, J.M., 2016. Stabilized nanosilver based antimicrobial poly(3-hydroxybutyrate-*co*-3-hydroxyvalerate) nanocomposites of interest in active food packaging. Innov. Food Sci. Emerg. Technol. 33, 524–533.

Cen, L., Neoh, K.G., Kang, E.T., 2003. Surface functionalization technique for conferring antibacterial properties to polymeric and cellulosic surfaces. Langmuir 19 (24), 10295–10303.

Cerkez, I., Worley, S.D., Broughton, R.M., Huang, T.S., 2013. Antimicrobial coatings for polyester and polyester/cotton blends. Prog. Org. Coat. 76 (7–8), 1082–1087.

Chakraborty, S., Kar, N., Kumari, L., De, A., Bera, T., 2017. Inhibitory effect of a new orally active cedrol-loaded nanostructured lipid carrier on compound 48/80-induced mast cell degranulation and anaphylactic shock in mice. Int. J. Nanomed. 12, 4849.

Chang, C., Duan, B., Cai, J., Zhang, L., 2010. Superabsorbent hydrogels based on cellulose for smart swelling and controllable delivery. Eur. Polym. J. 46 (1), 92–100.

Chen, C.Z., Cooper, S.L., 2002. Interactions between dendrimer biocides and bacterial membranes. Biomaterials 23 (16), 3359–3368.

Chen, C.Z., Beck-Tan, N.C., Dhurjati, P., van Dyk, T.K., LaRossa, R.A., Cooper, S.L., 2000. Quaternary ammonium functionalized poly(propylene imine) dendrimers as effective antimicrobials: structure–activity studies. Biomacromolecules (3), 473–480.

Chen, H., Yi, Z., Sun, L., Li, X., Shi, S., Hu, J., et al., 2018. Synthesis of chitosan-based micelles for pH responsive drug release and antibacterial application. Carbohydr. Polym. 189, 65–71.

Cheng, L., Zhang, K., Zhou, C.C., Weir, M.D., Zhou, X.D., Xu, H.H., 2016. One-year water-ageing of calcium phosphate composite containing nano-silver and quaternary ammonium to inhibit biofilms. Int. J. Oral Sci. 8 (3), 172–181.

Child, R., Evans, D., Allen, J., Arnold, G., 1993. Growth response in oilseed rape (*Brassica napus* L.) to combined applications of the triazole chemicals triapenthenol and tebuconazole and interactions with gibberelli. Plant Growth Regul. 13 (2), 203–212.

Chiriac, V., Stratulat, D.N., Calin, G., Nichitus, S., Burlui, V., Stadoleanu, C., et al., 2016. Antimicrobial property of zinc based nanoparticles. IOP Conf. Ser. Mater. Sci. Eng. 133 (1), 012055.

Chittasupho, C., Xie, S.X., Baoum, A., Yakovleva, T., Siahaan, T.J., Berkland, C.J., 2009. ICAM-1 targeting of doxorubicin-loaded PLGA nanoparticles to lung epithelial cells. Eur. J. Pharm. Sci. 37 (2), 141–150.

Christian, K.A., Ijaz, K., Dowell, S.F., Chow, C.C., Chitale, R.A., Bresee, J.S., et al., 2013. What we are watching—five top global infectious disease threats, 2012: a perspective from CDC's Global Disease Detection Operations Center. Emerg. Health Threats J. 6 (1), 20632.

Chu, H.L., Yu, H.Y., Yip, B.S., Chih, Y.H., Liang, C.W., Cheng, H.T., et al., 2013. Boosting salt resistance of short antimicrobial peptides. Antimicrob. Agents Chemother. 57 (8), 4050–4052.

Contini, C., Katsikogianni, M.G., O'Neill, F., O'Sullivana, M., Dowling, D.P., Monahana, F.J., 2011. Development of active packaging containing natural antioxidants. Procedia Food Sci. 1, 224–228.

Corcoran, L.M., 1998. Determining the Processing Parameters and Conditions to Apply Antimicrobial Finishes on 100% Cotton and 100% Polyester Dyed Knit Fabrics. Institute of Textile Technology, Charlottesville, VA.

Cornell, R.J., Donaruma, L.G., 1965. 2-Methacryloxytropones. Intermediates for the synthesis of biologically active polymers. J. Med. Chem. 8 (3), 388–390.

Costa, F.M., Maia, S.R., Gomes, P.A., Martins, M.C., 2015. Dhvar5 antimicrobial peptide (AMP) chemoselective covalent immobilization results on higher antiadherence effect than simple physical adsorption. Biomaterials 52, 531–538.

Dai, T., Tanaka, M., Huang, Y.Y., Hamblin, M.R., 2011. Chitosan preparations for wounds and burns: antimicrobial and wound-healing effects. Expert Rev. Anti-Infect. Ther. 9 (7), 857–879.

Dann, A.B., Hontela, A., 2011. Triclosan: environmental exposure, toxicity and mechanisms of action. J. Appl. Toxicol. 31 (4), 285–311.

Daraee, H., Etemadi, A., Kouhi, M., Alimirzalu, S., Akbarzadeh, A., 2016. Application of liposomes in medicine and drug delivery. Artif. Cells Nanomed. Biotechnol. 44 (1), 381–391.

Dizman, B., Elasri, M.O., Mathias, L.J., 2004. Synthesis and antimicrobial activities of new water-soluble bis-quaternary ammonium methacrylate polymers. J. Appl. Polym. Sci. 94 (2), 635–642.

Dong, Y.S., Xiong, X.H., Lu, X.W., Wu, Z.Q., Chen, H., 2016. Antibacterial surfaces based on poly(cationic liquid) brushes: switchability between killing and releasing via anion counterion switching. J. Mater. Chem. B 4 (36), 6111–6116.

Duce, G., Fabry, J., Nicolle, L., 2000. Prevention of Hospital Acquired Infections: A Practical Guide. World Health Organization, Geneva.

Duday, D., Vreuls, C., Moreno, M., Frache, G., Boscher, N.D., Zocchi, G., et al., 2013. Atmospheric pressure plasma modified surfaces for immobilization of antimicrobial nisin peptides. Surf. Coat. Technol. 218, 152–161.

Dutta, S., Shome, A., Kar, T., Das, P.K., 2011. Counterion-induced modulation in the antimicrobial activity and biocompatibility of amphiphilic hydrogelators: influence of in-situ-synthesized Ag − nanoparticle on the bactericidal property. Langmuir 27 (8), 5000−5008.

Edwards, R.H., 2001. Drug delivery via the blood−brain barrier. Nat. Neurosci. 4 (3), 221−222.

Farhangi, M., Kobarfard, F., Mahboubi, A., Vatanara, A., Martazavi, S.A., 2018. Preparation of an optimized ciprofloxacin loaded chitosan nanomicelle with enhanced antibacterial activity. Drug Dev. Ind. Pharm. 44 (8), 1273−1284.

Feiertag, P., Albert, M., Ecker-Eckhofen, E.M., Hayn, G., Hönig, H., Oberwalder, H.W., et al., 2003. Structural characterization of biocidal oligoguanidines. Macromol. Rapid Commun. 24 (9), 567−570.

Ferrer, M.C.C., Dastgheyb, S., Hickok, N.J., Eckmann, D.M., Composto, R.J., 2014. Designing nanogel carriers for antibacterial applications. Acta Biomater. 10, 2105−2111.

Fidkowski, C., Kaazempur-Mofrad, M.R., Borenstein, J., Vacanti, J.P., Langer, R., Wang, Y., 2005. Endothelialized microvasculature based on a biodegradable elastomer. Tissue Eng. 11 (1−2), 302−309.

Fik, C.P., Konieczny, S., Pashley, D.H., Waschinski, C.J., Ladisch, R.S., Salz, U., et al., 2014. Telechelic poly(2-oxazoline) s with a biocidal and a polymerizable terminal as collagenase inhibiting additive for long-term active antimicrobial dental materials. Macromol. Biosci. 14 (11), 1569−1579.

Francolini, I., Donelli, G., Crisante, F., Taresco, V., Piozzi, A., 2015. Antimicrobial polymers for anti-biofilm medical devices: state-of-art and perspectives. Adv. Exp. Med. Biol. 831, 93−117.

Gabriel, G.J., Madkour, A.E., Dabkowski, J.M., Nelson, C.F., Nüsslein, K., Tew, G.N., 2008. Synthetic mimic of antimicrobial peptide with nonmembrane-disrupting antibacterial properties. Biomacromolecules 9, 2980−2983.

Ganewatta, M.S., Tang, C., 2015. Controlling macromolecular structures towards effective antimicrobial polymers. Polymer 63, A1−A29.

Gao, B., Zhang, X., Zhu, Y., 2007. Studies on the preparation and antibacterial properties of quaternized polyethyleneimine. J. Biomater. Sci. Polym. 18 (5), 531−544.

Gatoo, M.A., Naseem, S., Arfat, M.Y., Mahmood Dar, A., Qasim, K., Zubair, S., 2014. Physicochemical properties of nanomaterials: implication in associated toxic manifestations. BioMed. Res. Int. 2014, 1−8.

Gnanadhas, D.P., Thomas, M.B., Elango, M., Raichur, A.M., Chakravortty, D., 2013. Chitosan−dextran sulphate nanocapsule drug delivery system as an effective therapeutic against intraphagosomal pathogen *Salmonella*. J. Antimicrob. Chemother. 68 (11), 2576−2586.

Gottenbos, B., Grijpma, D.W., van der Mei, H.C., Feijen, J., Busscher, H.J., 2001. Antimicrobial effects of positively charged surfaces on adhering Gram-positive and Gram-negative bacteria. J. Antimicrob. Chemother. 48 (1), 7−13.

Guittard, F., Geribaldi, S., 2001. Highly fluorinated molecular organised systems: strategy and concept. J. Fluorine Chem. 107 (2), 363−374.

Hajji, S., Chaker, A., Jridi, M., Maalej, H., Jellouli, K., Boufi, S., et al., 2016. Structural analysis, and antioxidant and antibacterial properties of chitosan-poly(vinyl alcohol) biodegradable films. Environ. Sci. Pollut. Res. Int. 23 (15), 15310−15320.

Hamley, I.W., 2014. PEG−peptide conjugates. Biomacromolecules 15 (5), 1543−1559.

He, C., Wang, M., Cai, X., Huang, X., Li, L., Zhu, H., et al., 2011. Chemically induced graft copolymerization of 2-hydroxyethyl methacrylate onto polyurethane surface for improving blood compatibility. Appl. Surf. Sci. 258 (2), 755–760.

Hedden, P., Croker, S.J., Rademacher, W., Jung, J., 1989. Effect of the triazole plant growth retardant BAS 111W on gibberellin levels in oilseed rape, *Brassica napus*. Physiol. Plant. 75 (4), 445–451.

Hippius, C., Butun, V., Erel-Goktepe, I., 2014. Bacterial anti-adhesive properties of a monolayer of zwitterionic block copolymer micelles. Mater. Sci. Eng. C 41, 354–362.

Hoagland, P.D., 1999. Inventor; The United States of America, as Represented by The Secretary of Agriculture, Assignee, Biodegradable Laminated Films Fabricated From Pectin and Chitosan.

Hong, S.I., Lee, J.W., Son, S.M., 2005. Properties of polysaccharide coated polypropylene films as affected by biopolymer and plasticizer types. Packag. Technol. Sci. 18 (1), 1–9.

Hoogenboom, R., 2009. Poly(2-oxazoline)s: a polymer class with numerous potential applications. Angew. Chem. Int. Ed. 48 (43), 7978–7994.

Hou, Z., Shankar, Y.V., Liu, Y., Ding, F., Subramanion, J.L., Ravikumar, V., et al., 2017. Nanoparticles of short cationic peptidopolysaccharide self-assembled by hydrogen bonding with antibacterial effect against multidrug-resistant bacteria. ACS Appl. Mater. Interface 9 (44), 38288–38303.

Hu, F.X., Neoh, K.G., Cen, L., Kang, E.T., 2005. Antibacterial and antifungal efficacy of surface functionalized polymeric beads in repeated applications. Biotechnol. Bioeng. 89 (4), 474–484.

Huang, J., Murata, H., Koepsel, R.R., Russell, A.J., Matyjaszewski, K., 2007. Antibacterial polypropylene via surface-initiated atom transfer radical polymerization. Biomacromolecules 8 (5), 1396–1399.

Huang, K.S., Yang, C.H., Huang, S.L., Chen, C.Y., Lu, Y.Y., Lin, Y.S., 2016. Recent advances in antimicrobial polymers: a mini-review. Int. J. Mol. Sci. 17 (9), 1578.

Huang, Y., Mei, L., Chen, X., Wang, Q., 2018. Recent developments in food packaging based nanomaterials. Nanomaterials 8 (10), 1–29.

Huh, A.J., Kwon, Y.J., 2011. "Nanoantibiotics": a new paradigm for treating infectious diseases using nanomaterials in the antibiotics resistant era. J. Controlled Release 156 (2), 128–145.

Ikeda, T.O., Yamaguchi, H.I., Tazuke, S.H., 1984. New polymeric biocides: synthesis and antibacterial activities of polycations with pendant biguanide groups. Antimicrob. Agents Chemother. 26 (2), 139–144.

Ilker, M.F., Nüsslein, K., Tew, G.N., Coughlin, E.B., 2004. Tuning the hemolytic and antibacterial activities of amphiphilic polynorbornene derivatives. J. Am. Chem. Soc. 126 (48), 15870–15875.

Ismail, N.S., Gopinath, S.C.B., 2017. Enhanced antibacterial effect by antibiotic loaded starch nanoparticle. J. Assoc. Arab Univ. Basic Appl. Sci. 24, 136–140.

Iyisan, B., Landfester, K., 2019. Polymeric nanocarriers. In: Gehr, P., Zellner, R. (Eds.), Biological Responses to Nanoscale Particles, Nanoscience and Technology. Springer, Cham, pp. 53–84.

Jain, A., Duvvuri, L.S., Farah, S., Beyth, N., Domb, A.J., Khan, W., 2014. Antimicrobial polymers. Adv. Healthcare Mater. 3 (12), 1969–1985.

Jang, Y.S., Amna, T., Hassan, M.S., 2015. Nanotitania/mulberry fibers as novel textile with anti-yellowing and intrinsic antimicrobial properties. Ceram. Int. 41 (5), 6274–6280.

Jansen, K.U., Knirsch, C., Anderson, A.S., 2018. The role of vaccines in preventing bacterial antimicrobial resistance. Nat. Med. 24 (1), 10.

Jayakumar, R., Prabaharan, M., Kumar, P.S., Nair, S.V., Tamura, H., 2011. Biomaterials based on chitin and chitosan in wound dressing applications. Biotechnol. Adv. 29 (3), 322–337.

Joerger, R.D., 2007. Antimicrobial films for food applications: a quantitative analysis of their effectiveness and science. Packag. Technol. Sci. 20 (4), 231–273.

Jones, A., Mandal, A., Sharma, S., 2015. Protein-based bioplastics and their antibacterial potential. J. Appl. Polym. Sci. 132 (18), 1–11.

Jung, J., Kasi, G., Seo, J., 2018. Development of functional antimicrobial papers using chitosan/starch-silver nanoparticles. Int. J. Biol. Macromol. 112, 530–536.

Kalhapure, R.S., Suleman, N., Mocktar, C., Seedat, N., Govender, T., 2015. Nanoengineered drug delivery systems for enhancing antibiotic therapy. J. Pharm. Sci. 104 (3), 872–905.

Kanazawa, A., Ikeda, T., Endo, T., 1993a. Polymeric phosphonium salts as a novel class of cationic biocides. IV. Synthesis and antibacterial activity of polymers with phosphonium salts in the main chain. J. Polym. Sci. A Polym. Chem. 31 (12), 3031–3038.

Kanazawa, A., Ikeda, T., Endo, T., 1993b. Polymeric phosphonium salts as a novel class of cationic biocides. II. Effects of counter anion and molecular weight on antibacterial activity of polymeric phosphonium salts. J. Polym. Sci. A Polym. Chem. 31 (6), 1441–1447.

Katas, H., Alpar, H.O., 2006. Development and characterisation of chitosan nanoparticles for siRNA delivery. J. Controlled Release 115 (2), 216–225.

Kenawy, E.R., Abdel-Hay, F.I., El-Shanshoury, A.E.R., El Newehy, M.H., 2002. Biologically active polymers. V. Synthesis and antimicrobial activity of modified poly (glycidyl methacrylate-*co*-2-hydroxyethyl methacrylate) derivatives with quaternary ammonium and phosphonium salts. J. Polym. Sci. A Polym. Chem. 40 (14), 2384–2393.

Kenawy, E.R., Worley, S.D., Broughton, R., 2007. The chemistry and applications of antimicrobial polymers: a state-of-the-art review. Biomacromolecules 8 (5), 1359–1384.

Kim, K., Yu, M., Zong, X., Chiu, J., Fang, D., Seo, Y.S., et al., 2003. Control of degradation rate and hydrophilicity in electrospun non-woven poly(D,L-lactide) nanofiber scaffolds for biomedical applications. Biomaterials 24 (27), 4977–4985.

Klibanov, A.M., 2007. Permanently microbicidal materials coatings. J. Mater. Chem. 17 (24), 2479–2482.

Kolambkar, Y.M., Dupont, K.M., Boerckel, J.D., Huebsch, N., Mooney, D.J., Hutmacher, D.W., et al., 2011. An alginate-based hybrid system for growth factor delivery in the functional repair of large bone defects. Biomaterials 32 (1), 65–74.

Kugel, A.J., Jarabek, L.E., Daniels, J.W., Wal, L.J.V., Ebert, S.M., Jepperson, M.J., et al., 2009. Combinatorial materials research applied to the development of new surface coatings XII: Novel, environmentally friendly antimicrobial coatings derived from biocide-functional acrylic polyols and isocyanates. J. Coat. Technol. Res. 6, 107–121.

Kumar, G., Sharma, S., Shafiq, N., Khuller, G.K., Malhotra, S., 2012. Optimization, in vitro–in vivo evaluation, and short-term tolerability of novel levofloxacin-loaded PLGA nanoparticle formulation. J. Pharm. Sci. 101 (6), 2165–2176.

Kumar, S.V., Bafana, A.P., Pawar, P., Rahman, A., Dahoumane, S.A., Jeffryes, C.S., 2018. High conversion synthesis of <10 nm starch-stabilized silver nanoparticles using microwave technology. Sci. Rep. 8, 1–10.

Kumarasamy, K.K., Toleman, M.A., Walsh, T.R., Bagaria, J., Butt, F., Balakrishnan, R., et al., 2010. Emergence of a new antibiotic resistance mechanism in India, Pakistan, and the UK: a molecular, biological, and epidemiological study. Lancet Infect. Dis. 10 (9), 597–602.

Kumari, L., Al Hoque, A., Sakure, K., Ramachandra Badwaik, H., 2019. Recent advancements in the lipid polymer hybrid nanoparticles for drug delivery: an overview. Acta Sci. Pharm. Sci. 3 (2), 21–28.

Ladd, J., Zhang, Z., Chen, S., Hower, J.C., Jiang, S., 2008. Zwitterionic polymers exhibiting high resistance to nonspecific protein adsorption from human serum and plasma. Biomacromolecules 9 (5), 1357–1361.

Lam, S.J., O'Brien-Simpson, N.M., Pantarat, N., Sulistio, A., Wong, E.H., Chen, Y.Y., et al., 2016. Combating multidrug resistant gram-negative bacteria with structurally nanoengineered antimicrobial peptide polymers. Nat. Microbiol. 1, 16162.

Lee, S., Voros, J., 2005. An aqueous-based surface modification of poly(dimethylsiloxane) with poly(ethylene glycol) to prevent biofouling. Langmuir 21 (25), 11957–11962.

Lee, C.H., An, D.S., Park, H.J., Lee, D.S., 2003. Wide-spectrum antimicrobial packaging materials incorporating nisin and chitosan in the coating. Packag. Technol. Sci. 16 (3), 99–106.

Lee, I.J., Kim, H.S., Yoo, H.S., 2009. DNA nanogels composed of chitosan and pluronic with thermo-sensitive and photo-crosslinking properties. Int. J. Pharm. 373 (1–2), 93–99.

Li, H., Bao, H., Bok, K.X., Lee, C.Y., Li, B., Zin, M.T., et al., 2016. High durability and low toxicity antimicrobial coatings fabricated by quaternary ammonium silane copolymers. Biomater. Sci. 4 (2), 299–309.

Lin, W.C., Lien, C.C., Yeh, H.J., Yu, C.M., Hsu, S.H., 2013. Bacterial cellulose and bacterial cellulose–chitosan membranes for wound dressing applications. Carbohydr. Polym. 94 (1), 603–611.

Liu, Z., Deshazer, H., Rice, A.J., Chen, K., Zhou, C., Kallenbach, N.R., 2006. Multivalent antimicrobial peptides from a reactive polymer scaffold. J. Med. Chem. 49 (12), 3436–3439.

Liu, L., Li, W., Liu, Q., 2014. Recent development of antifouling polymers: structure, evaluation, and biomedical applications in nano/micro-structures. Wiley Interdiscip. Rev. Nanomed. Nanotechnol. 6 (6), 599–614.

Liu, G., Wu, G., Jin, C., Kong, Z., 2015. Preparation and antimicrobial activity of terpene-based polyurethane coatings with carbamate group-containing quaternary ammonium salts. Prog. Org. Coat. 80, 150–155.

Lubasova, D., Netravali, A., Parker, J., Ingel, B., 2014. Bacterial filtration efficiency of green soy protein based nanofiber air filter. J. Nanosci. Nanotechnol. 14 (7), 4891–4898.

Magalhaes, A.P.R., Moreira, F.C.L., Alves, D.R.S., Estrela, C.R.A., Estrela, C., Bakuzis, A.F., et al., 2016. Silver nanoparticles in resin luting cements: antibacterial and physiochemical properties. J. Clin. Exp. Dent. 8 (4), e415–e422.

Majumdar, P., Lee, E., Gubbins, N., Stafslien, S.J., Daniels, J., Thorson, C.J., et al., 2009. Synthesis and antimicrobial activity of quaternary ammonium-functionalized POSS (Q-POSS) and polysiloxane coatings containing Q-POSS. Polymer 50 (5), 1124–1133.

Malafaya, P.B., Stappers, F., Reis, R.L., 2006. Starch-based microspheres produced by emulsion crosslinking with a potential media dependent responsive behavior to be used as drug delivery carriers. J. Mater. Sci. Mater. Med. 17 (4), 371–377.

Malzahn, K., Jamieson, W.D., Droge, M., Mailander, V., Jenkins, A.T.A., Weiss, C.K., et al., 2014. Advanced dextran based nanogels for fighting *Staphylococcus aureus* infections by sustained zinc release. J. Mater. Chem. B 2 (15), 2175–2183.

Maness, P.C., Smolinski, S., Blake, D.M., Huang, Z., Wolfrum, E.J., Jacoby, W.A., 1999. Bactericidal activity of photocatalytic TiO_2 reaction: toward an understanding of its killing mechanism. Appl. Environ. Microbiol. 65 (9), 4094–4098.

Mao, J., Li, Y., Wu, T., Yuan, C., Zeng, B., Xu, Y., et al., 2016. A simple dual-pH responsive prodrug-based polymeric micelles for drug delivery. ACS Appl. Mater. Interface 8 (27), 17109–17117.

Markovic, D., Milovanovic, S., Radeti, M., Jokic, B., Zizovic, I., 2015. Impregnation of corona modified polypropylene non-woven material with thymol in supercritical carbon dioxide for antimicrobial application. J. Supercrit. Fluids 101, 215–221.

Masood, F., 2016. Polymeric nanoparticles for targeted drug delivery system for cancer therapy. Mater. Sci. Eng. C 60, 569–578.

Matejka, V., Tokarsky, J., 2014. Photocatalytical nanocomposites: a review. J. Nanosci. Nanotechnol. 14 (2), 1597–1616.

Melo, M.N., Ferre, R., Castanho, M.A., 2009. Antimicrobial peptides: linking partition, activity and high membrane-bound concentrations. Nat. Rev. Microbiol. 7 (3), 245.

Michl, T.D., Locock, K.E., Stevens, N.E., Hayball, J.D., Vasilev, K., Postma, A., et al., 2014. RAFT-derived antimicrobial polymethacrylates: elucidating the impact of end-groups on activity and cytotoxicity. Polym. Chem. 5 (19), 5813–5822.

Moon, W.S., Chul Kim, J., Chung, K.H., Park, E.S., Kim, M.N., Yoon, J.S., 2003. Antimicrobial activity of a monomer and its polymer based on quinolone. J. Appl. Polym. Sci. 90 (7), 1797–1801.

Muriel-Galet, V., Cerisuelo, J.P., Lopez-Carballo, G., Lara, M., Gavara, R., Hernandez-Munoz, P., 2012. Development of antimicrobial films for microbiological control of packaged salad. Int. J. Food Microbiol. 157 (2), 195–201.

Nam, S., Ali, D.M., Kim, J., 2016. Characterization of alginate/silver nanobiocomposites synthesized by solution plasma process and their antimicrobial properties. J. Nanomater. 2016, 1–9.

Nassimi, M., Schleh, C., Lauenstein, H.D., Hussein, R., Hoymann, H.G., Koch, W., et al., 2010. A toxicological evaluation of inhaled solid lipid nanoparticles used as a potential drug delivery system for the lung. Eur. J. Pharm. Biopharm. 75 (2), 107–116.

Nath, D., Banerjee, P., 2013. Green nanotechnology—a new hope for medical biology. Environ. Toxicol. Pharmacol. 36 (3), 997–1014.

Nathan, C., Cunningham-Bussel, A., 2013. Beyond oxidative stress: an immunologist's guide to reactive oxygen species. Nat. Rev. Immunol. 13 (5), 349.

Neely, A.N., Maley, M.P., 2000. Survival of enterococci and staphylococci on hospital fabrics and plastic. J. Clin. Microbiol. 38 (2), 724–726.

Nonaka, T., Hua, L., Ogata, T., Kurihara, S., 2003. Synthesis of water-soluble thermosensitive polymers having phosphonium groups from methacryloyloxyethyl trialkyl phosphonium chlorides–*N*-isopropylacrylamide copolymers and their functions. J. Appl. Polym. Sci. 87 (3), 386–393.

Nootsuwan, N., Sukthavorn, K., Wattanathana, W., Jongrungruangchok, S., Veranitisagul, C., Koonsaeng, N., et al., 2018. Development of antimicrobial hybrid materials from polylactic acid and nano-silver coated chitosan. Orient. J. Chem. 34 (2), 683–692.

Oh, J.W., Chun, S.C., Chandrasekaran, M., 2019. Article preparation and in vitro characterization of chitosan nanoparticles and their broad-spectrum antifungal action compared to antibacterial activities against phytopathogens of tomato. Agronomy 9 (21), 1–21.

Palermo, E.F., Kuroda, K., 2010. Structural determinants of antimicrobial activity in polymers which mimic host defense peptides. Appl. Microbiol. Biotechnol. 87 (5), 1605–1615.

Pan, X., Redding, J.E., Wiley, P.A., Wen, L., McConnell, J.S., Zhang, B., 2010. Mutagenicity evaluation of metal oxide nanoparticles by the bacterial reverse mutation assay. Chemosphere 79 (1), 113–116.

Panaitescu, D.M., Ionita, E.R., Nicolae, C.A., Gabor, A.R., Ionita, Roxana Trusca, M.D., et al., 2018. Poly(3-hydroxybutyrate) modified by nanocellulose and plasma treatment for packaging applications. Polymers 10 (11), 1–24.

Panarin, E.F., Solovskii, M.V., Ekzemplyarov, O.N., 1971. Synthesis and antimicrobial properties of polymers containing quaternary ammonium groups. Pharm. Chem. J. 5 (7), 406–408.

Panyam, J., Labhasetwar, V., 2003. Biodegradable nanoparticles for drug and gene delivery to cells and tissue. Adv. Drug Deliv. Rev. 55 (3), 329–347.

Park, E.S., Moon, W.S., Song, M.J., Kim, M.N., Chung, K.H., Yoon, J.S., 2001. Antimicrobial activity of phenol and benzoic acid derivatives. Int. Biodeterior. Biodegrad. 47 (4), 209–214.

Park, E.S., Kim, H.K., Shim, J.H., Kim, M.N., Yoon, J.S., 2004a. Synthesis and properties of polymeric biocides based on poly(ethylene-*co*-vinyl alcohol). J. Appl. Polym. Sci. 93 (2), 765–770.

Park, E.S., Kim, H.S., Kim, M.N., San Yoon, J., 2004b. Antibacterial activities of polystyrene-block-poly(4-vinyl pyridine) and poly(styrene-random-4-vinyl pyridine). Eur. Polym. J. 40 (12), 2819–2822.

Parveen, S., Sahoo, S.K., 2008. Polymeric nanoparticles for cancer therapy. J. Drug Target. 16 (2), 108–123.

Pascual, A.M.D., Vicente, A.L.D., 2014. Poly(3-hydroxybutyrate)/ZnO bionanocomposites with improved mechanical, barrier and antibacterial properties. Int. J. Mol. Sci. 15 (6), 10950–10973.

Pasquier, N., Keul, H., Heine, E., Moeller, M., Angelov, B., Linser, S., et al., 2008. Amphiphilic branched polymers as antimicrobial agents. Macromol. Biosci. 8 (10), 903–915.

Patel, M.B., Patel, S.A., Ray, A., Patel, R.M., 2003. Synthesis, characterization, and antimicrobial activity of acrylic copolymers. J. Appl. Polym. Sci. 89 (4), 895–900.

Patel, J.N., Patel, M.V., Patel, R.M., 2005. Copolymers of 2,4-dichlorophenyl methacrylate with styrene: synthesis, thermal properties, and antimicrobial activity. J. Macromol. Sci. A 42 (1), 71–83.

Patel, J.N., Dolia, M.B., Patel, M.B., Patel, R.M., 2006. 4-Chloro-3-methylphenyl methacrylate copolymers with 2,4-dichlorophenyl methacrylate: synthesis, characterization, and antimicrobial activity. J. Appl. Polym. Sci. 100 (1), 439–448.

Patel, A., Patel, R.J., Patel, K.H., Patel, R.M., 2009. Synthesis, characterization, thermal properties and antimicrobial activity of acrylic copolymers derived from 2,4-dichlorophenyl acrylate. J. Chil. Chem. Soc. 54 (3), 228–233.

Pelgrift, R.Y., Friedman, A.J., 2013. Nanotechnology as a therapeutic tool to combat microbial resistance. Adv. Drug Deliv. Rev. 65 (13–14), 1803–1815.

Pietrokovski, Y., Nisimov, I., Kesler-Shvero, D., Zaltsman, N., Beyth, N., 2016. Antibacterial effect of composite resin foundation material incorporating quaternary ammonium polyethyleneimine nanoparticles. J. Prosthet. Dent. 116 (4), 603–609.

Ramos, J., Forcada, J., Hidalgo-Alvarez, R., 2013. Cationic polymer nanoparticles and nanogels: from synthesis to biotechnological applications. Chem. Rev. 114 (1), 367–428.

Ren, X., Akdag, A., Kocer, H.B., Worley, S.D., Broughton, R.M., Huang, T.S., 2009. *N*-Halamine-coated cotton for antimicrobial and detoxification applications. Carbohydr. Polym. 78 (2), 220–226.

Renton, A., 2006. Welcome to the World of Nano Foods. Available at: http://observer.guardian.co.uk/foodmonthly/futureoffood/story/0,1971266,00.html

Restrepoa, I., Floresa, P., Rodriguez-Llamazaresc, S., 2018. Antibacterial nanocomposite of poly(lactic acid) and ZnO nanoparticles stabilized with poly(vinyl alcohol): thermal and morphological characterization. Polym. Plast. Technol. Eng. 58 (1), 1–8.

Rhim, J.W., Ng, P.K., 2007. Natural biopolymer-based nanocomposite films for packaging applications. Crit. Rev. Food Sci. Nutr. 47 (4), 411–433.

Rodič, P., Bratuša, M., Lukšič, M., Vlachy, V., Hribar-Lee, B., 2013. Influence of the hydrophobic groups and the nature of counterions on ion-binding in aliphatic ionene solutions. Colloids Surf. A Physicochem. Eng. Aspects 424, 18–25.

Rodriguez, B.M., Figueroa-Lopez, K.J., Bernardos, A., Martinez-Manez, R., Cabedo, L., Torres-Giner, S., et al., 2019. Electrospun antimicrobial films of poly(3-hydroxybutyrate-*co*-3-hydroxyvalerate) containing eugenol essential oil encapsulated in mesoporous silica nanoparticles. Nanomaterials 9 (2), 1–24.

Roman, M., Dong, S., Hirani, A., Lee, Y.W., 2009. Cellulose nanocrystals for drug delivery. ACS Symp. Ser. 1017, 81–91.

Rowley, J.A., Madlambayan, G., Mooney, D.J., 1999. Alginate hydrogels as synthetic extracellular matrix materials. Biomaterials 20 (1), 45–53.

Russo, R., Malinconico, M., Petti, L., Romano, G., 2005. Physical behavior of biodegradable alginate–poly(vinyl alcohol) blends films. J. Polym. Sci. B Polym. Phys. 43 (10), 1205–1213.

Saafan, A., Zaazou, M.H., Sallam, M.K., Mosallam, O., El Danaf, H.A., 2018. Assessment of photodynamic therapy and nanoparticles effects on caries models. Open Access Maced. J. Med. Sci. 6 (7), 1289.

Sampathkumar, S.G., Yarema, K.J., 2007. Dendrimers in cancer treatment and diagnosis. Nanotechnol. Life Sci.: Online 7, 1–43.

Sannino, A., Pappada, S., Giotta, L., Maffezzoli, A., 2007. Spin coating cellulose derivatives on quartz crystal microbalance plates to obtain hydrogel-based fast sensors and actuators. J. Appl. Polym. Sci. 106 (5), 3040–3050.

Sapalidis, A., Sideratou, Z., Panagiotaki, K.N., Sakellis, E., Kouvelos, E.P., Papageorgiou, S., et al., 2018. Fabrication of antibacterial poly(vinyl alcohol) nanocomposite films containing dendritic polymer functionalized multi-walled carbon nanotubes. Front. Mater. 5, 11.

Sari, P., Mann, B., Kumar, R., Singh, R.R.B., Sharma, R., Bhardwaj, M., et al., 2015. Preparation and characterization of nanoemulsion encapsulating curcumin. Food Hydrocolloids 43, 540–546.

Sawada, H., Umedo, M., Kawase, T., Tomita, T., Baba, M., 1999. Synthesis and properties of fluoroalkylated end-capped betaine polymers. Eur. Polym. J. 35 (9), 1611–1617.

Saxena, A.K., Marler, J., Benvenuto, M., Willital, G.H., Vacanti, J.P., 1999. Skeletal muscle tissue engineering using isolated myoblasts on synthetic biodegradable polymers: preliminary studies. Tissue Eng. 5 (6), 525–531.

Seol, Y.J., Lee, J.Y., Park, Y.J., Lee, Y.M., Rhyu, I.C., Lee, S.J., et al., 2004. Chitosan sponges as tissue engineering scaffolds for bone formation. Biotechnol. Lett. 26 (13), 1037–1041.

Shahzad, M., Millhouse, E., Culshaw, S., Edwards, C.A., Ramage, G., Combet, E., 2015. Selected dietary (poly)phenols inhibit periodontal pathogen growth and biofilm formation. Food Funct. 6 (3), 719–729.

Shawki, M.M., Hereba, A.M., Ghazal, A., 2010. Formation and characterisation of antimicrobial dextran nanofibers. Rom. J. Biophys. 20 (4), 335–346.

Shi, Z., Neoh, K.G., Kang, E.T., 2004. Surface-grafted viologen for precipitation of silver nanoparticles and their combined bactericidal activities. Langmuir 20 (16), 6847–6852.

Siedenbiedel, F., Tiller, J.C., 2012. Antimicrobial polymers in solution and on surfaces: overview and functional principles. Polymers 4 (1), 46–71.

Siriwardena, T.N., Stach, M., He, R., Gan, B.H., Javor, S., Heitz, M., et al., 2017. Lipidated peptide dendrimers killing multidrug-resistant bacteria. J. Am. Chem. Soc. 140 (1), 423–432.

Soykan, C., Coşkun, R., Delibaş, A., 2005. Microbial screening of copolymers of *N*-vinylimidazole with phenacyl methacrylate: synthesis and monomer reactivity ratios. J. Macromol. Sci. A 42 (12), 1603–1619.

Stoleru, E., Dumitriu, R.P., Munteanub, B.S., Zaharescuc, T., Tanased, E.E., Mitelutd, A., et al., 2016. Novel procedure to enhance PLA surface properties by chitosan irreversible immobilization. Appl. Surf. Sci. 367, 407–417.

Subramanyam, E., Mohandoss, S., Shin, H.W., 2009. Synthesis, characterization, and evaluation of antifouling polymers of 4-acryloyloxybenzaldehyde with methyl methacrylate. J. Appl. Polym. Sci. 112 (5), 2741–2749.

Sun, Y., Sun, G., 2001. Novel regenerable *N*-halamine polymeric biocides. III. Grafting hydantoin-containing monomers onto synthetic fabrics. J. Appl. Polym. Sci. 81 (6), 1517–1525.

Sung, S.Y., Sin, L.T., Tee, T.T., Bee, S.T., Rahmat, A.R., Rahman, W.A.W.A., et al., 2013. Antimicrobial agents for food packaging applications. Trends Food Sci. Technol. 33 (2), 110–123.

Talbot, G.H., Bradley, J., Edwards Jr, J.E., Gilbert, D., Scheld, M., Bartlett, J.G., 2006. Bad bugs need drugs: an update on the development pipeline from the Antimicrobial Availability Task Force of the Infectious Diseases Society of America. Clin. Infect. Dis. 42 (5), 657–668.

Tamami, M., Salas-de la Cruz, D., Winey, K.I., Long, T.E., 2012. Structure–property relationships of water-soluble ammonium–ionene copolymers. Macromol. Chem. Phys. 213 (9), 965–972.

Tang, S., Wang, Z., Li, P., Li, W., Li, C., Wang, Y., et al., 2018. Degradable and photocatalytic antibacterial Au-TiO_2/sodium alginate nanocomposite films for active food packaging. Nanomaterials 8 (11), 1–11.

Taresco, V., Crisante, F., Francolini, I., Martinelli, A., D'Ilario, L., Ricci-Vitiani, L., et al., 2015. Antimicrobial and antioxidant amphiphilic random copolymers to address medical device-centered infections. Acta Biomater. 22, 131–140.

Tashiro, T., 2001. Antibacterial and bacterium adsorbing macromolecules. Macromol. Mater. Eng. 286 (2), 63–87.

Taylor, M., McCollister, B., Park, D., 2015. Highly bactericidal polyurethane effective against both normal and drug-resistant bacteria: potential use as an air filter coating. Appl. Biochem. Biotechnol. 178 (5), 1053–1067.

Tiller, J.C., Liao, C.J., Lewis, K., Klibanov, A.M., 2001. Designing surfaces that kill bacteria on contact. Proc. Natl. Acad. Sci. U.S.A. 98 (11), 5981–5985.

Timofeeva, L., Kleshcheva, N., 2011. Antimicrobial polymers: mechanism of action, factors of activity, and applications. Appl. Microbiol. Biotechnol. 89 (3), 475–492.

Timofeeva, L.M., Kleshcheva, N.A., Moroz, A.F., Didenko, L.V., 2009. Secondary and tertiary polydiallylammonium salts: novel polymers with high antimicrobial activity. Biomacromolecules 10 (11), 2976–2986.

Tosi, G., Costantino, L., Ruozi, B., Forni, F., Vandelli, M.A., 2008. Polymeric nanoparticles for the drug delivery to the central nervous system. Expert Opin. Drug Deliv. 5 (2), 155–174.

Turalija, M., Bischof, S., Budimir, A., Gaan, S., 2016. Antimicrobial PLA films from environment friendly additives. Compos. B Eng. 102, 94–99.

Uddin, F., Aman, W., Ullah, I., Qureshi, O.S., Mustapha, O., Shafique, S., et al., 2017. Effective use of nanocarriers as drug delivery systems for the treatment of selected tumors. Int. J. Nanomed. 12, 7291.

Varona, S., Kareth, S., Martin, A., Cocero, M.J., 2010. Formulation of lavandin essential oil with biopolymers by PGSS for application as biocide in ecological agriculture. J. Supercrit. Fluids 54 (3), 369–377.

Vasile, C., Baican, M.C., Tibirna, C.M., Tuchilus, C., Debarnot, D., Paslaru, E., et al., 2011. Microwave plasma activation of a polyvinylidene fluoride surface for protein immobilization. J. Phys. D Appl. Phys. 44 (47), 1–15.

Vinatier, C., Gauthier, O., Fatimi, A., Merceron, C., Masson, M., Moreau, A., et al., 2009. An injectable cellulose-based hydrogel for the transfer of autologous nasal chondrocytes in articular cartilage defects. Biotechnol. Bioeng. 102 (4), 1259–1267.

Vogl, O., Tirrell, D., 1979. Functional polymers with biologically active groups. J. Macromol. Sci. Chem. 13 (3), 415–439.

Volova, T., Zhila, N., Vinogradova, O., Shumilova, A., Prudnikova, S., Shishatskaya, E., 2015. Characterization of biodegradable poly-3-hydroxybutyrate films and pellets loaded with the fungicide tebuconazole. Environ. Sci. Pollut. Res. 23 (6), 5243–5254.

Wang, S., Lawson, R., Ray, P.C., Yu, H., 2011. Toxic effects of gold nanoparticles on *Salmonella typhimurium* bacteria. Toxicol. Ind. Health 27 (6), 547–554.

Wang, R., Wang, L., Zhou, L., Su, Y., Qiu, F., Wang, D., et al., 2012a. The effect of a branched architecture on the antimicrobial activity of poly(sulfone amines) and poly (sulfone amine)/silver nanocomposites. J. Mater. Chem. 22 (30), 15227–15234.

Wang, Z., Sun, B., Zhang, M., Ou, L., Che, Y., Zhang, J., et al., 2012b. Functionalization of electrospun poly(ε-caprolactone) scaffold with heparin and vascular endothelial growth factors for potential application as vascular grafts. J. Bioact. Compat. Polym. 28 (2), 154–166.

Waschinski, C.J., Tiller, J.C., 2005. Poly(oxazoline)s with telechelic antimicrobial functions. Biomacromolecules 6 (1), 235–243.

Waschinski, C.J., Zimmermann, J., Salz, U., Hutzler, R., Sadowski, G., Tiller, L.C., 2008. Design of contact active antimicrobial acrylate based materials using biocidal macromers. Adv. Mater. 20 (1), 104–108.

Weiss, J., Takhistov, P., McClements, D.J., 2006. Functional materials in food nanotechnology. J. Food Sci. 71 (9), R107–R116.

Xie, J., Zhao, Q., Li, S., Yan, Z., Li, J., Li, Y., et al., 2017. Novel antimicrobial peptide CPF-C1 analogs with superior stabilities and activities against multidrug-resistant bacteria. Chem. Biol. Drug Des. 90 (5), 690–702.

Xiong, X., Zhang, L., Wang, Y., 2005. Polymer fractionation using chromatographic column packed with novel regenerated cellulose beads modified with silane. J. Chromatogr. A 1063 (1–2), 71–77.

Xu, R., Fisher, M., Juliano, R.L., 2011. Targeted albumin-based nanoparticles for delivery of amphipathic drugs. Bioconjugate Chem. 22 (5), 870–878.

Xue, Y., Xiao, H., Zhang, Y., 2015. Antimicrobial polymeric materials with quaternary ammonium and phosphonium salts. Int. J. Mol. Sci. 16 (2), 3626–3655.

Yang, W.W., Pierstorff, E., 2012. Reservoir-based polymer drug delivery systems. J. Lab. Autom. 17 (1), 50–58.

Yang, J.M., Lin, H.T., Wu, T.H., Chen, C.C., 2003. Wettability and antibacterial assessment of chitosan containing radiation-induced graft nonwoven fabric of polypropylene-*g*-acrylic acid. J. Appl. Polym. Sci. 90 (5), 1331–1336.

Ye, Q., Zhou, F., 2015. Antifouling surfaces based on polymer brushes. In: Zhou, F. (Ed.), Antifouling Surfaces and Materials. Springer, Berlin, Germany, pp. 55–81.

Ye, S.H., Watanabe, J., Iwasaki, Y., Ishihara, K., 2003. Antifouling blood purification membrane composed of cellulose acetate and phospholipid polymer. Biomaterials 24, 4143–4152.

Yu, K., Mei, Y., Hadjesfandiari, N., Kizhakkedathu, J.N., 2014. Engineering biomaterials surfaces to modulate the host response. Colloids Surf. B Biointerfaces 124, 69–79.

Yudovin-Farber, I., Beyth, N., Nyska, A., Weiss, E.I., Golenser, J., Domb, A.J., 2008. Surface characterization and biocompatibility of restorative resin containing nanoparticles. Biomacromolecules 9 (11), 3044–3050.

Yuen, J., Chung, T., Loke, A., 2015. Methicillin-resistant *Staphylococcus aureus* (MRSA) contamination in bedside surfaces of a hospital ward and the potential effectiveness of enhanced disinfection with an antimicrobial polymer surfactant. Int. J. Environ. Res. Public. Health 12 (3), 3026–3041.

Zahedi, P., Rezaeian, I., Ranaei-Siadat, S.O., Jafari, S.H., Supaphol, P., 2010. A review on wound dressings with an emphasis on electrospun nanofibrous polymeric bandages. Polym. Adv. Technol. 21 (2), 77–95.

Zhang, H., Chiao, M., 2015. Anti-fouling coatings of poly(dimethylsiloxane) devices for biological and biomedical applications. J. Med. Biol. Eng. 35 (2), 143–155.

Zhang, Y., Jiang, J., Chen, Y., 1999. Synthesis and antimicrobial activity of polymeric guanidine and biguanidine salts. Polymer 40 (22), 6189–6198.

Zhang, F., Kang, E.T., Neoh, K.G., Wang, P., Tan, K.L., 2001. Surface modification of stainless steel by grafting of poly(ethylene glycol) for reduction in protein adsorption. Biomaterials 22 (12), 1541–1548.

Zhang, L., Gu, F.X., Chan, J.M., Wang, A.Z., Langer, R.S., Farokhzad, O.C., 2008. Nanoparticles in medicine: therapeutic applications and developments. Clin. Pharmacol. Ther. 83 (5), 761–769.

Zhang, L., Pornpattananangkul, D., Hu, C.M., Huang, C.M., 2010. Development of nanoparticles for antimicrobial drug delivery. Curr. Med. Chem. 17 (6), 585–594.

Zhang, W., Zhang, Z., Zhang, Y., 2011. The application of carbon nanotubes in target drug delivery systems for cancer therapies. Nanoscale Res. Lett. 6 (1), 555.

Zhao, C., Tan, A., Pastorin, G., Ho, H.K., 2013. Nanomaterial scaffolds for stem cell proliferation and differentiation in tissue engineering. Biotechnol. Adv. 31 (5), 654–668.

Zhou, C., Wang, M., Zou, K., Chen, J., Zhu, Y., Du, J., 2013. Antibacterial polypeptide-grafted chitosan-based nanocapsules as an "armed" carrier of anticancer and antiepileptic drugs. ACS macro. Lett. 2 (11), 1021–1025.

Zhou, F., Qin, X., Li, Y., Ren, L., Zhao, Y., Yuan, X., 2015. Fluorosilicone multi-block copolymers tethering quaternary ammonium salt groups for antimicrobial purpose. Appl. Surf. Sci. 347, 231–241.

CHAPTER

Polymeric nanomaterials for targeting the cellular suborganelles

9

Mengjiao Zhou[1], Fang Fang[2] and Jinfeng Zhang[2]

[1]*School of Pharmacy, Nantong University, Nantong, P.R. China*

[2]*Key Laboratory of Molecular Medicine and Biotherapy, School of Life Sciences, Beijing Institute of Technology, Beijing, P.R. China*

9.1 Introduction

In the past years, advanced nanotechnology based on various nanomaterials has emerged as the most cutting-edge tool and played important roles in disease treatments at cellular level (Björnmalm et al., 2017). Nanomaterial is a powerful platform to across physiological barriers and selectively delivers therapeutic or diagnostic agents to intracellular target sites (Zhang et al., 2015). The specifically targeted delivery of traditional drugs by using nanomaterials could relieve many inevitable problems associated with random drug distribution in whole cells (Qin et al., 2018). First, delivering therapeutic agents to their subcellular target sites of action could prevent their potential off-target toxic and side effects on normal tissues (Chen et al., 2019b). Second, the specific distribution of therapeutic agents in cellular suborganelles ensures high efficiency of subcellular compartments damage and cell apoptosis, which can realize the optimal therapeutic performance with low-dose agent (von Roemeling et al., 2017). Third, the multidrug resistance (MDR) phenomenon, which is frequently emerged in cancer therapy, can be overcome by the organelles-targeted cancer therapy since drug molecules are difficult to efflux in subcellular compartments (Zhou et al., 2016; Ma et al., 2016a). Finally, each subcellular organelle possesses different characteristics and functions (Liang et al., 2018; Pearce et al., 2017). It is well known that each organelle is responsible for versatile cellular functions including cell growth, proliferation, differentiation, or death (Ma et al., 2016b). For example, nucleus regulates gene expression and cell proliferation (Liu et al., 2018a); mitochondria are responsible for adenosine triphosphate (ATP) synthesis, apoptosis regulation, and calcium ion cycle (Deng et al., 2017); lysosomes are related to digestion, autophagy, and cell defense (Zhao et al., 2017); Golgi and endoplasmic reticulum (ER) are associated with the production and transport of proteins (Rosenblum et al., 2018). Owing to the special biological effects of cellular organelles, the introduction of appropriate therapies into specific organelles will bring new opportunities for effective

Advances in Polymeric Nanomaterials for Biomedical Applications. DOI: https://doi.org/10.1016/B978-0-12-814657-6.00009-4

disease treatments, such as cancers, diabetes, Alzheimer's, autoimmune diseases, and infectious, in a more precise and controlled manner (Cheng et al., 2019b).

Up to now, polymeric nanomaterials have received considerable attention and emerged as the most widely developed nanomaterials because of their excellent synthetic flexibility, good light-harvesting property, high photostability, and great biocompatibility (Zhang et al., 2018). In particular, a variety of polymeric nanomaterials such as polymer-drug conjugates, micelles, dendrimers, polymersomes, and semiconducting polymer nanoparticles (NPs) have been explored in drug delivery, fluorescence and photoacoustic imaging (PAI), as well as photodynamic and photothermal therapy (Zhang et al., 2017a; Shen et al., 2018). Given the abovementioned advantages of suborganelle-targeting approach, considerable efforts have been made in developing therapeutic/diagnostic polymeric nanomaterials for specific subcellular targeting and subsequently treating various diseases (Yao et al., 2017; Gao et al., 2019).

This chapter summarizes the recent advances in smart design and construction of polymeric nanomaterials for targeting the cellular suborganelles. Fig. 9.1 illustrates

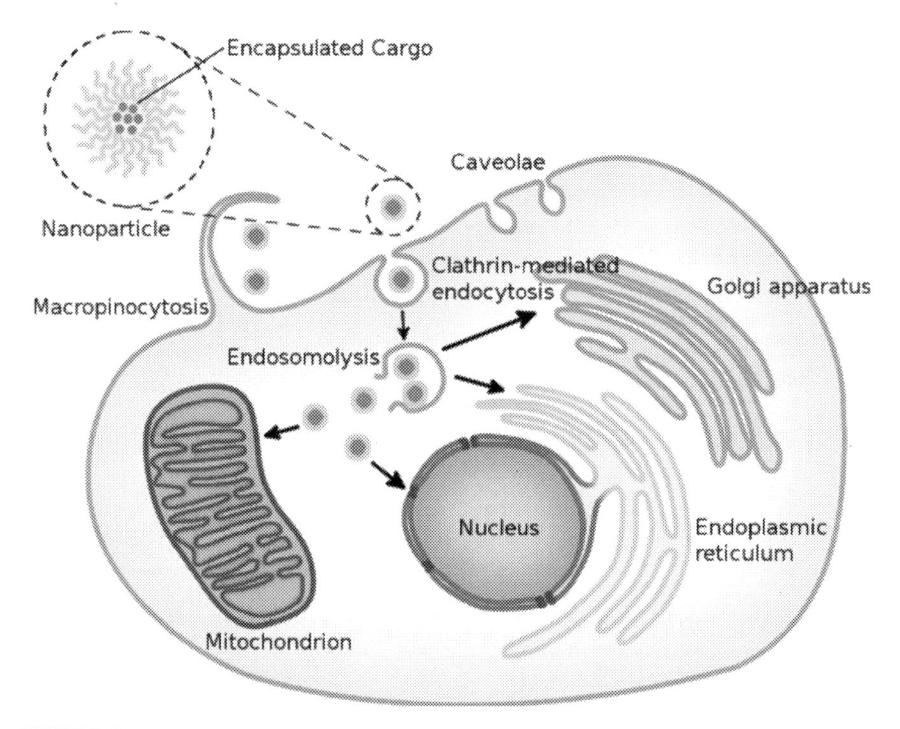

FIGURE 9.1

Major endocytic pathways and the potential target sites for the internalization of nanomaterials (Huang et al., 2011).

Reproduced with permission from Huang, J.G., Leshuk, T., Gu, F.X., 2011. Emerging nanomaterials for targeting subcellular organelles. Nano Today 6 (5), 478–492.

major endocytic pathways and subcellular target sites (plasma membrane, lysosomes/endosomes, mitochondria, nucleus, Golgi, ER, and cytoplasm) for the internalization of nanomaterials. Moreover, the interactions between nanomaterials and intracellular specific organelles based on different delivery strategies will also be presented with recent examples (Nurunnabi et al., 2019). Finally, some opinions on future perspectives of subcellular-targeted polymeric nanomaterials for biomedical applications will be shared. This chapter may not only offer valuable information for researchers to enhance the therapeutic/diagnostic efficiency of various disease treatments but also attract more interests in different fields of chemistry, materials, biological sciences, and medicine, promoting further development of polymeric nanomaterials for biomedical applications.

9.2 Different suborganelle-targeting strategies based on polymeric nanomaterials

9.2.1 Cytoplasm

A number of therapeutic/diagnostic agents need to be transported into the cytosol because their receptors are expressed in the cytosol or their target sites are cellular suborganelles (Ulbrich et al., 2016). Until now, various nanomaterials have been developed to transport small molecules or biologics [small-interfering RNA (siRNA), DNA, proteins, antibodies] for cytosolic delivery (Zhou et al., 2019). However, some research have found that it is difficult to transport macromolecules into the cells because cytosol is extremely viscous (Fang et al., 2020a). In fact, there are many cellular organelles involved in the cytosolic delivery (Wang et al., 2017). Actin filaments have been verified to participate in the endocytic process of polymeric nanomaterials, and microtubules have been proved to deliver polyplexes from the cytosolic to perinuclear region via vesicle transport (Bar-Zeev et al., 2017). In the meantime, the diffusion ability of nanomaterials into the cytoplasm will be influenced by several factors. For example, size and shape of nanomaterials play crucial roles in their diffusion efficiency (Zhang et al., 2020). Smaller spherical NPs exhibited much higher diffusivity than the larger nonspherical ones (Azevedo et al., 2018). Surface modification is another important factor influencing the diffusion ability in cytosolic delivery (Liu et al., 2018b). Owing to the weak interaction with cytosolic organelles, nanomaterials could be surface coated with polyethylene glycol (PEG), called "PEGylation," aimed at enhancing their ability to transport agents into the cytoplasm (Zhou et al., 2013).

It is well known that compared with normal tissues, solid tumors exhibit distinguishing tumor microenvironments, such as decreased interstitial pH values, increased glutathione (GSH) concentrations, and elevated levels of certain enzymes (Grzybowski et al., 2018). These specific biological factors differentiating between tumor and normal tissues could be utilized as stimuli to trigger specific changes of polymeric nanomaterials (Yu et al., 2018). Recently, numerous stimuli-responsive polymeric nanomaterials have been developed as temporal-, spatial-, and dosage-controlled delivery systems, showing great promise in disease treatments (Zhou et al., 2019). Specifically, physicochemical properties, such as morphology, size, hydrophobicity, or surface charge, of these stimuli-responsive polymeric nanomaterials could be changed to achieve additional merits including deeper tumor penetration, enhanced cellular endocytosis, efficient endosomal escape, as well as controlled drug release, thus boosting the eventual therapeutic efficacy of polymeric nanomaterials and making them be promising in various disease treatments (Wei et al., 2017).

9.2.1.1 pH-responsive polymeric nanomaterials

Among all these stimuli-responsive nanomaterials, pH-sensitive nanomaterials have gained much more attentions for two main reasons (Zhou et al., 2020). One reason is that nanomaterials are commonly taken up via endocytosis where endosomes are one of the inevitable stops which would develop into obvious acidified lumens (pH 4.5−5.5) and then degrade therapeutic/diagnostic agents (Guo et al., 2018). Specific functional groups including pH-sensitive and positively charged moieties could be involved in polymeric nanomaterials to promote the escape of therapeutic/diagnostic agents from the endocytic pathway (Yuba et al., 2017). pH-sensitive nanomaterials are always stable at physiological environment (pH 7.4) but unstable in the acidic environment (such as lysosome, endosomes), thereby releasing encapsulated agents into the cytoplasm away from the transmembrane efflux pumps (Kanamala et al., 2016). Endosome escape can increase available drug concentration in the cytoplasm (Xue et al., 2018). The other reason is that acidification in tumor tissue could be exploited for specifically targeting the tumor sites rather than normal tissues, therefore improving the selectivity of passive targeting (enhanced permeability and retention effect, or EPR effect) (Koren et al., 2012).

In 2018 Tang et al. reported pH-sensitive hybrid polymeric nanomaterials based on reversibly activatable cell-penetrating peptides for cytoplasmic targeting, by which oligoarginine was connected to a highly pH-sensitive sequence through polyglycine linker (HE-CPP) (Fig. 9.2). The surface of polyethyleneglycol-polylactic acid (PEG-PLA) polymeric micelles was coupled by HE-CPP sequence (PMs-HE-CPP) to achieve enhanced tumor-selective delivery of paclitaxel (PTX). PTX/PMs-HE-CPP NPs exhibited high drug-loading capacity, excellent size distribution, and reversible charge conversion triggered by the surrounding acidic microenvironment. PMs-HE-CPP NPs possessed negative charged at pH 7.4, moderately positive charged at tumor extracellular (pH 6.5), and more positive charged at lower intracellular pH microenvironment. Coumarin 6 loading PMs-HE-CPP NPs improved uptake into cancer cells at acidic tumor microenvironment via clathrin-mediated and energy-mediated endocytosis. Moreover, PTX/PMs-HE-CPP NPs showed much higher cytotoxicity at pH 6.5 than at pH 7.4 toward mouse breast cancer (4T1) cells. The tumor-targeted capacity of PMs-HE-CPP NPs has been demonstrated by in vivo imaging studies in 4T1 tumor−bearing BALB/c models. PMs-HE-CPP NPs could exhibit great potential for realizing tumor-targeted drug delivery and advanced cancer treatments.

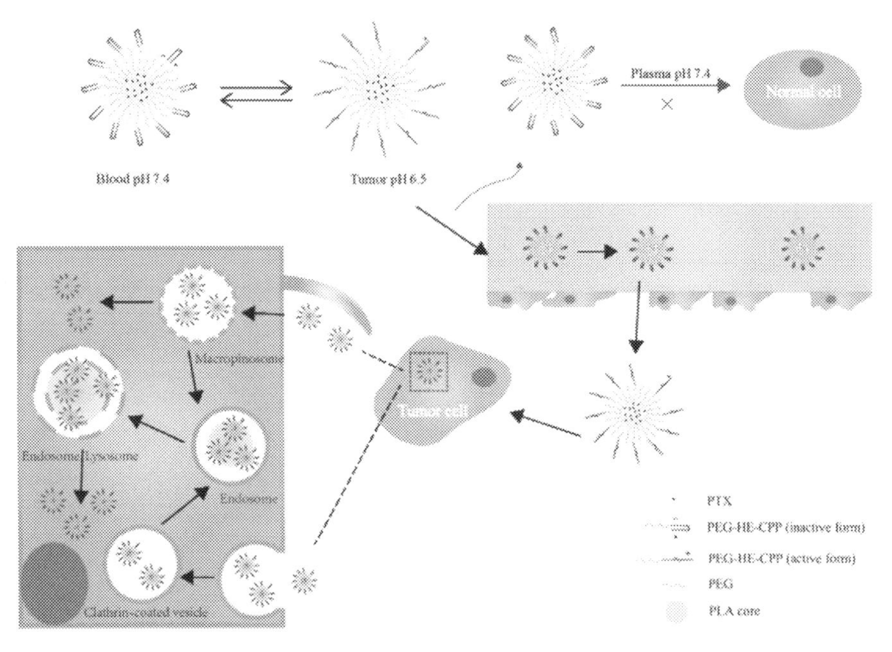

FIGURE 9.2

Schematic representation of designing pH-sensitive PMs-HE-CPP responding to tumor extracellular pH to achieve tumor-specific cytoplasm-targeting and enhanced antitumor efficacy (Tang et al., 2018).

Reproduced with permission from Tang, B., Zaro, J. L., Shen, Y., Chen, Q., Yu, Y., Sun, P., Sun, C., 2018. Acid-sensitive hybrid polymeric micelles containing a reversibly activatable cell-penetrating peptide for tumor-specific cytoplasm targeting. J. Controlled Release 279, 147–156.

9.2.1.2 Redox-responsive polymeric nanomaterials

In the past decades a variety of redox-responsive polymeric nanomaterials have also been developed for drug delivery to achieve superior efficacy in disease treatments (Yan et al., 2018). Compared to the low GSH (a typical reductive agent) concentration in the extracellular fluids (2–20 μmol/L), an obvious higher GSH concentration is found in the cytoplasm (2–20 mmol/L) in tumor tissues (Li et al., 2015). Many redox-responsive polymeric nanomaterials have been successfully fabricated for both in vitro and in vivo drug delivery to achieve a better therapeutic effect (Chen et al., 2018a). One of the most commonly used redox-responsive polymeric nanomaterials is the self-assembly amphiphilic copolymers bearing disulfide bonds, which could be rapid degraded in the cytoplasm under high concentration of GSH (Liu et al., 2018d). When redox-responsive nanomaterials enter the tumor cells, their disulfide bonds can be prone to rapid cleavage by intracellular GSH, resulting in prompt cytosolic release of drugs for further therapeutic outcome.

For example, Xu et al. developed pillar[5]arenes-based redox-responsive single molecular layer polymeric nanocapsules for cytoplasm-targeted delivery (Fig. 9.3). The polymeric nanocapsules possessed thin shell which consisted of covalent cross-linked pillar[5]arenes, and the disulfide group was set as linkers. Owing to high concentration of GSH in intracellular space, the functional nanosystem could be internalized into the target sites effectively and trigger release of drugs in the cytoplasm. Besides this, smart nanocapsules showed excellent inhibitory effect on tumor cells and low side effects on normal cells. This work develops a novel redox-responsive single molecular layer nanocapsule for antitumor drug delivery, extending the biomedical applications of stimuli-responsive polymeric nanomaterials.

9.2.1.3 Enzyme-responsive polymeric nanomaterials

Enzyme-responsive nanomaterials exhibit specific enzyme stimuli ability in the cytoplasm, providing a tremendous opportunity to improve cytosolic drug delivery and corresponding tumor accumulation (Callmann et al., 2015). Compared

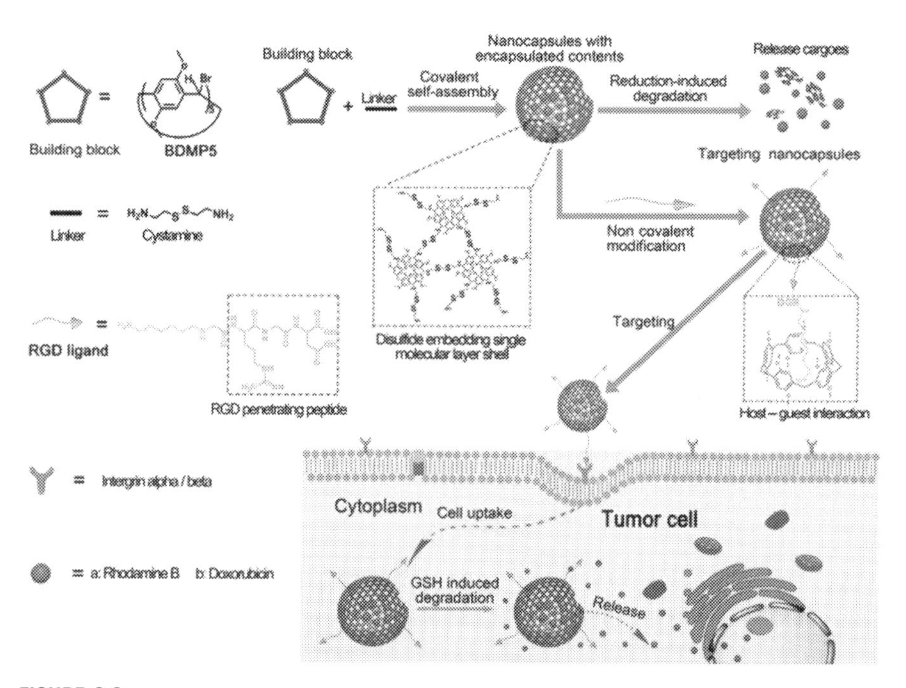

FIGURE 9.3

Design of redox-responsive pillar[5]arene-based single molecular layer polymer nanocapsules for cytoplasm-targeted drug delivery (Xu et al., 2018).

Reproduced with permission from Xu, X., Wu, J., Liu, S., Saw, P.E., Tao, W., Li, Y., Farokhzad, O.C., 2018. Redox-responsive nanoparticle-mediated systemic RNAi for effective cancer therapy. Small 14 (41), e1802565.

with other types of stimuli, enzymes exhibit several distinct but significant advantages for biomedical applications. First, enzymes are endogenous, which do not require addition of external stimuli (such as light, ultrasound, or magnetic fields), thus providing inherent biocompatibility and biosafety (Mu et al., 2018). Moreover, many reactions based on enzyme-responsive materials possess a fast reaction rate, high efficiency, and moderate reaction conditions, such as mild pH, temperature, and aqueous solution. Besides, enzymes always exhibit extraordinary specificity on their substrates, allowing controllable biological reactions in the cytoplasm (Wilkes, 2018). Therefore more and more enzyme-responsive nanomaterials have been developed to selectively deliver therapeutic/diagnose agents to their target sites (Lian et al., 2018).

Matrix metalloproteinases (MMPs), a family of zinc-dependent proteolytic enzyme, can regulate various tumor cell behaviors. MMPs are served as important endogenous stimuli for enzyme-responsive drug delivery since their expression is dramatically high in almost all human tumor cells. Among them, type IV collagenases metalloprotease 2 (MMP-2) is low concentration in normal cells but overexpressed in tumor cells, which have been demonstrated to exhibit a good capacity for enzyme-responsive delivery of polymeric nanomaterials. Zhu et al. (2014) developed multifunctional nanomaterials based on MMP-2 sensitive copolymer, which is prepared by a simple self-assembly method to deliver siRNA and PTX concurrently. The as-designed polymeric nanomaterials presented obvious advantages for tumor therapy, including good stability, efficient polyethylenimine (PEI) condensation for siRNA, passive targeting by EPR effect, active targeting activated by increasing intracellular MMP-2, as well as enhanced internalization due to MMP-2 mediated linker cleavage. All these functions have greatly improved cellular internalization, synergistically integrated the therapeutic efficiency of siRNA/PTX, and eventually realized excellent antitumor performance.

9.2.2 Nucleus

Cell nucleus, one of the most important cellular organelles, contains various transcriptional receptors, growth factors, and proteins (Yang et al., 2018b; Chen et al., 2019a). As the key regulator of cell reproduction, metabolism, gene activation, and cell cycle management, nucleus is supposed to be the most desired target site of different therapeutics especially for malignant tumors (Liu et al., 2018c). In chemotherapy, a large number of first-line anticancer drugs including platinum compounds, doxorubicin, and camptothecin kill cancer cells by interacting with DNA inside the nucleus (Cao et al., 2019). In addition, gene therapy can deliver siRNA into the nucleus, interfere the expression of specific genes, and subsequently prevent the translation process, aiming at achieving disease treatments at the genetic level (Li et al., 2017a). Besides chemotherapy and gene therapy, cell nucleus has also been considered as the most hypersensitive subcellular organelle for effective photodynamic therapy (PDT), in which reactive oxygen species (ROS) can be generated by photoexcitation of photosensitizer (PS). ROS can break DNA strands or induce DNA repair enzymes inactivation by reacting with DNA and proteins in the immediate vicinity (Cheng et al., 2019c).

Delivery of different molecules from cytoplasm to nucleus usually occurs through the nuclear pore complexes (NPCs) which is typically 40 nm in diameter (Li et al., 2018a). In particular, small molecules and ions (with molecular weight <40 kDa) could freely and passively diffuse into/out the nucleus via the central pore of NPCs, while macromolecules with diameter >90 nm or molecular weight >40 kDa need targeting signals to successfully transport into the nucleus (Tang et al., 2017). Attractively, nuclear localization signal (NLS) can be recognized by nuclear transport receptors; therefore various nuclear transport receptors are always used for active translocating larger exogenous agents into the nucleus (Pan et al., 2018).

In the past few years, great efforts have been made to design efficient nuclear-targeted strategies for transporting various therapeutic agents (Cheng et al., 2019a). Typically, pathways of entering the cell nucleus efficiently include passive diffusion, active targeting, and opening the nuclear envelope. As mentioned earlier, only ultra-small molecules can access the cell nucleus freely, most nanomaterials will be away from the nucleus because of their large size (Karandish et al., 2018). Fortunately, active nuclear targeting of nanomaterials could be achieved by surface modification, such as ligand modification, switchable surface charge, or changeable particle size (Yang et al., 2018a; Vankayala et al., 2015). Accordingly, the main strategies explored for nucleus-targeted delivery of polymeric nanomaterials are summarized into three main categories: (1) ligand modification, (2) switchable surface charge, (3) changeable particle size, and (4) opening the nuclear envelope.

9.2.2.1 Ligand modification

Surface ligand modification plays an important role in active nuclear penetration, aiming at transporting exogenous polymeric nanomaterials larger than the sizes of NPCs. Recently, NLSs are widely served as ligands for transporting exogenous polymeric nanomaterials into nucleus via the importin α/β pathway (Ding et al., 2018). Specifically, trans-activating transcription (TAT) peptide, adenoviral, and large T antigen are the commonly used NLSs in nucleus-targeted therapy for various diseases.

TAT peptides, a nuclear target peptide, are derived from transactivator of human immunodeficiency virus type 1 (HIV-1) transcription (Benhamou et al., 2018). As far, a variety of nucleus-targeted polymeric nanomaterials based on TAT peptides have been developed. Wang et al. have designed a highly efficient TAT-targeted polymeric micelle (^{S}TAT-NP$_{IR\&DOX}$) for photo-switchable anticancer therapy (Fig. 9.4). The hydrophilic shell of ^{S}TAT-NP$_{IR\&DOX}$ consisted of a TAT-modified short-chain PEG and a thermo-responsive long-chain polyphosphoester (PPE). Without near-infrared (NIR) irradiation the TAT peptide of ^{S}TAT-NP$_{IR\&DOX}$ was masked by long-chain PPE to minimize nonspecific cellular uptake of nanocarriers. Upon NIR irradiation the TAT-targeting peptide was ultrafastly reexposed (within 60 s) via the collapse of thermo-responsive long-chain PPE, resulting in significantly enhanced cellular uptake of nanocarriers. In normal tissues the TAT peptide of ^{S}TAT-NP$_{IR\&DOX}$ was camouflaged by the long-chain PPE, which could minimize the nonspecific uptake of nanomaterials. In tumor tissues the TAT peptide would be reexposed through the broken of thermo-responsive PPE upon ultrafast NIR photoactivation, leading to obviously enhanced cellular accumulation and anticancer efficacy. This as-prepared photo-responsive TAT-targeted polymeric nanomaterial provided new avenues for nucleus-target drug delivery.

9.2.2.2 Switchable surface charge

Surface charge of the polymeric nanomaterials may influence their molecular interaction with cells to a large extent. It is worth noting that intracellular

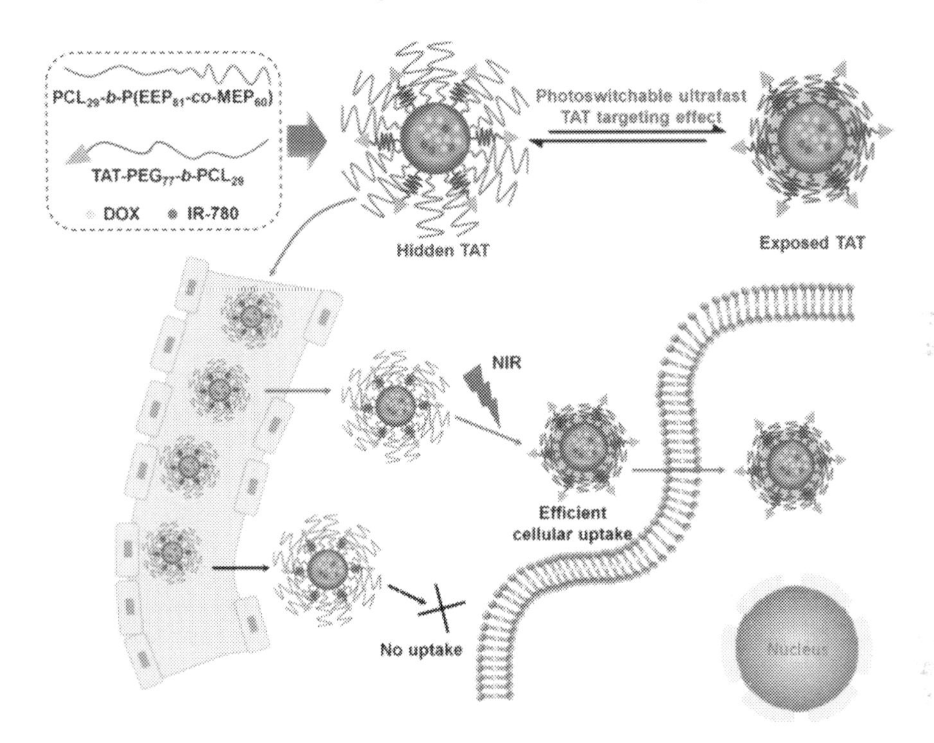

FIGURE 9.4

Schematic illustration of polymeric micelles ^{S}TAT-NP$_{IR\&DOX}$ for on-demand drug delivery by photo-switchable ultrafast TAT-targeting effect. The ^{S}TAT-NP$_{IR\&DOX}$ encapsulated IR-780 and DOX was self-assembled from the TAT-functionalized copolymer TAT-PEG$_{77}$-*b*-PCL$_{29}$ and thermo-responsive copolymer PCL$_{29}$-*b*-P(EEP$_{81}$-*co*-MEP$_{60}$) (Wang et al., 2018b). *TAT*, Trans-activating transcription.

Reproduced with permission from Wang, J., Shen, S., Li, D., Zhan, C., Yuan, Y., Yang, X., 2018. Photoswitchable ultrafast transactivator of transcription (TAT) targeting effect for nanocarrier-based on-demand drug delivery. Adv. Funct. Mater. 28 (3), 1704806.

transport, final localization, and further biological functions of the polymeric nanomaterials primarily depend on the interactions between nanomaterials and cells (Wang et al., 2018a). Since cell membranes mainly consist of phospholipid bilayer membranes and are inherently negatively charged, therefore positively charged polymeric nanomaterials are more likely to bind in cells (Chen et al., 2018c). In fact, most NLSs containing large amounts of lysine and arginine residues also possess positive charges, and such characteristics will improve their ability to increase nuclear uptake of those positively charged nanomaterials (Peng et al., 2017).

Han et al. developed dual pH-sensitive polypeptide micelles with switchable charge for delivering drugs to cancer cells. The polymeric nanomaterials could be transported to nucleus via stepwise pH response to extracellular mildly acidic pH (≈ 6.5) and intracellular lysosomal pH (≈ 5.0) in tumor sites (Han et al, 2015). Polypeptides containing β-carboxylic amide were first synthesized and subsequently self-assembled into micelles with negatively charged. TAT peptide was further combined with the polypeptides via a click reaction. Under the acidic extracellular environment the micelles would transform to positively charged nanomaterials owing to the hydrolyzation of amide, which would be easily internalized by cancer cells. After nanomaterials were transported into acidic intracellular lysosomes, TAT peptide succinyl amide would be hydrolyzed and the nucleus-targeted functions will be reactivated, thereby enhancing drug accumulation in the cell nucleus. Overall, this surface charge switchable strategy can improve nuclear uptake and enhance anticancer efficacy, providing a promising strategy for nucleus-target therapy.

9.2.2.3 Changeable particle size

Apart from ligand modification and surface charge, particle size also plays an important role in transporting nanomaterials into cells. The change of particle size caused by different stimuli (such as pH, redox) provides an alternative way to overcome the main obstacles for therapeutic/diagnose agents delivery from blood circulation to cell nucleus (Ji et al., 2018). As mentioned earlier, nanomaterials of small size can directly pass through the NPCs and transport into nucleus, which is commonly utilized for efficient nuclear uptake. Although nanomaterials with small size show a good capacity of tumor penetration, they may be rapid eliminated in bloodstream via renal clearance due to their small size, leading to poor tumor accumulation (Zhai et al., 2018). In contrast, larger nanomaterials can passively target and accumulate in tumor tissues by EPR effect (Fang et al., 2020b). However, these nanomaterials with large size cannot penetrate deeply into the tumors and achieve nuclear internalization owing to the compact tumor extracellular matrix (Wan et al., 2020). Therefore it is highly desirable that the size of nanomaterials could be changed by a multistage stimuli response. In detail, the size of nanomaterials could be large enough at the initial stage to reduce renal excretion and simultaneously trigger EPR effects and then be decreased by further stimuli to penetrate into tumor deeply for nuclear entry (Li et al., 2018b).

Guo et al. have designed a size changeable micelle with PLA as core which linked with methoxy polyethylene glycol (mPEG) and PEI via a disulfide bond (PELEss-DA), which could promote nuclear uptake of therapeutic agents (Guo et al., 2015). The as-prepared micelle possessed a typical core-corona structure, in which the PLA segment acted as the core material because of its good biodegradability and biocompatibility. One end of PLA segment was conjugated with mPEG; the other end was linked with PEI via a disulfide bond. Both hydrophilic mPEG and PEI were served as the corona layer of the polymeric nanomaterials. Anticancer drugs doxorubicin (DOX) were finally loaded in the PELEss-DA micelles. The positive charge of NPs was shielded by the amidation of PEI, ensuring their excellent physiological stability (at pH 7.4) and a long blood circulation time. Once the NPs accumulated in the tumor tissues, switching surface charge from negative to positive would occur under the acidic pH environment, which was beneficial for their following internalization via electrostatic interaction. Afterward, the size of NPs would change from large to small under intracellular high GSH concentration, leading to enhanced nuclear accumulation. In contrast, the mPEG-PLA-PEI-DMMA NPs of GSH-insensitive were set as control, which were unable to deshield the PEI shell and thus limited their nuclear uptake. In short, the PELEss-DA micelles exhibited superior antitumor effect against MDR in tumors with low systemic toxicity.

9.2.2.4 Opening the nuclear envelope

In addition to designing functional polymeric nanomaterials to satisfy various criteria of nuclear targeting, modifying the NPCs themselves rather than the nanomaterials is another interesting approach to enhance nuclear translocation of exogenous nanomaterials. For example, to increase permeability of the nuclear membrane, a method of enlarging NPCs has been put forward for improving nucleus transportation (Steinke et al., 2018).

Zhu et al. have developed light/pH-responsive polymeric nanomaterials for delivering therapeutic agents to the nucleus. This nanoplatform was self-assembled by a polyamine-containing polyhedral oligomeric silsesquioxane unit, hydrophilic PEG chains, and hydrophobic molecular PSs (Zhu et al., 2018). The positively charged amine enhanced drug accumulation in the cancer cells. Under light irradiation, considerable singlet oxygen was generated and disrupted the structure of lysosomes. After escaping from endosome/lysosomes the nanomaterials accumulated onto the nuclear membranes, destroyed the integrity of nuclear membranes, and facilitated the nuclear entry of molecular drugs. Since the nuclear membrane was broken, the penetration ability and uptake of therapeutic agents were greatly enhanced. This nuclear membrane opening strategy provides an attractive platform for intelligent nanomaterials for efficient nucleus-target delivery.

9.2.3 Mitochondria

Mitochondria, the "powerhouse" of cells which are responsible for generating energy as energy supply, have been applied as a promising therapeutic target for highly efficient disease treatments (Jung et al., 2017). As one of the most crucial subcellular organelles in cells, mitochondria are not only involved in many metabolic pathways including citrate cycle, fatty acids oxidation, gluconeogenesis synthesis, and steroid hormones but also undertake other important biological functions, such as electron transport, ATP synthesis, ROS generation, calcium metabolism, and apoptotic pathways initiation (Zielonka et al., 2017). Furthermore, mitochondrial ROS are also associated with a variety of diseases covering diabetes, obesity, neurodegenerative diseases, and cancers (Wang et al., 2018c). In fact, many clinically approved drugs act directly toward mitochondria by triggering cell apoptosis (Chan et al., 2017). Moreover, mitochondria-targeted treatments can help to overcome MDR and further realize a superior therapeutic efficiency (Wan et al., 2019). Attractively, many mitochondria-targeted nanomaterials have been developed to regulate metabolism and manage diseases associated with mitochondrial dysfunction (Rui et al., 2017).

Until now, a number of mitochondria-specific anticancer drugs have been discovered to kill cancer cells according to different mechanisms of action, mainly including targeting mitochondrial metabolism (such as biosynthetic function, bioenergetics capacity, and redox capacity) and regulating abnormal mitochondrial genes (Tan et al., 2018). However, obstacles are always encountered during the process of delivering therapeutic agents to the mitochondria (Tan et al., 2017). One of the most important challenges is that many therapeutic molecules are impermeable to traverse the two membranes of mitochondria. To solve this problem, many advanced nanotechnologies based on polymeric nanomaterials have been increasingly developed in mitochondrial-targeted drug delivery, for example, engineering the polymeric nanomaterials with delocalized lipophilic cations (DLCs), mitochondria-penetrating peptides (MPPs), and mitochondrial-targeting sequences (MTSs) (Wu et al., 2018).

9.2.3.1 Delocalized lipophilic cations

To achieve specific delivery of mitochondria-targeted nanomaterials, DLCs including triphenylphosphine (TPP), cetyl trimethyl ammonium bromide, rhodamine 123, substituted benzoquinone derivatives, and MKT-077 (rhodacyanine derivative) have been extensively utilized for targeting mitochondria (Pathak et al., 2015). The high negative potential (-180 to -200 mV) of mitochondrial membrane provides a favorable opportunity to make lipophilic cations selectively transport and accumulate into the mitochondria (Zhang et al., 2017b). Because of the negative transmembrane charge, polymeric nanomaterials with delocalized positive charge and adequate lipophilicity can penetrate mitochondrial membrane and achieve high local accumulation in the mitochondria (Yang 2016).

Li et al. have fabricated mitochondria-targeted polydopamine (PDA) NPs, where TPP was used as the mitochondrial penetrating unit (Li et al., 2017b). They prepared two kinds of PEG-modified PDA NPs, and only one was functionalized with TPP (PDA-PEG-TPP NPs vs PDA-PEG NPs). Both of these NPs were then loaded with a chemotherapeutic drug (DOX). To simulate repeated anticancer therapy in clinical trials, MDA-MD-231 cells were treated with DOX-loaded NPs for long-term investigations. The experimental results indicated that mitochondria-targeted PDA-PEG-TPP-DOX NPs exhibited obviously higher tumor internalization and antitumor efficacy than PDA-PEG-DOX NPs. PDA-PEG-TPP-DOX NPs could also effectively overcome the drug resistance in cancer therapy; therefore it is a promising strategy for mitochondria-targeted cancer delivery.

9.2.3.2 Mitochondria-penetrating peptides

MPPs are identified as cationic and lipophilic peptides which can target the inner membrane of mitochondria (Rodrigues and Bernardes, 2018). More importantly, MPPs basically do not affect the potential of mitochondrial membrane. Acting as antioxidant peptides, MPPs can prevent ROS formation in tumor cells and protect mitochondria from oxidative damage. MPPs also exhibit good pharmacokinetic properties including excellent water solubility, good stability, and long elimination half-life time (Alta et al., 2017). Although the penetration mechanism is not fully clear, MPPs still exhibit great potential in mitochondria-targeted therapy due to the abovementioned unique advantages. The development and optimization of MPPs based on mitochondrial-targeted polymeric nanomaterials have made breakthroughs in mitochondrial function and dysfunction related disease treatments.

Selmin et al. (2017) have developed novel hybrid poly(lactide-*co*-glycolide) nanomaterials modified with 6-mer MPPs, which composed of alternating arginine and cyclohexylalanine. Due to the characteristics of cationic and lipophilic, MPPs can transport into the mitochondria sites and link to bioactive molecules, resulting in enhanced intracellular internalization of therapeutic/diagnose agents. The as-developed polymeric nanomaterials containing MPPs showed very low toxicity in 3-(4, 5-dimethylthiazolyl-2)-2, 5-diphenyltetrazolium bromide (MTT) cell ability assay, demonstrating their promising potential for mitochondria-targeted disease diagnosis and therapy.

9.2.3.3 Mitochondrial-targeting sequences

MTS, a multirole sorting sequence, is derived from mitochondrial proteins synthesized in the cytosol. MTSs possess an amphipathic α-helix structure and hydrophobic surface with higher positive charged, allowing recognition via the protein import pores of mitochondria and transporting therapeutic agents to the mitochondria sites (Moretton et al., 2017). These mitochondrial proteins are synthesized as larger precursors, containing a cleavable amino-terminal presequence as the matrix-targeting signal of mitochondria. Typically, MTSs always consist of 10–80 amino acid residues that are mostly hydrophobic and positively charged (Krainz et al., 2016). These amino acid residues can be specifically recognized by the surface receptor of mitochondria. Recently, MTSs have been successfully exploited for constructing mitochondria-targeted polymeric nanomaterial delivery systems to transport different agents, such as proteins, nucleic acids, and highly catalytic enzymes.

In 2015 Jiang et al. reported PTX-loaded liposomes with both pH-responsive and mitochondria-targeted functions, aiming at enhancing drug uptake in mitochondria and eventually improving therapeutic efficiency against drug-resistant cancer cells (Fig. 9.5). In this case, one kind of MTS peptide, $_D$[KLAKLAK]$_2$ (KLA) was first conjugated with 1,2-distearoyl-sn-glycero-3-phosphoethanolamine (DSPE), then functioned with 2,3-dimethylmaleic anhydride (DMA), and finally constructed into DSPE–KLA–DMA liposomes. The surface charge of liposomes could be reversed from negative to positive charge under tumor extracellular pH ($\sim$6.8), which would promote internalization of nanomaterials. After cellular uptake, positively charged KLA peptide selectively transported liposomes into mitochondria and released PTX in the target sites. The as-developed PTX-loaded liposomes are promising mitochondria-targeted delivery systems which can enhance anticancer efficacy for both in vitro and in vivo cancer therapy.

9.2.4 Lysosomes

Similar to the mitochondrial, lysosomes play a crucial role in many important processes of cell homeostasis, such as intracellular and extracellular degradation, cholesterol homeostasis, cell membrane repair, and cell death signaling (He et al., 2015). As the terminal of the endocytic process and the main digestive unit of cell, dysfunction of lysosome is related to the pathogenesis of many severe diseases including cancers, cardiovascular diseases, and neurodegenerative disorders (Park et al., 2019). Compared with other subcellular organelles, targeting lysosome is relatively easier to achieve for nanomaterials (Tian et al., 2018). Many polymeric nanomaterials have been reported to exhibit superior ability of targeting and accumulating in lysosome sites (Rathore et al., 2019). More importantly, lysosomes display an acidic environment characteristic and contain a large variety of hydrolytic enzymes, and thus many researchers have taken advantages of these two features to design various nanomaterials for lysosome-targeted smart drug delivery (Zhu et al., 2017).

Although cancer cells make use of many mechanisms to evade death, cell death could still be easily caused by hydrolytic enzymes releasing from lysosomes under endogenous or exogenous stress (Chen et al., 2018b). When lysosomal membrane is damaged, lysosomal membrane permeabilization (LMP) will occur (Guan et al., 2017). Subsequently, the contents (especially lysosomal hydrolases) inside will be released into the cytoplasm, establishing an important cell apoptosis pathway: the released enzymes of cytoplasm can digest the whole cell and trigger cell death pathways (Niu et al., 2019). Therefore besides lysosome-targeted smart drug delivery, lysosome is also an ideally potential target site for enhanced disease treatments via LMP-mediated cell death pathway.

In 2016 Hu et al. have constructed an NIR dye (boron dipyrromethene, BODIPY)-based polymeric NPs by a simple nanoprecipitation method for lysosome-targeted PAI and acid-activatable PDT (Fig. 9.6). The as-fabricated BODIPY-based polymeric NPs not only possessed outstanding biocompatibility, excellent photostability, and physiological stability but also exhibited high potential for acid-activatable and

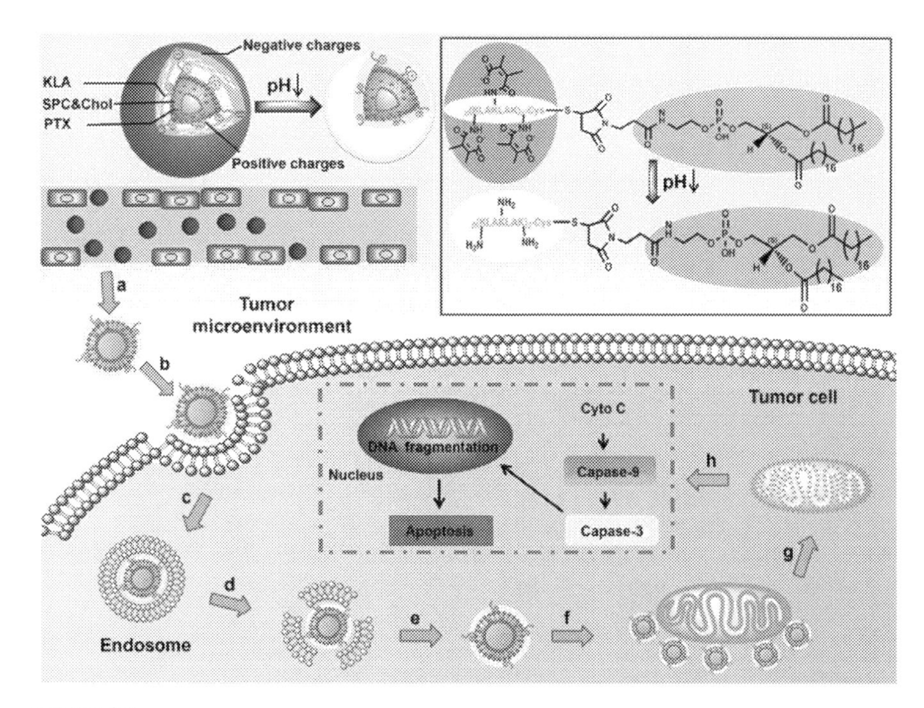

FIGURE 9.5

Scheme of dual-functional liposome (DKD-Lip) with pH response to the tumor microenvironment and mitochondrial-targeted anticancer drug delivery. (a) Surface charge conversion via pH response to mildly acidic tumor microenvironment. (b) Positive charged liposome improved cellular uptake. (c) Internalization into tumor cells. (d) Endosomal escape. (e) Release in the cytoplasm. (f) Binding to mitochondria. (g) Mitochondria damage. (h) Cell death via mitochondria apoptotic pathway (Jiang et al., 2015). *DKD*, 1,2-Distearoyl-sn-glycero-3-phosphoethanolamine–$_{D}$[KLAKLAK]$_2$–2,3-dimethylmaleic anhydride.

Reproduced with permission from Jiang, L., Li, L., He, X., Yi, Q., He, B., Cao, J., Gu, Z., 2015. Overcoming drug-resistant lung cancer by paclitaxel loaded dual-functional liposomes with mitochondria targeting and pH-response. Biomaterials 52, 126–139.

lysosome-targeted theranostic applications. The lysosome-targeted capability of such polymeric NPs is based on the specific response to lysosomes of bis-styryl BODIPY dye. High-performance lysosomal PAI and acid-activatable PDT could be simultaneously triggered by pulsed NIR laser. More importantly, this work furnished a new example with concurrent PAI and PDT for effectively lysosome-targeted delivery.

9.2.5 Golgi and endoplasmic reticulum

In addition to the organelles discussed earlier, other subcellular organelles such as Golgi and ER have also been emerging as newly attractive target sites for polymeric nanomaterials due to their individual roles in cells (Son et al., 2016). Golgi is responsible for posttranslational modifications of the synthesized proteins and participates in synthesis process of carbohydrate structures including glycosaminoglycans and polysaccharides (Luo et al., 2019). Changes in the Golgi apparatus would cause the emergence of various neurodegenerative diseases (such as Alzheimer's disease, Niemann–Pick disease, Parkinson's disease) and cancers. ER, complex folded membrane-wrapped tubules and sacs, extends from the nuclear membrane to the cytoplasm (Sneh-Edri et al., 2011). Importantly, ER can participate in lots of signaling pathways as well as many intracellular stress responses, including calcium signaling, calcium storage, hypoxia, ischemia, exposure to free radicals, elevated protein synthesis, oxidative stress, and genetic mutations. The ER stress is associated with a variety of diseases, such as diabetes, neurodegenerative diseases, cardiovascular, and cancers. In short, both Golgi and ER could deliver agents to the plasma membrane through vesicular trafficking. Therefore the Golgi and ER can be served as important sites for polymeric nanomaterials based suborganelles targeted therapy.

For example, Wan et al. (2018) constructed an ER-targeted polymer based on Ca(II) ion–rich ER lumen and carboxyl group of poly(aspartic acid) (PAsp-*g*-(PEG-ICG)) for enhanced cancer therapy. PAsp-*g*-(PEG-ICG) NPs were designed and developed successfully by grafting modified PEG and ICG onto modified PAsp via the copper(I)-catalyzed alkyne-azide cycloaddition. ICG could not only monitor the distribution of PAsp-*g*-(PEG-ICG) NPs as imaging agent but also produce ROS as protein destructive agent, leading to protein denaturation. In addition, chemotherapeutic drugs, for example, PTX, could be encapsulated in the

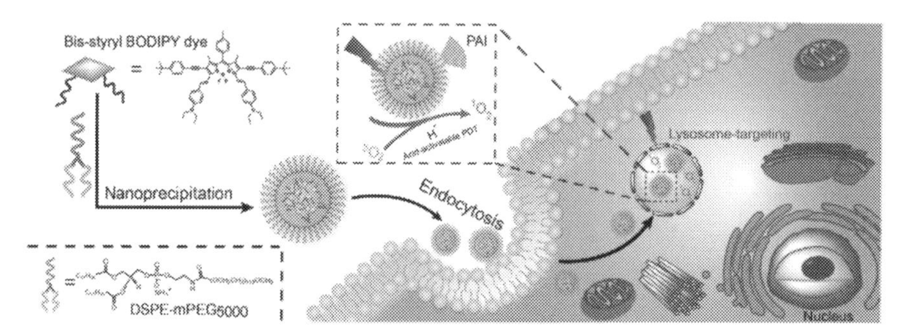

FIGURE 9.6

Schematically illustrating the preparation of lysosome-targeting BODIPY based polymeric NPs with concurrent PAI and PDT for effectively lysosome-targeted delivery (Hu et al., 2016). *BODIPY*, Boron dipyrromethene; *NP*, nanoparticle; *PAI*, photoacoustic imaging; *PDT*, photodynamic therapy.

Reproduced with permission from Hu, W., Ma, H., Hou, B., Zhao, H., Ji, Y., Jiang, R., Huang, W., 2016. Engineering lysosome-targeting BODIPY nanoparticles for photoacoustic imaging and photodynamic therapy under near-infrared light. ACS Appl. Mater. Interfaces 8 (19), 12039–12047.

PAsp-*g*-(PEG-ICG) NPs and possess high drug-loading efficacy and good stability. Because of the coordination interaction with Ca^{2+} of ER lumen, PTX@PAsp-*g*-(PEG-ICG) NPs could selectively target and accumulate in the ER of cancer cells. Moreover, PTX@PAsp-*g*-(PEG-ICG) NPs showed enhanced synergistic effect on in vivo cancer therapy, proving the potential application of ER-targeted disease treatments.

9.3 Conclusion and future perspectives

In this chapter, various polymeric nanomaterials have been developed and modified aiming at transporting therapeutic/diagnostic agents to target and accumulate in specific organelles. Cellular suborganelles are crucial components for survival and proliferation of all cells. Polymeric nanomaterials targeting the cellular organelles exhibit significant advantages over traditional therapeutic agents, including improving therapeutic index, overcoming MDR, and avoiding side effects. Cellular organelles–targeted therapeutics (chemotherapy, gene therapy, PDT, photothermal therapy, etc.)-based polymeric nanomaterials have been widely studied in recent years. These advanced strategies for cellular organelles–targeted disease treatments can improve the efficacy and safety of nanomaterials. However, the problem of fully understanding the targeted mechanisms still need to be resolved, which is of high significance for achieving smart and rational designs of subcellular-targeted delivery systems, thereby avoiding preparation of unnecessary complex structures. In conclusion, the future of cellular organelles–targeted polymeric nanomaterials looks promising for biomedical applications.

References

Alta, R.Y.P., Vitorino, H.A., Goswami, D., Liria, C.W., Wisnovsky, S.P., Kelley, S.O., et al., 2017. Mitochondria-penetrating peptides conjugated to desferrioxamine as chelators for mitochondrial labile iron. PLoS One 12 (2), e0171729.

Azevedo, C., Macedo, M.H., Sarmento, B., 2018. Strategies for the enhanced intracellular delivery of nanomaterials. Drug Discov. Today 23 (5), 944–959.

Bar-Zeev, M., Livney, Y.D., Assaraf, Y.G., 2017. Targeted nanomedicine for cancer therapeutics: towards precision medicine overcoming drug resistance. Drug Resist. Updates 31, 15–30.

Benhamou, R.I., Bibi, M., Berman, J., Fridman, M., 2018. Localizing antifungal drugs to the correct organelle can markedly enhance their efficacy. Angew. Chem. Int. Ed. 57 (21), 6230–6235.

Björnmalm, M., Thurecht, K.J., Michael, M., Scott, A.M., Caruso, F., 2017. Bridging bio-nano science and cancer nanomedicine. ACS Nano 11 (10), 9594–9613.

Callmann, C.E., Barback, C.V., Thompson, M.P., Hall, D.J., Mattrey, R.F., Gianneschi, N.C., 2015. Therapeutic enzyme-responsive nanoparticles for targeted delivery and accumulation in tumors. Adv. Mater. 27 (31), 4611–4615.

Cao, Y., Wu, T.T., Zhang, K., Meng, X.D., Dai, W.H., Wang, D.D., et al., 2019. Engineered exosome-mediated near-infrared-II region V_2C quantum dot delivery for nucleus-target low-temperature photothermal therapy. ACS Nano 13 (2), 1499–1510.

Chan, M.S., Liu, L.S., Leung, H.M., Lo, P.K., 2017. Cancer-cell-specific mitochondria-targeted drug delivery by dual-ligand-functionalized nanodiamonds circumvent drug resistance. ACS Appl. Mater. Interfaces 9 (13), 11780–11789.

Chen, W.H., Luo, G.F., Vazquez-Gonzalez, M., Cazelles, R., Sohn, Y.S., Nechushtai, R., et al., 2018a. Glucose-responsive metal-organic-framework nanoparticles act as "smart" sense-and-treat carriers. ACS Nano 12 (8), 7538–7545.

Chen, X.M., Chen, Y., Yu, Q.L., Gu, B.H., Liu, Y., 2018b. Supramolecular assemblies with near-infrared emission mediated in two stages by cucurbituril and amphiphilic calixarene for lysosome-targeted cell imaging. Angew. Chem. Int. Ed. 57 (38), 12519–12523.

Chen, Y.L., Liu, H.P., Xiong, Y.Y., Ju, H.X., 2018c. Quantitative screening of cell-surface gangliosides by nondestructive extraction and hydrophobic collection. Angew. Chem. Int. Ed. 57 (3), 785–789.

Chen, W.H., Liu, J.H., Wang, Y., Jiang, C.H., Yu, B., Sun, Z., et al., 2019a. A C_5N_2 nano-particle based direct nucleus delivery platform for synergistic cancer therapy. Angew. Chem. Int. Ed. 58 (19), 6290–6294.

Chen, W.H., Luo, G.F., Zhang, X.Z., 2019b. Recent advances in subcellular targeted cancer therapy based on functional materials. Adv. Mater. 31 (3), e1802725.

Cheng, H., Fan, J.H., Zhao, L.P., Fan, G.L., Zheng, R.R., Qiu, X.Z., et al., 2019a. Chimeric peptide engineered exosomes for dual-stage light guided plasma membrane and nucleus targeted photodynamic therapy. Biomaterials 211, 14–24.

Cheng, H., Zheng, R.R., Fan, G.L., Fan, J.H., Zhao, L.P., Jiang, X.Y., et al., 2019b. Mitochondria and plasma membrane dual-targeted chimeric peptide for single-agent synergistic photodynamic therapy. Biomaterials 188, 1–11.

Cheng, Y., Sun, C.L., Liu, R., Yang, J.L., Dai, J., Zhai, T.Y., et al., 2019c. A multifunctional peptide-conjugated AIEgen for efficient and sequential targeted gene delivery into the nucleus. Angew. Chem. Int. Ed. 58 (15), 5049–5053.

Deng, J.J., Wang, K., Wang, M., Yu, P., Mao, L.Q., 2017. Mitochondria targeted nanoscale zeolitic imidazole framework-90 for ATP imaging in live cells. J. Am. Chem. Soc. 139 (16), 5877–5882.

Ding, F., Mou, Q.B., Ma, Y., Pan, G.F., Guo, Y.Y., Tong, G.S., et al., 2018. A crosslinked nucleic acid nanogel for effective siRNA delivery and antitumor therapy. Angew. Chem. Int. Ed. 57 (12), 3064–3068.

Fang, F., Li, M., Zhang, J.F., Lee, C.S., 2020a. Different strategies for organic nanoparticle preparation in biomedicine. ACS Mater. Lett. 2, 531–549.

Fang, F., Zhao, D.X., Zhang, Y.F., Li, M., Ye, J., Zhang, J.F., 2020b. Europium-doped nanoparticles for cellular luminescence lifetime imaging via multiple manipulations of aggregation state. ACS Appl. Bio Mater. 3, 5103–5110.

Gao, P., Pan, W., Li, N., Tang, B., 2019. Boosting cancer therapy with organelle-targeted nanomaterials. ACS Appl. Mater. Interfaces 11 (30), 26529–26558.

Grzybowski, M., Taki, M., Senda, K., Sato, Y., Ariyoshi, T., Okada, Y., et al., 2018. A highly photostable near-infrared labeling agent based on a phospha-rhodamine for long-term and deep imaging. Angew. Chem. Int. Ed. 57 (32), 10137–10141.

Guan, Y., Lu, H.G., Li, W., Zheng, Y.D., Jiang, Z., Zou, J.L., et al., 2017. Near-infrared triggered upconversion polymeric nanoparticles based on aggregation-induced emission and mitochondria targeting for photodynamic cancer therapy. ACS Appl. Mater. Interfaces 9 (32), 26731–26739.

Guo, X., Wei, X., Jing, Y.T., Zhou, S.B., 2015. Size changeable nanocarriers with nuclear targeting for effectively overcoming multidrug resistance in cancer therapy. Adv. Mater. 27 (41), 6450–6456.

Guo, X., Wang, L., Duval, K., Fan, J., Zhou, S.B., Chen, Z., 2018. Dimeric drug polymeric micelles with acid-active tumor targeting and fret-traceable drug release. Adv. Mater. 30 (3), 1705436.

Han, S.S., Li, Z.Y., Zhu, J.Y., Han, K., Zeng, Z.Y., Hong, W., et al., 2015. Dual-pH sensitive charge-reversal polypeptide micelles for tumor-triggered targeting uptake and nuclear drug delivery. Small 11 (21), 2543–2554.

He, L., Li, Y., Tan, C.P., Ye, R.R., Chen, M.H., Cao, J.J., et al., 2015. Cyclometalated iridium(III) complexes as lysosome-targeted photodynamic anticancer and real-time tracking agents. Chem. Sci. 6 (10), 5409–5418.

Hu, W.B., Ma, H.H., Hou, B., Zhao, H., Ji, Y., Jiang, R.C., et al., 2016. Engineering lysosome-targeting BODIPY nanoparticles for photoacoustic imaging and photodynamic therapy under near-infrared light. ACS Appl. Mater. Interfaces 8 (19), 12039–12047.

Huang, J.G., Leshuk, T., Gu, F.X., 2011. Emerging nanomaterials for targeting subcellular organelles. Nano Today 6 (5), 478–492.

Ji, C.D., Gao, Q., Dong, X.H., Yin, W.Y., Gu, Z.J., Gan, Z.H., et al., 2018. A size-reducible nanodrug with an aggregation-enhanced photodynamic effect for deep chemo-photodynamic therapy. Angew. Chem. Int. Ed. 57 (35), 11384–11388.

Jiang, L., Li, L., He, X.D., Yi, Q.Y., He, B., Cao, J., et al., 2015. Overcoming drug-resistant lung cancer by paclitaxel loaded dual-functional liposomes with mitochondria targeting and pH-response. Biomaterials 52, 126–139.

Jung, H.S., Lee, J.H., Kim, K., Koo, S., Verwilst, P., Sessler, J.L., et al., 2017. A mitochondria-targeted cryptocyanine-based photothermogenic photosensitizer. J. Am. Chem. Soc. 139 (29), 9972–9978.

Kanamala, M., Wilson, W.R., Yang, M.M., Palmer, B.D., Wu, Z.M., 2016. Mechanisms and biomaterials in pH-responsive tumour targeted drug delivery: a review. Biomaterials 85, 152–167.

Karandish, F., Mamnoon, B., Feng, L., Haldar, M.K., Xia, L., Gange, K.N., et al., 2018. Nucleus-targeted, echogenic polymersomes for delivering a cancer stemness inhibitor to pancreatic cancer cells. Biomacromolecules 19 (10), 4122–4132.

Koren, E., Apte, A., Jani, A., Torchilin, V.P., 2012. Multifunctional PEGylated 2C5-immunoliposomes containing pH-sensitive bonds and TAT peptide for enhanced tumor cell internalization and cytotoxicity. J. Controlled Release 160 (2), 264–273.

Krainz, T., Gaschler, M.M., Lim, C., Sacher, J.R., Stockwell, B.R., Wipf, P., 2016. A mitochondrial-targeted nitroxide is a potent inhibitor of ferroptosis. ACS Cent. Sci. 2 (9), 653–659.

Li, Y., Lin, J.Y., Huang, Y., Li, Y.X., Yang, X.R., Wu, H.J., et al., 2015. Self-targeted, shape-assisted, and controlled-release self-delivery nanodrug for synergistic targeting/anticancer effect of cytoplasm and nucleus of cancer cells. ACS Appl. Mater. Interfaces 7 (46), 25553–25559.

Li, L., Li, X., Wu, Y.Z., Song, L.J., Yang, X., He, T., et al., 2017a. Multifunctional nucleus-targeting nanoparticles with ultra-high gene transfection efficiency for *in vivo* gene therapy. Theranostics 7 (6), 1633–1649.

Li, W.Q., Wang, Z.G., Hao, S.J., He, H.Z., Wan, Y., Zhu, C.D., et al., 2017b. Mitochondria-targeting polydopamine nanoparticles to deliver doxorubicin for overcoming drug resistance. ACS Appl. Mater. Interfaces 9 (20), 16793–16802.

Li, N., Sun, Q.Q., Yu, Z.Z., Gao, X.N., Pan, W., Wan, X.Y., et al., 2018a. Nuclear-targeted photothermal therapy prevents cancer recurrence with near-infrared triggered copper sulfide nanoparticles. ACS Nano 12 (6), 5197–5206.

Li, W., Suzuki, T., Minami, H., 2018b. A facile method for preparation of polymer particles having a "cylindrical" shape. Angew. Chem. Int. Ed. 57 (31), 9936–9940.

Lian, X.Z., Huang, Y.Y., Zhu, Y.Y., Fang, Y., Zhao, R., Joseph, E., et al., 2018. Enzyme-MOF nanoreactor activates nontoxic paracetamol for cancer therapy. Angew. Chem. Int. Ed. 57 (20), 5725–5730.

Liang, T.X.Z., Yao, Z.G., Ding, J., Min, Q.H., Jiang, L.P., Zhu, J.J., 2018. Cascaded aptamers-governed multistage drug-delivery system based on biodegradable envelope-type nanovehicle for targeted therapy of HER2-overexpressing breast cancer. ACS Appl. Mater. Interfaces 10 (40), 34050–34059.

Liu, Q., Das, M., Liu, Y., Huang, L., 2018a. Targeted drug delivery to melanoma. Adv. Drug Deliver. Rev. 127, 208–221.

Liu, S.C., Pan, J.M., Liu, J.X., Ma, Y., Qiu, F.X., Mei, L., et al., 2018b. Dynamically PEGylated and borate-coordination-polymer-coated polydopamine nanoparticles for synergetic tumor-targeted, chemo-photothermal combination therapy. Small 14 (13), e1703968.

Liu, X.T., Wang, L., Xu, X.W., Zhao, H.Y., Jiang, W., 2018c. Endogenous stimuli-responsive nucleus-targeted nanocarrier for intracellular mRNA imaging and drug delivery. ACS Appl. Mater. Interfaces 10 (46), 39524–39531.

Liu, Y., Zhen, W.Y., Jin, L.H., Zhang, S.T., Sun, G.Y., Zhang, T.Q., et al., 2018d. All-in-one theranostic nanoagent with enhanced reactive oxygen species generation and modulating tumor microenvironment ability for effective tumor eradication. ACS Nano 12 (5), 4886–4893.

Luo, J.W., Zhang, P., Zhao, T., Jia, M.D., Yin, P., Li, W.H., et al., 2019. Golgi apparatus-targeted chondroitin-modified nanomicelles suppress hepatic stellate cell activation for the management of liver fibrosis. ACS Nano 13 (4), 3910–3923.

Ma, X.W., Gong, N.Q., Zhong, L., Sun, J.D., Liang, X.J., 2016a. Future of nanotherapeutics: targeting the cellular sub-organelles. Biomaterials 97, 10–21.

Ma, Y.F., Huang, J., Song, S.J., Chen, H.B., Zhang, Z.J., 2016b. Cancer-targeted nanotheranostics: recent advances and perspectives. Small 12 (36), 4936–4954.

Moretton, A., Morel, F., Macao, B., Lachaume, P., Ishak, L., Lefebvre, M., et al., 2017. Selective mitochondrial DNA degradation following double-strand breaks. PLoS One 12 (4), e0176795.

Mu, J., Lin, J., Huang, P., Chen, X.Y., 2018. Development of endogenous enzyme-responsive nanomaterials for theranostics. Chem. Soc. Rev. 47 (15), 5554–5573.

Niu, N., Zhou, H.P., Liu, N., Jiang, H., Hussain, E., Hu, Z.Z., et al., 2019. A smart perylene derived photosensitizer for lysosome-targeted and self-assessed photodynamic therapy. Chem. Commun. 55 (8), 1036–1039.

Nurunnabi, M., Khatun, Z., Badruddoza, A.Z.M., McCarthy, J.R., Lee, Y.K., Huh, K.M., 2019. Biomaterials and bioengineering approaches for mitochondria and nuclear targeting drug delivery. ACS Biomater. Sci. Eng. 5 (4), 1645–1660.

Pan, L.M., Liu, J.N., Shi, J.L., 2018. Cancer cell nucleus-targeting nanocomposites for advanced tumor therapeutics. Chem. Soc. Rev. 47 (18), 6930–6946.

Park, G.K., Lee, J.H., Levitz, A., El Fakhri, G., Hwang, N.S., Henary, M., et al., 2019. Lysosome-targeted bioprobes for sequential cell tracking from macroscopic to microscopic scales. Adv. Mater. 31 (14), e1806216.

Pathak, R.K., Kolishetti, N., Dhar, S., 2015. Targeted nanoparticles in mitochondrial medicine. Wiley Interdiscip. Rev. Nanomed. Nanobiotechnol. 7 (3), 315–329.

Pearce, A.K., Simpson, J.D., Fletcher, N.L., Houston, Z.H., Fuchs, A.V., Russell, P.J., et al., 2017. Localised delivery of doxorubicin to prostate cancer cells through a PSMA-targeted hyperbranched polymer theranostic. Biomaterials 141, 330–339.

Peng, H.B., Tang, J., Zheng, R., Guo, G.N., Dong, A.G., Wang, Y.J., et al., 2017. Nuclear-targeted multifunctional magnetic nanoparticles for photothermal therapy. Adv. Healthcare Mater. 6 (7), 1704806.

Qin, S.Y., Zhang, A.Q., Zhang, X.Z., 2018. Recent advances in targeted tumor chemotherapy based on smart nanomedicines. Small 14 (45), e1802417.

Rathore, B., Sunwoo, K., Jangili, P., Kim, J., Kim, J.H., Huang, M., et al., 2019. Nanomaterial designing strategies related to cell lysosome and their biomedical applications: a review. Biomaterials 211, 25–47.

Rodrigues, T., Bernardes, G.J.L., 2018. Development of antibody-directed therapies: *quo vadis*? Angew. Chem. Int. Ed. 57 (8), 2032–2034.

Rosenblum, D., Joshi, N., Tao, W., Karp, J.M., Peer, D., 2018. Progress and challenges towards targeted delivery of cancer therapeutics. Nat. Commun. 9 (1), 1410.

Rui, L.L., Xue, Y.D., Wang, Y., Gao, Y., Zhang, W.A., 2017. A mitochondria-targeting supramolecular photosensitizer based on pillar[5]arene for photodynamic therapy. Chem. Commun. 53 (21), 3126–3129.

Selmin, F., Magri, G., Gennari, C.G.M., Marchiano, S., Ferri, N., Pellegrino, S., 2017. Development of poly(lactide-*co*-glycolide) nanoparticles functionalized with a mitochondria penetrating peptide. J. Pept. Sci. 23 (2), 182–188.

Shen, Y.T., Liang, L.J., Zhang, S.Q., Huang, D.S., Deng, R., Zhang, J., et al., 2018. Organelle-targeting gold nanorods for macromolecular profiling of subcellular organelles and enhanced cancer cell killing. ACS Appl. Mater. Interfaces 10 (9), 7910–7918.

Sneh-Edri, H., Likhtenshtein, D., Stepensky, D., 2011. Intracellular targeting of PLGA nanoparticles encapsulating antigenic peptide to the endoplasmic reticulum of dendritic cells and its effect on antigen cross-presentation *in vitro*. Mol. Pharm. 8 (4), 1266–1275.

Son, S.H., Seko, A., Daikoku, S., Fujikawa, K., Suzuki, K., Ito, Y., et al., 2016. Endoplasmic reticulum (ER)-targeted, galectin-mediated retrograde transport by using a halotag carrier protein. ChemBioChem 17 (7), 630–639.

Steinke, M., Zunhammer, F., Chatzopoulou, E.I., Teller, H., Schutze, K., Walles, H., et al., 2018. Rapid analysis of cell-nanoparticle interactions using single-cell Raman trapping microscopy. Angew. Chem. Int. Ed. 57 (18), 4946–4950.

Tan, X., Luo, S.L., Long, L., Wang, Y., Wang, D.C., Fang, S.T., et al., 2017. Structure-guided design and synthesis of a mitochondria-targeting near-infrared fluorophore with multimodal therapeutic activities. Adv. Mater. 29 (43), 1704196.

Tan, Y.N., Zhu, Y., Zhao, Y., Wen, L.J., Meng, T.T., Liu, X., et al., 2018. Mitochondrial alkaline pH-responsive drug release mediated by celastrol loaded glycolipid-like micelles for cancer therapy. Biomaterials 154, 169–181.

Tang, R., Wang, M., Ray, M., Jiang, Y., Jiang, Z.W., Xu, Q.B., et al., 2017. Active targeting of the nucleus using nonpeptidic boronate tags. J. Am. Chem. Soc. 139 (25), 8547–8551.

Tang, B.Q., Zaro, J.L., Shen, Y., Chen, Q., Yu, Y.L., Sun, P.P., et al., 2018. Acid-sensitive hybrid polymeric micelles containing a reversibly activatable cell-penetrating peptide for tumor-specific cytoplasm targeting. J. Controlled Release 279, 147–156.

Tian, Z.Z., Li, J.J., Zhang, S.M., Xu, Z.S., Yang, Y.L., Kong, D.L., et al., 2018. Lysosome-targeted chemotherapeutics: half-sandwich ruthenium(II) complexes that are selectively toxic to cancer cells. Inorg. Chem. 57 (17), 10498–10502.

Ulbrich, K., Hola, K., Subr, V., Bakandritsos, A., Tucek, J., Zboril, R., 2016. Targeted drug delivery with polymers and magnetic nanoparticles: covalent and noncovalent approaches, release control, and clinical studies. Chem. Rev. 116 (9), 5338–5431.

Vankayala, R., Kuo, C.L., Nuthalapati, K., Chiang, C.S., Hwang, K.C., 2015. Nucleus-targeting gold nanoclusters for simultaneous *in vivo* fluorescence imaging, gene delivery, and NIR-light activated photodynamic therapy. Adv. Funct. Mater. 25 (37), 5934–5945.

von Roemeling, C., Jiang, W., Chan, C.K., Weissman, I.L., Kim, B.Y.S., 2017. Breaking down the barriers to precision cancer nanomedicine. Trends Biotechnol. 35 (2), 159–171.

Wan, Y.P., Lu, G.H., Wei, W.C., Huang, Y.H., Li, S.L., Chen, J.X., et al., 2020. Stable organic photosensitizer nanoparticles with absorption peak beyond 800 nanometers and high reactive oxygen species yield for multimodality phototheranostics. ACS Nano 14, 9917–9920.

Wan, Y.P., Lu, G.H., Zhang, J.F., Wang, Z.Y., Li, X.Z., Chen, R., et al., 2019. A biocompatible free radical nanogenerator with real-time monitoring capability for high performance sequential hypoxic tumor therapy. Adv. Funct. Mater. 29, 1903436.

Wan, J.X., Sun, L.Y., Wu, P., Wang, F., Guo, J., Cheng, J.J., et al., 2018. Synthesis of indocyanine green functionalized comblike poly(aspartic acid) derivatives for enhanced cancer cell ablation by targeting the endoplasmic reticulum. Polym. Chem. 9 (10), 1206–1215.

Wang, Y.Y., Deng, Y.B., Luo, H.H., Zhu, A.J., Ke, H.T., Yang, H., et al., 2017. Light-responsive nanoparticles for highly efficient cytoplasmic delivery of anticancer agents. ACS Nano 11 (12), 12134–12144.

Wang, H.M., Feng, Z.Q.Q., Qin, Y.N., Wang, J.Q., Xu, B., 2018a. Nucleopeptide assemblies selectively sequester ATP in cancer cells to increase the efficacy of doxorubicin. Angew. Chem. Int. Ed. 57 (18), 4931–4935.

Wang, J.X., Shen, S., Li, D.D., Zhan, C.Y., Yuan, Y.Y., Yang, X.Z., 2018b. Photoswitchable ultrafast transactivator of transcription (TAT) targeting effect for nanocarrier-based on-demand drug delivery. Adv. Funct. Mater. 28 (3), 1704806.

Wang, Z., Chen, Y.Z., Zhang, H., Li, Y.W., Ma, Y.F., Huang, J., et al., 2018c. Mitochondria-targeting polydopamine nanocomposites as chemophotothermal therapeutics for cancer. Bioconjugate Chem. 29 (7), 2415–2425.

Wei, M.L., Gao, Y.F., Li, X., Serpe, M.J., 2017. Stimuli-responsive polymers and their applications. Polym. Chem. 8 (1), 127–143.

Wilkes, G.M., 2018. Targeted therapy: attacking cancer with molecular and immunological targeted agents. Asia-Pac. J. Oncol. Nurs. 5 (2), 137–155.

Wu, J., Li, J., Wang, H., Liu, C.B., 2018. Mitochondrial-targeted penetrating peptide delivery for cancer therapy. Expert Opin. Drug Del. 15 (10), 951–964.

Xu, X.D., Wu, J., Liu, S.S., Saw, P.E., Tao, W., Li, Y.J., et al., 2018. Redox-responsive nanoparticle-mediated systemic RNAi for effective cancer therapy. Small 14 (41), e1802565.

Xue, F.F., Wei, P., Ge, X.T., Zhong, Y.P., Cao, C.Y., Yu, D.P., et al., 2018. A pH-responsive organic photosensitizer specifically activated by cancer lysosomes. Dyes Pigm 156, 285–290.

Yan, J., He, W.X., Yan, S.Q., Niu, F., Liu, T.Y., Ma, B.H., et al., 2018. Self-assembled peptide-lanthanide nanoclusters for safe tumor therapy: overcoming and utilizing biological barriers to peptide drug delivery. ACS Nano 12 (2), 2017–2026.

Yang, H., 2016. Targeted nanosystems: advances in targeted dendrimers for cancer therapy. Nanomedicine 12 (2), 309–316.

Yang, Y., Xu, L.G., Zhu, W.J., Feng, L.Z., Liu, J.J., Chen, Q., et al., 2018a. One-pot synthesis of pH-responsive charge-switchable PEGylated nanoscale coordination polymers for improved cancer therapy. Biomaterials 156, 121–133.

Yang, Y., Zhu, W.J., Feng, L.Z., Chao, Y., Yi, X., Dong, Z.L., et al., 2018b. G-quadruplex-based nanoscale coordination polymers to modulate tumor hypoxia and achieve nuclear-targeted drug delivery for enhanced photodynamic therapy. Nano Lett. 18 (11), 6867–6875.

Yao, Q., Choi, J.H., Dai, Z., Wang, J., Kim, D., Tang, X., et al., 2017. Improving tumor specificity and anticancer activity of dasatinib by dual-targeted polymeric micelles. ACS Appl. Mater. Interfaces 9 (42), 36642–36654.

Yu, B., Wei, H., He, Q.J., Ferreira, C.A., Kutyreff, C.J., Ni, D.L., et al., 2018. Efficient uptake of ^{177}Lu-porphyrin-PEG nanocomplexes by tumor mitochondria for multimodal-imaging-guided combination therapy. Angew. Chem. Int. Ed. 57 (1), 218–222.

Yuba, E., Yamaguchi, A., Yoshizaki, Y., Harada, A., Kono, K., 2017. Bioactive polysaccharide-based pH-sensitive polymers for cytoplasmic delivery of antigen and activation of antigen-specific immunity. Biomaterials 120, 32–45.

Zhai, J., Jia, Y.W., Zhao, L.N., Yuan, Q., Gao, F.P., Zhang, X.C., et al., 2018. Turning on/off the anti-tumor effect of the Au cluster *via* atomically controlling its molecular size. ACS Nano 12 (5), 4378–4386.

Zhang, Y.F., Fang, F., Li, L., Zhang, J.F., 2020. Self-assembled organic nanomaterials for drug delivery, bioimaging, and cancer therapy. ACS Biomater. Sci. Eng. 6, 4816–4833.

Zhang, J.F., Li, S.L., An, F.F., Liu, J., Jin, S.B., Zhang, J.C., et al., 2015. Self-carried curcumin nanoparticles for *in vitro* and *in vivo* cancer therapy with real-time monitoring of drug release. Nanoscale 7 (32), 13503–13510.

Zhang, J.F., Yang, C.X., Zhang, R., Chen, R., Zhang, Z.Y., Zhang, W.J., et al., 2017a. Biocompatible D-A semiconducting polymer nanoparticle with light-harvesting unit for highly effective photoacoustic imaging guided photothermal therapy. Adv. Funct. Mater. 27 (13), 1605094.

Zhang, Y., Zhang, C.J., Chen, J., Liu, L., Hu, M.Y., Li, J., et al., 2017b. Trackable mitochondria-targeting nanomicellar loaded with doxorubicin for overcoming drug resistance. ACS Appl. Mater. Interfaces 9 (30), 25152–25163.

Zhang, J.F., Chen, J., Ren, J.K., Guo, W.S., Li, X.L., Chen, R., et al., 2018. Biocompatible semiconducting polymer nanoparticles as robust photoacoustic and photothermal agents revealing the effects of chemical structure on high photothermal conversion efficiency. Biomaterials 181, 92–102.

Zhao, S.J., Niu, G.L., Wu, F., Yan, L., Zhang, H.Y., Zhao, J.F., et al., 2017. Lysosome-targetable polythiophene nanoparticles for two-photon excitation photodynamic therapy and deep tissue imaging. J. Mater. Chem. B 5 (20), 3651–3657.

Zhou, M.J., Xie, Y.Q., Xu, S.J., Xin, J.Q., Wang, J., Han, T., et al., 2020. Hypoxia-activated nanomedicines for effective cancer therapy. Eur. J. Med. Chem. 195, 112274.

Zhou, M.J., Zhang, X.J., Yang, Y.L., Liu, Z., Tian, B.S., Jie, J.S., et al., 2013. Carrier-free functionalized multidrug nanorods for synergistic cancer therapy. Biomaterials 34 (35), 8960–8967.

Zhou, M.J., Zhang, X.J., Yu, C.T., Nan, X.Y., Chen, X.F., Zhang, X.H., 2016. Shape regulated anticancer activities and systematic toxicities of drug nanocrystals *in vivo*. Nanomedicine 12 (1), 181–189.

Zhou, M.J., Wei, W.J., Chen, X.F., Xu, X.Z., Zhang, X.H., Zhang, X.J., 2019. pH and redox dual responsive carrier-free anticancer drug nanoparticles for targeted delivery and synergistic therapy. Nanomedicine: NBM 20, 102008.

Zhu, L., Perche, F., Wang, T., Torchilin, V.P., 2014. Matrix metalloproteinase 2-sensitive multifunctional polymeric micelles for tumor-specific co-delivery of siRNA and hydrophobic drugs. Biomaterials 35 (13), 4213–4222.

Zhu, X.D., Sun, Y., Chen, D., Li, J.F., Dong, X., Wang, J., et al., 2017. Mastocarcinoma therapy synergistically promoted by lysosome dependent apoptosis specifically evoked by 5-Fu@nanogel system with passive targeting and pH activatable dual function. J. Controlled Release 254, 107–118.

Zhu, Y.X., Jia, H.R., Pan, G.Y., Ulrich, N.W., Chen, Z., Wu, F.G., 2018. Development of a light-controlled nanoplatform for direct nuclear delivery of molecular and nanoscale materials. J. Am. Chem. Soc. 140 (11), 4062–4070.

Zielonka, J., Joseph, J., Sikora, A., Hardy, M., Ouari, O., Vasquez-Vivar, J., et al., 2017. Mitochondria-targeted triphenylphosphonium-based compounds: syntheses, mechanisms of action, and therapeutic and diagnostic applications. Chem. Rev. 117 (15), 10043–10120.

CHAPTER

Polymeric nanomaterials in neuroscience

10

Maria Bohra[1], Ankan Sarkar[1], Swapnil Raut[1], Upasna Singh[1], Priya Jagtap[1], Birva Shah[1], Falguni Baidya[1], Aishika Datta[1], Harpreet Kaur[1], Deepaneeta Sarmah[1], Anupom Borah[2], Kunjan R. Dave[3] and Pallab Bhattacharya[1]

[1]*Department of Pharmacology and Toxicology, National Institute of Pharmaceutical Education and Research (NIPER), Ahmedabad, Gandhinagar, India*

[2]*Cellular and Molecular Neurobiology Laboratory, Department of Life Science and Bioinformatics, Assam University, Silchar, India*

[3]*Department of Neurology, University of Miami Miller School of Medicine, Miami, FL, United States*

10.1 Introduction

Neuropathologies have influenced humanity from time immemorial thus causing a deleterious effect on day-to-day life. Hitherto, there is no permanent treatment to overcome numerous devastating diseases, and researchers are continuously trying to find out a way to cope up with these by using several different techniques (Li and Mezzenga, 2013). Many formulations have been made for managing neuropathologies, but none of them has proven to be satisfactory. The major concerning issue is the blood–brain barrier (BBB), which restricts the entry of many drugs and makes the permanent treatment of neuropathologies unattainable (Gilmore et al., 2008). Even nontargeted delivery of the drug is a matter of concern (in the case of cancer) that may cause a nuisance to nonpathological entities (Coates et al., 1983). Prior diagnosis of various neurological disorders can be sufficient to combat it.

Nanoparticles (NPs) are the particles of 1–100 nm (Arruebo et al., 2007) being popular in recent times for broader application in neuropathological disorders due to several reasons such as NPs, as quantum dots (QDs), magnetic NPs, carbon nanotubes (CNTs), etc. may play a major role in overcoming the obstacles of current interventions. Being nano in size, they can be useful in curbing the demerits of entry constraint of molecules to the brain via BBB. Nanoparticles are being used as nanocarriers for facilitating the delivery of drugs to the targeted site (Saeedi et al., 2019). NPs have shown to improve various neural pathological conditions upon preliminary detection. NPs such as nanospheres and CNT are found to reduce the infarct volume and help in early

Advances in Polymeric Nanomaterials for Biomedical Applications. DOI: https://doi.org/10.1016/B978-0-12-814657-6.00006-9

detection of glucose and lactate concentration changes (Lin et al., 2009) in global or focal ischemia, respectively. CNTs and QDs have shown neural cell regeneration and differentiation (Jan and Kotov, 2007). These NPs have been found to reach their target sites by crossing BBB via the olfactory nerve pathway (Wu et al., 2016). Drug loaded gold nanoparticles, dendrimers and osmotin loaded iron magnetic nanoparticles, were found to reduce hyperphosphorylation of tau proteins (Amin et al., 2017; Xu et al., 2013) along with the aggregation of amyloid-beta plaques exhibiting improved memory and spatial learning (Sanati et al., 2019) in Alzheimer's patients (AD). PEGylated liposomal formulation of existing drugs shows safety and better plasma and brain concentration (Montesinos, 2017). Some of these NPs are polymerized with various polymers for stability and targeted delivery, making these NPs more robust and particular. By coating magnetic NPs with CpG oligodeoxynucleotides (Nunes et al., 2012) helps to curb cancers such as glioblastomas (Shevtsov et al., 2018) and causing magnetic hyperthermia and destruction of cancer (Fig. 10.1). NPs have also shown efficacy in Parkinson's disease (PD) by reducing oxidative stress, Lewy body degradation, and SNCA gene silencing and inhibiting dopamine apoptosis (Hu et al., 2018). The use of these nanomaterials to deliver drugs to brain are found to be useful in various other neurological disorders such as Amyotrophic lateral sclerosis (ALS), Bell's palsy, Prion diseases etc. (Xu et al., 2013; Cordes et al., 2007).

The peculiar properties of nanomaterials captivate researchers to go beyond it that has proven to be a boon for medical science for defeating neuropathologies affecting mankind and making them more resilient. Table 10.1 lists the various applications of nanomaterials in neuroscience.

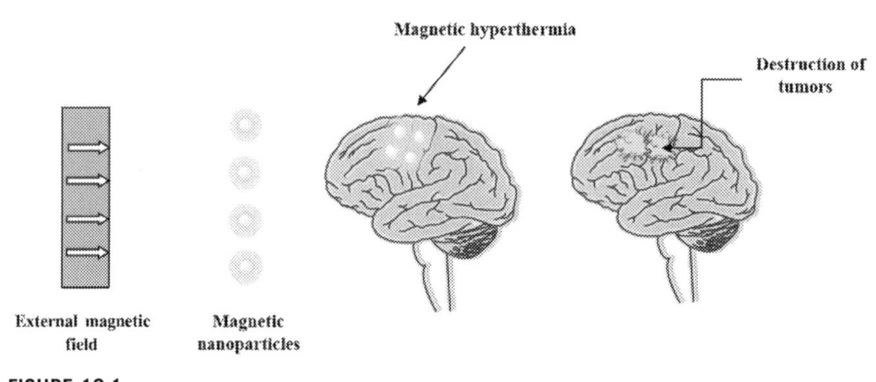

FIGURE 10.1

Destruction of glioblastoma by chitosan-based magnetic nanoparticle on application of external magnetic field by magnetic hyperthermia.

(Adapted from ChemBioDraw Ultra. Version:14.0.0.117.)

Table 10.1 Implementation of nanomaterials in neuropathologies.

Sr. no.	Nanomaterials	Drugs loaded	Coating materials	Disease treatment	References
1.	Nanosphere	Erythropoietin (HMG-CoA reductase inhibitors)	Chitosan	Brain targeting for CNS disease	Aderibigbe and Naki, 2019; Soni et al., 2016; Karatas et al., 2009
		NMDA-NR1 vaccine	PLGA	Alzheimer's disease	
		Caspase-3 inhibitor		Stroke	
2.	Gold nanoparticles	SNCA siRNA		Parkinson's disease	Hu et al., 2018
3.	CNT	Stem cells	PEG	Alzheimer's disease	Zhao et al., 2011; John et al., 2015
		CpG oligodeoxynucleotides		Parkinson's disease, and ischemia	
				Glioma	
4.	Magnetic nanoparticles	α-Synuclein RNAi plasmid	Ferrite	Parkinson's disease	Niu et al., 2017
5.	Dendrimers	Sialic acid		Alzheimer's disease	Patel et al., 2007
6.	Liposomes	Memantine, rivastigmine, donepezil, galantamine	PEG	Alzheimer disease	Ross et al., 2018; Gunay et al., 2017; Bruch et al., 2019
		Levodopa	PEG	Parkinson's disease	
		tPA	Actin	Stroke	
7.	Quantum dot	Graphene oxide		Reduces neurotoxicity	Ren et al., 2018

CNT, *Carbon nanotube;* PEG, *polyethylene glycol;* PLGA, *poly(lactide-co-glycolic acid);* tPA, *tissue plasminogen activator.*

10.2 The gamut of nanomaterials in neurological disorders

10.2.1 Nanospheres

Nanospheres are the homogenous spheres in which a dispersed active compound or drug is adsorbed on the surface, or it may be entrapped within the polymeric matrix structure through the solid sphere. The size of the nanospheres ranges from 100 to 1000 nm. It is prepared through the microemulsion polymerization technique, solvent evaporation, solvent displacement technique, and phase inversion method (Singh et al., 2010). The drug is released by passive diffusion from the polymeric matrix. The polymers used may be synthetic polymers such as poly (lactide-*co*-glycolic acid), poly(butylcyano-acrylate), poly(glycolic acid), and poly (lactic acid). Sometimes, natural polymers such as chitosan, gelatin, sodium alginate, and albumin may also use in the preparation of nanospheres (Shah, 2016).

To prepare nanospheres, a monodisperse nanosphere solution composed of the polymer is delivered to a flat substrate. Under specified optimum condition, when the solvent evaporates, the nanospheres self-assemble and form a hexagonal, close-packed monolayer structure; this leads to creation of voids between the nanospheres where the underlying substrate or drug is exposed (Colson et al., 2013).

Nanospheres are found beneficial in many disorders such as ischemic stroke, glioblastoma, and multiple sclerosis. A reduced infarct volume is observed in mice with focal ischemia when a transferrin-targeted nanospheres loaded with the irreversible caspase-3 inhibitor is delivered to the transient ischemic stroke patient (Soni et al., 2016). It was observed that the drug penetration across the blood–tumor barrier (BTB) is poor in the case of glioblastoma brain or spinal cord. The BTB, although considered leakier than the BBB, is very heterogeneous, has non uniform permeability and presence of active efflux transporters (Arvanitis et al., 2019, 2020). Soni et al. carried out a study in which a liposome loaded with a drug is chemically linked with a nano chain composed of three iron oxide (IO) nanospheres, which form a linear chain–like assembly. This linear chain–like assembly possesses a unique ability to have rapid access to brain and deposits the drug in brain tumor sites through the $\alpha v\beta 3$ integrin receptor (Soni et al., 2016). In the case of multiple sclerosis the insulating covers of nerve cells in the brain and spinal cord get damaged, which leads to disruption of the ability of the nervous system to communicate. Ultra-sized cerium oxide nanospheres reduce oxidative stress and alleviate motor deficit in multiple sclerosis brain (Soni et al., 2016).

The primacy of nanosphere is extensive. Due to their ultra-tiny size, nanospheres can easily pass through the smallest capillary vessels; hence, it can be used for targeted drug delivery. In addition, nanospheres may be able to avoid rapid phagocyte clearance, and so it remains in the bloodstream for a prolonged duration (Singh et al., 2010).

Nanospheres possess some negative aspects such as during drug loading of nanospheres and rapid release of the drug; there are higher chances of particle aggregation as they have a smaller size and larger surface area (Singh et al., 2010).

Nanospheres may generate immune response due to off-target effect, which may lead to tissue toxicity due to inadequate removal from the body (Singh et al., 2010).

10.2.2 Carbon nanotubes

Iijima first discovered CNTs for their scientific use in 1991. They are principally the allotropes of carbon present in the form of a small cylinder (Pampaloni et al., 2018). CNTs are fabricated from graphene sheets and can be categorized as single-walled CNTs (SWCNTs) and multiwalled CNTs (MWCNTs). Double-walled CNTs are intermedial form between SWCNTs and MWCNTs made up of two coaxial graphene cylinders (Malarkey and Parpura, 2010). The size of CNTs ranges from 0.4 to 2 nm for SWCNTs; for MWCNTs, the outer diameter is 2–100 nm and the inner diameter is 1–3 nm and their length varies from 1 to many micrometers. The various methods of CNTs synthesis are electric arc, laser ablation, and chemical vapor deposition utilizing diverse metal catalysts such as Fe, Ni, and Co (Gottipati et al., 2014).

CNTs are acceptable to use for treatment and detection purposes because of their electrical and thermal conductivity, inert nature, and property to undergo chemical and functional moderation based on their use (Komane et al., 2016).

Contemporarily approaches are available for the observation of electrophysiological processes, but the major shortcoming is unwanted interference in detection. Encrustation of electrodes with MWCNTs enhances the recording of electrophysiological signals and also reduces the signal-to-noise ratio (Keefer et al., 2008). SWCNTs can be used for the live detection of glucose and lactate concentration during focal or global ischemia by developing a biosensor in which methylene blue is adsorbed into SWCNTs along with dehydrogenases (Lin et al., 2009).

In neurological disorders, remedy preference can either be neurogenesis (formation of new neurons) or healing the damaged neurons (Nunes et al., 2012). CNTs can be layered on to neural stem cells to improve neuronal injury and enhance differentiation of neuronal and nonneuronal cells (Jan and Kotov, 2007). SWCNTs, when functionalized with polyethylene glycol (PEG), can be benefited in cases of neuronal injury for tissue repair (Roman et al., 2011).

CNTs can be used as a drug carrier and transverse BBB and persuasively deliver the drug at the site of injury. Prior studies have shown that amine-functionalized CNTs can be used in middle cerebral artery occlusion stroke model to reduce the neuronal damage, and it showed enhanced motor functions in rodents (Lee et al., 2011). The use of CNT incorporated with CpG oligodeoxynucleotides showed better results in glioma treatment and also prevented tumor rechallenge (Nunes et al., 2012). According to recent reports, administration of functionalized CNTs incorporated with caspase-3 siRNA in the perilesional area reduced the ischemic damage to the motor cortex of rodents both before and after ischemia (Nair et al., 2012).

CNTs are harmonious to the nerve cell and thus are useful in neurite resurgence, in complementing the neuronal functions and in reinforcing the neuronal connections. For example, coating of MWCNTs with substrate (polyethylene-diamine) showed a large number of neurite resurgence, MWCNTs also invigorate neuronal growth and differentiation when coated with growth factors such as nerve growth factors, brain-derived nerve growth (BDNF), CNTs also affect neuronal information processing due to their electrical conductive property (Nunes et al., 2012).

Considerable toxicity coupled with CNTs is due to the potentiality of a metal catalyst (Fe, Ni), which can influence the ion levels in the neuronal cells. The functionalized CNTs can amass in the cells culminating in oxidative stress and reactive oxygen species (ROS) generation and liberation of inflammatory mediators (Nunes et al., 2012; Komane et al., 2016).

10.2.3 Quantum dots

QDs are semiconductor NP with sizes ranging from 5 to 8 nm (Pathak et al., 2006). Mostly, QD is made up of cadmium and other metalloids (such as selenium, sulfur, and tellurium) as they have very high luminescence (Kovtun et al., 2018). They are extensively used in the medical field as fluorescence probe due to their optical properties (such as wide absorption spectra and narrow emission spectra), photostability, and reduced photobleaching. Due to their optical properties, they can give multiple colors in the sample at the same time, and hence, they are superior to the traditional fluorophores (Pathak et al., 2006; Wu et al., 2016). By virtue of their selective probing ability, we can selectively tag a protein in a sample containing protein mixture (Pathak et al., 2006). Sometimes, the QD is not compatible for particular biomedical application, and hence, they need to be modified to functionalized QD (15–20 nm) by coating them with specific material (such as amphiphilic polymer and a ligand) and making them compatible with that particular application (Leary et al., 2006; Wu et al., 2016).

QD can be delivered to the brain either by a systemic route or by the intranasal route. By systemic route, they can reach their target site by their receptor–ligand interaction property, that is, receptor-mediated endocytosis by using adenosine triphosphate (ATP) as an energy source (actively) or they can get accumulate into the specific organ by their biophysical property and enhanced permeability and retention effect (passively) (Leary et al., 2006).

Silica-coated QD can easily cross the BBB and can reach the neurons. They can be delivered through the nose to the brain via the olfactory nerve pathway (Wu et al., 2016). QD can be encapsulated in PEG-PE2 (PEG–phosphatidyl ethanolamine) and can be delivered in aerosol form from nose to brain via olfactory nerve pathway (Hopkins et al., 2014).

QDs are mostly used for imaging and diagnostic purposes. In conventional methods, imaging of synapses was difficult due to their limited space, but that problem has been overcome by QD because of their extremely small size and high optical resolution (Pathak et al., 2006). Due to their photostability and biostability property, QD can give us the real-time imaging of the dynamic changes of membrane and protein and allow us for efficient tagging and long-term tracking of cells (Kosaka et al., 2010). QD is the most suitable tool for single-particle tracking because of the less photobleaching property (Kovtun et al., 2018).

QD might have a beneficial role in neuroscience, but it also has its detrimental effect, which should be considered while using it for diagnostic purposes. QD has neurotoxic, cytotoxic, immunotoxic, and hepatotoxic effects because of cadmium. QD may increase oxidative stress by increasing the level of ROS in ischemia, AD, PD, and Huntington's disease making it difficult for the neuronal cell to survive. It makes the cells more susceptible to necrosis, apoptosis, or necroptosis and leads to the neurodegeneration (Foster et al., 2006). QD may also increase the calcium level, which may lead to calcium-dependent excitotoxicity, and it may regulate the voltage-dependent sodium channel (Tang et al., 2008). QD may hamper synaptic transmission in the hippocampus area leading to impaired learning and memory (Tang et al., 2009). These toxicities mostly occur due to cadmium-containing QD; this problem can be overcome by replacing cadmium with graphene oxide QD. QD can reduce the neurotoxicity by reducing the oxidative stress through regulation of catalase and metabolic activity. It may also help in neuronal growth and regeneration (Bramini et al., 2018; Ren et al., 2018).

10.2.4 Gold nanoparticle

Gold NPs are small gold particles of diameter ranging from 1 to 100 nm. When dissolved in water, it leads to the formation of colloidal gold (Thomas et al., 2015). They possess exclusive chemical and physical characteristics because of electronic properties and large surface areas (Alaqad and Saleh, 2016). In vitro cellular uptake of AuNP takes place through clathrin-mediated endocytosis and receptor-mediated endocytosis (Papasani et al., 2012) (Fig. 10.2).

The principle is based on the application of white light, which causes oscillation of electrons resulting in polarization and formation of dipole moment, which constitute a resonance called surface plasmon resonance (SPR) (Paviolo and Stoddart, 2017). By using thiolated alkyl chain, SPR is responsible for measuring the shift in the wavelength and also for the detection of analytes used in the functionalization of surface (Odom and Nehl, 2008).

The standard methods for aqueous and organic synthesis are Turkevich and Brust–Schiffrin methods. The Turkevich method results in hydrophilic and citrate-capped Au NPs with a diameter of 15–150 nm. In contrast, the Brust–Schiffrin method results in hydrophobic and stable AuNP ranging from 1 to 5 nm (Mieszawska et al., 2013). Agglomeration of the particles while synthesis has some lacunas that can be corrected by using stabilizers (Polte et al., 2010).

The extraordinary properties of the gold aid its use in diagnostic and mitigation. For example, first, in X-rays imaging, the immense electron density and huge atomic number cause adequate adsorption of X-ray when compared to typical iodine contrast, also the prolonged circulation of AuNP facilitates imaging and specific targeting. Further, in fluorescence imaging, AuNP with aspect ratio 2 have an emission of 540 nm and AuNP with aspect ratio 5.9 leads to an emission of 750 nm. This benefit

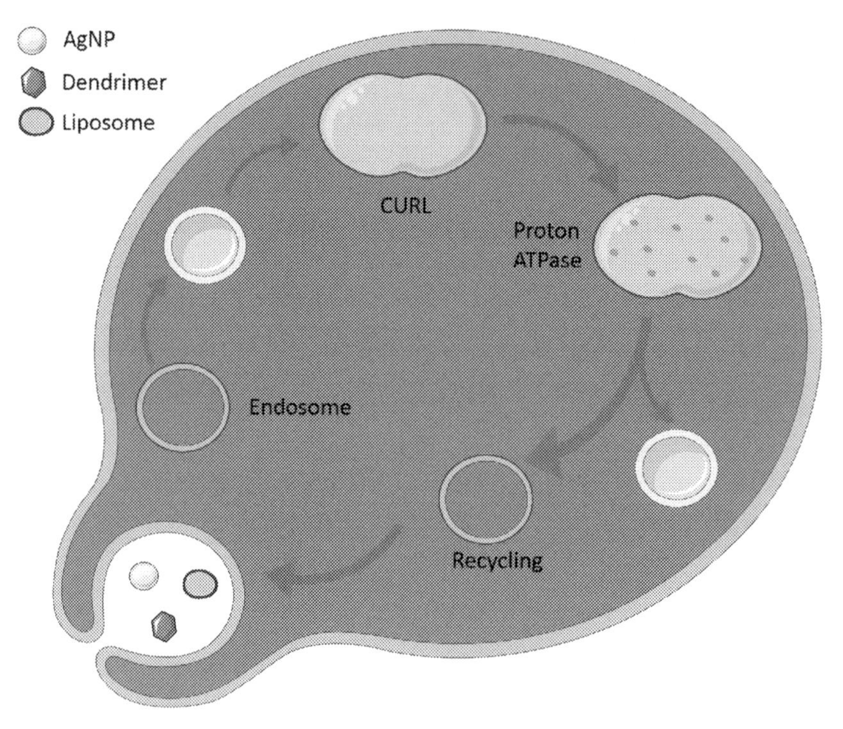

FIGURE 10.2

Entry of nanoparticles. Clathrin-mediated endocytosis leads to invagination of the membrane to form vesicles which fuse to form CURL. The surrounding H-ATPase then diffuses inside the compartment of uncoupling ligand from receptor (CURL). This leads to repulsion due to the positive charge and further leads to bursting of the endosome that results in the release of nanoparticles and the receptor will be recycled.

(Adapted from Servier Medical Art by Servier is licensed under a Creative Commons Attribution 3.0 Unported License (https://smart.servier.com/)).

of fluorescence is indicated in DNA biosensing (Mieszawska et al., 2013). In magnetic resonance imaging, AuNP is used in in vivo envision of the transplanted human neural cell using modified deoxythymidine oligonucleotide having gadolinium(III) chelate and red fluorescent CY3 moiety (Nicholls et al., 2016). AuNP by pulsing near-infrared, inflect the axonal growth in primary neuronal cells by the transmission of chitosan siRNA from NP present on the neuronal wall (Paviolo et al., 2013). Dissociation of amyloid-beta in AD by administrating intrahippocampal and intraperitoneal injection of AuNP in rat acknowledges enhancement in memory and spatial learning due to hike in the expression of BDNF and STIM (Sanati et al., 2019). Silencing of SNCA gene in PD by delivering siRNA through plasmid DNA loaded in AuNP inhibits the apoptosis of dopamine neurons and promotes the silencing of SNCA (Hu et al., 2018). In photothermal therapy the attribution of AuNP to convert absorption of a photon to heat energy is widely used in tumor eradication.

Besides the diverse attribution of AuNP, distinct pitfalls like an accumulation of 5–10 and 60 nm PEG AuNP in the liver and spleen, respectively, result in a deleterious effect on cells (Jia et al., 2017). Accumulation of AuNP leads to damage of DNA in the rat cerebral cortex (Cardoso et al., 2014). Another lacuna of AuNP is lipopolysaccharide induced hike in the expression of IL-6 and iNOS in RAW264.7 cells (Jia et al., 2017).

10.2.5 Magnetic nanoparticles

Magnetic NPs have fascinated scientists since the last few decades for being propitious on neurological pathologies. Initially, it was used for separation catalysts, wastewater treatment (Koehler et al., 2009), nuclear waste, etc. (Lu et al., 2007). Nowadays, researchers are anticipating it as being preeminent in dealing with various neurological disorders.

These are particles of size ranging between 1 and 100 nm (Arruebo et al., 2007) composed of various metals such as iron, ferrites, and plastic magnets (Zaidi et al., 2004), enclosed in a polymer having superparamagnetic property (Laurent et al., 2011) on applying external magnetic field having less coercivity. These are coated with polymers for better stability and targeted delivery.

It has been extensively used in the treatment of cancer by locally targeting cancer cells with superparamagnetic iron oxide NPs, which upon application of external magnetic field causes magnetic hyperthermia destroying tumors efficiently (Shevtsov et al., 2018).

The BBB restricts the entry of various molecules to the brain, causing failure to treat multiple pathologies. Magnetic NPs have found to reach the hippocampal area for the delivery of a drug (Thomsen et al., 2015) by crossing BBB in AD. It has been known that iron is accumulated in amyloid plaques and hence magnetic NPs having antibodies attached to it and can be used as an early diagnostic method to detect ferritin (protein enclosing iron) levels (Fernández et al., 2018). This can be a diagnostic target for AD. Magnetic NPs have also been found to show a reduction in the accumulation of Aβ, hyperphosphorylation of tau, deleterious effect of memory (Amin et al., 2017).

Ferrite magnetic NPs loaded with α-synuclein RNAi plasmid are used to inhibit the expression of α-synuclein (Niu et al., 2017) ameliorate PD. Kaushik et al. (2018) reported that cerium oxide magnetic NPs are found to provide neuroprotection and reduce oxidative stress and Lewy body degradation. Overall, magnetic NPs can be used as an early diagnostic method for motor neuron diseases such as amyotrophic lateral sclerosis (Ambesh and Angeli, 2015).

10.2.6 Dendrimers

Dendrimers are in the blossoming phase of drug delivery in micro and nanosystems for local or systemic brain administration (Yu et al., 2018). Dendrimers are three-dimensional molecules that contain structural symmetry (Xu et al., 2013).

They have continuously branched molecules that contain a central unit called core and branching points. In dendrimers, branching points are essential for functioning and deciding branching generations. The more the number of branching points, the more is the generation number (Xu et al., 2013; Yu et al., 2018). Dendrimers synthesized are classified as polyamidoamine (PAMAM) dendrimers, polylysine dendrimers, carbosilane dendrimers, phosphorus-containing dendrimers, etc. (Florendo et al., 2018). Some researchers classify dendrimers as polycationic and polyionic dendrimers, but polyanionic dendrimers are preferred due to its less toxicity (Xu et al., 2013). PAMAM class of dendrimers is popular and most widely used due to its reproducibility, safety, biocompatibility, stability, small size, and precision (Florendo et al., 2018). They contain tertiary amine branches and alkyldiamine core and are polycationic. Dendrimer entry inside the cells like neurons and astrocytes is said to take place via receptor-mediated endocytosis and macropinocytosis (Kesharwani et al., 2014).

The main advantage of dendrimers is the drug-loading ability within the cavities of dendrimers, which acts as the main site by the encapsulation process. They have wide applications in neurodegenerative disorders such as cerebral palsy, AD, PD, prions disease, and also in CNS imaging and diagnosis. Cationic phosphorous–containing dendrimers were found to interact with the aggregation of plaques and tangles. It has been reported that sialic acid–conjugated dendrimers are able to inhibit the hyperphosphorylation of tau tangles at a micromolar concentration, which is lower than soluble sialic acid (Xu et al., 2013). PPI and G5 PAMAM dendrimers show antiprion activity in neuroblastoma ScN2 cells (Cordes et al., 2007). It was recently revealed that conjugation of CY5-labeled free activable cell-penetrating peptides to PAMAM dendrimers is able to differentiate the tumor and adjacent tissues and hence increased tumor resects in a mouse xenograft model (Nguyen et al., 2010). Researchers suggested that the intravenous route of administration effectively penetrates CNS with wide biodistribution for extended therapy (Zhang et al., 2017).

The toxicity of dendrimers markedly depends on factors such as a number of generations, core, and surface properties (Duncan and Izzo, 2005). Amino-terminated dendrimers were found to be toxic due to shielding of internal cationic charge by surface modification (Xu et al., 2013). To overcome the toxicity of dendrimers, increase in generation and conjugation with biocompatible groups like PEG is done (Xu et al., 2013).

10.2.7 Liposomes

Liposomes are small synthetic spherical vesicles, having a particle size less than 200 nm, made up of uni- or multilamellar phospholipid bilayer of natural origin like phosphatidylcholine, which surrounds internal aqueous core (Torchilin, 2005). Liposomes have distinctive characteristics such as biocompatibility, biodegradability, low toxicity, site-specific delivery, nonimmunogenicity, and ability to deliver both hydrophilic and lipophilic drug molecules. Due to these characteristics, they have procured substantial attention as carriers of diagnostic as well as therapeutic compounds. Besides these, liposomes also have shown to possess disadvantages such as neurotoxicity, physicochemical instability, rapid clearance, difficulty in sterilization (Teleanu et al., 2019). The coating of polymers like PEG, polyvinylpyrrolidone, and polyacrylamide within the phospholipid bilayer of traditional liposomes significantly extends the half-life of liposomal content by protecting it from gastrointestinal contents. In addition, the coupling of targeting elements such as peptides or monoclonal antibodies on the liposomal surface has increased the accumulation of liposomal content in the brain (Montesinos, 2017). Some proposed mechanisms through which liposomes can interact with the cells include adsorption of liposomes on to the cell membrane, engulfment, and internalization of liposome, also called endocytosis, followed by fusion of lipid bilayers of liposomes with the lipoidal cell membrane and intermixing of lipids resulting in delivery of the liposomal content into the cytoplasm (Çağdaş et al., 2014).

Liposomes have wide applications in neurodegenerative disorders, for example, PD, AD, epilepsy, and stroke. AD is one of the most common neurodegenerative diseases. For symptomatic relief of AD, there are four FDA-approved drugs: donepezil, galantamine, memantine, and rivastigmine (Tan et al., 2014). When actively targeted PEGylated liposomal formulation of these drugs was administered by the intranasal route, they exhibited safety, nontoxicity, higher plasma, and brain concentration as compared to the free drug (Al Asmari et al., 2016; Yang et al., 2013).

In PD, when levodopa is delivered alone, it is converted to dopamine by peripheral dopamine decarboxylase enzyme resulting in side effects such as dyskinesia and nausea (Nagatsu and Sawada, 2009). When the encapsulated levodopa in PEGylated and chlorotoxin-functionalized liposomes was given by intraperitoneal injection, it has been shown that dopamine distribution in the substantia nigra pars compacta is significantly increased and also reduced behavioral side effects (Xiang et al., 2012). In epilepsy the liposomal encapsulation of the nimodipine, curcumin, and gossypin, which are neuroprotective agents and inhibitors of permeability glycoprotein, significantly delayed the onset and decreased the time span of epileptic seizures as compared to the free drug (Cavalcanti et al., 2015; Agarwal et al., 2013; Dheeraj et al., 2016). In ischemic stroke, there is a blockage in the blood vessel, which supplies blood to the brain by a blood clot (Iadecola and Anrather, 2011). The only FDA-approved drug for ischemic stroke is tPA (tissue plasminogen activator), which causes hemorrhage in high doses. When the actin-targeted liposomal encapsulated form of tPA was given intravenously by the internal carotid artery, there was a reduction in hemorrhage caused by tPA (Koudelka et al., 2016).

10.3 Conclusions

Polymeric nanomaterials are in the developmental phase for diagnosis, mitigation, and treatment of neuropathologies. In this chapter, we have discussed the role of nanotools in neural regeneration, neuroprotection, and targeted delivery of drugs. Altogether, these applications lay down an essential foundation for future studies in neuroscience.

References

Aderibigbe, B.A., Naki, T., 2019. Chitosan-Based Nanocarriers for Nose to Brain Delivery. Applied Sciences 9, 2219.

Agarwal, N.B., Jain, S., Nagpal, D., Agarwal, N.K., Mediratta, P.K., Sharma, K.K., 2013. Liposomal formulation of curcumin attenuates seizures in different experimental models of epilepsy in mice. Fundam. Clin. Pharmacol. 27, 169–172.

Al Asmari, A.K., Ullah, Z., Tariq, M., Fatani, A., 2016. Preparation, characterization, and in vivo evaluation of intranasally administered liposomal formulation of donepezil. Drug Des. Dev. Ther. 10, 205.

Alaqad, K., Saleh, T.A., 2016. Gold and silver nanoparticles: synthesis methods, characterization routes and applications towards drugs. J. Environ. Anal. Toxicol. 6, 525–2161.

Ambesh, P., Angeli, D.G., 2015. Nanotechnology in neurology: genesis, current status, and future prospects. Ann. Indian Acad. Neurol. 18, 382.

Amin, F.U., Hoshiar, A.K., Do, T.D., Noh, Y., Shah, S.A., Khan, M.S., et al., 2017. Osmotin-loaded magnetic nanoparticles with electromagnetic guidance for the treatment of Alzheimer's disease. Nanoscale 9, 10619–10632.

Arruebo, M., Fernández-Pacheco, R., Ibarra, M.R., Santamaría, J., 2007. Magnetic nanoparticles for drug delivery. Nano Today 2, 22–32.

Arvanitis, C.D., Ferraro, G.B., Jain, R.K., 2019. The blood–brain barrier and blood–tumour barrier in brain tumours and metastases. Nat. Rev. Cancer 1–16.

Arvanitis, C.D., Ferraro, G.B., Jain, R.K., 2020. The blood-brain barrier and blood-tumour barrier in brain tumours and metastases. Nat Rev Cancer 1474-1768, 20 (1), 26–41. Available from: https://doi.org/10.1038/s41568-019-0205-x.31601988.

Bramini, M., Alberini, G., Colombo, E., Chiacchiaretta, M., DiFrancesco, M.L., Maya-Vetencourt, J.F., et al., 2018. Interfacing graphene-based materials with neural cells. Front. Syst. Neurosci. 12, 12.

Bruch, G.E., Fernandes, L.F, Bassi, B.L.T., Alves, M.T.R., Pereira, I.O., Frézard, F., et al., 2019. Liposomes for drug delivery in stroke. Brain Res Bull 1873-2747, 152, 246–256. Available from: https://doi.org/10.1016/j.brainresbull.2019.07.015. 31323280.

Çağdaş, M., Sezer, A.D., Bucak, S., 2014. Liposomes as potential drug carrier systems for drug delivery. Application of Nanotechnology in Drug Delivery. IntechOpen.

Cardoso, E., Rezin, G.T., Zanoni, E.T., de Souza Notoya, F., Leffa, D.D., Damiani, A.P., et al., 2014. Acute and chronic administration of gold nanoparticles cause DNA damage in the cerebral cortex of adult rats. Mutat. Res./Fundam. Mol. Mech. Mutagen. 766, 25–30.

Cavalcanti, I.M.F., Satyal, P., Santos-Magalhães, N.S., Rolim, H.M.L., Freitas, R.M., 2015. Acute toxicity and anticonvulsant activity of liposomes containing nimodipine on pilocarpine-induced seizures in mice. Neurosci. Lett. 585, 38–42.

Coates, A., Abraham, S., Kaye, S.B., Sowerbutts, T., Frewin, C., Fox, R., et al., 1983. On the receiving end—patient perception of the side-effects of cancer chemotherapy. Eur. J. Cancer Clin. Oncol. 19, 203–208.

Colson, P., Henrist, C., Cloots, R., 2013. Nanosphere lithography: a powerful method for the controlled manufacturing of nanomaterials. J. Nanomater. 2013, 21.

Cordes, H., Boas, U., Olsen, P., Heegaard, P.M., 2007. Guanidino-and urea-modified dendrimers as potent solubilizers of misfolded prion protein aggregates under non-cytotoxic conditions. dependence on dendrimer generation and surface charge. Biomacromolecules 8, 3578–3583.

Dheeraj, N., Nidhi, A., Deepshikha, K., 2016. Evaluation of liposomal gossypin in animal models of epilepsy. Int. J. Pharm. Pharm. Sci. 8.

Duncan, R., Izzo, L., 2005. Dendrimer biocompatibility and toxicity. Adv. Drug Delivery Rev. 57, 2215–2237.

Fernández, T., Martínez-Serrano, A., Cussó, L., Desco, M., Ramos-Gómez, M., 2018. Functionalization and characterization of magnetic nanoparticles for the detection of ferritin accumulation in Alzheimer's disease. ACS Chem. Neurosci. 9, 912–924.

Florendo, M., Figacz, A., Srinageshwar, B., Sharma, A., Swanson, D., Dunbar, G., et al., 2018. Use of polyamidoamine dendrimers in brain diseases. Molecules 23, 2238.

Foster, K.A., Galeffi, F., Gerich, F.J., Turner, D.A., Müller, M., 2006. Optical and pharmacological tools to investigate the role of mitochondria during oxidative stress and neurodegeneration. Prog. Neurobiol. 79, 136–171.

Gilmore, J.L., Yi, X., Quan, L., Kabanov, A.V., 2008. Novel nanomaterials for clinical neuroscience. J. NeuroImmune Pharmacol. 3, 83–94.

Gottipati, M.K., Verkhratsky, A., Parpura, V., 2014. Probing astroglia with carbon nanotubes: modulation of form and function. Philos. Trans. R. Soc. B Biol. Sci. 369, 20130598.

Gunay, M.S., Ozer, A.Y., Erdogan, S., Baysal, I., Gulhan, Z., Guilloteau, D., et al., 2017. Development of nanosized, pramipexole-encapsulated liposomes and niosomes for the treatment of Parkinson's disease. J. Nanosci. Nanotechnol. 17, 5155–5167.

Hopkins, L.E., Patchin, E.S., Chiu, P.-L., Brandenberger, C., Smiley-Jewell, S., Pinkerton, K.E., 2014. Nose-to-brain transport of aerosolised quantum dots following acute exposure. Nanotoxicology 8, 885–893.

Hu, K., Chen, X., Chen, W., Zhang, L., Li, J., Ye, J., et al., 2018. Neuroprotective effect of gold nanoparticles composites in Parkinson's disease model. Nanomed. Nanotechnol. Biol. Med. 14, 1123–1136.

Iadecola, C., Anrather, J., 2011. Stroke research at a crossroad: asking the brain for directions. Nat. Neurosci. 14, 1363.

Jan, E., Kotov, N.A., 2007. Successful differentiation of mouse neural stem cells on layer-by-layer assembled single-walled carbon nanotube composite. Nano Lett. 7, 1123–1128.

Jia, Y.P., Ma, B.Y., Wei, X.-W., Qian, Z.Y., 2017. The in vitro and in vivo toxicity of gold nanoparticles. Chin. Chem. Lett. 28, 691–702.

John, A.A, Subramanian, A.P., Vellayappan, M.V., Balaji, A., Mohandas, H., Jaganathan, S.K., 2015. Carbon nanotubes and graphene as emerging candidates in neuroregeneration and neurodrug delivery. Int J Nanomedicine 1178-2013, 10, 4267–4277. Available from: https://doi.org/10.2147/IJN.S83777. 26170663.

Karatas, H., Aktas, Y., Gursoy-Ozdemir, Y., Bodur, E., Yemisci, M., Caban, S., et al., 2009. A nanomedicine transports a peptide caspase-3 inhibitor across the blood-brain barrier and provides neuroprotection. J Neurosci 1529-2401, 29 (44), 13761–13769. Available from: https://doi.org/10.1523/JNEUROSCI.4246-09.2009. 19889988.

Kaushik, A.C., Bharadwaj, S., Kumar, S., Wei, D.-Q., 2018. Nano-particle mediated inhibition of Parkinson's disease using computational biology approach. Sci. Rep. 8, 9169.

Keefer, E.W., Botterman, B.R., Romero, M.I., Rossi, A.F., Gross, G.W., 2008. Carbon nanotube coating improves neuronal recordings. Nat. Nanotechnol. 3, 434.

Kesharwani, P., Jain, K., Jain, N.K., 2014. Dendrimer as nanocarrier for drug delivery. Prog. Polym. Sci. 39, 268–307.

Koehler, F.M., Rossier, M., Waelle, M., Athanassiou, E.K., Limbach, L.K., Grass, R.N., et al., 2009. Magnetic EDTA: coupling heavy metal chelators to metal nanomagnets for rapid removal of cadmium, lead and copper from contaminated water. Chem. Commun. 4862–4864.

Komane, P.P., Choonara, Y.E., du Toit, L.C., Kumar, P., Kondiah, P.P., Modi, G., et al., 2016. Diagnosis and treatment of neurological and ischemic disorders employing carbon nanotube technology. J. Nanomater. 2016, 34.

Kosaka, N., McCann, T.E., Mitsunaga, M., Choyke, P.L., Kobayashi, H., 2010. Real-time optical imaging using quantum dot and related nanocrystals. Nanomedicine 5, 765–776.

Koudelka, S., Mikulik, R., Mašek, J., Raška, M., Knotigová, P.T., Miller, A.D., et al., 2016. Liposomal nanocarriers for plasminogen activators. J. Controlled Release 227, 45–57.

Kovtun, O., Tomlinson, I.D., Bailey, D.M., Thal, L.B., Ross, E.J., Harris, L., et al., 2018. Single quantum dot tracking illuminates neuroscience at the nanoscale. Chem. Phys. Lett. 706, 741–752.

Laurent, S., Dutz, S., Häfeli, U.O., Mahmoudi, M., 2011. Magnetic fluid hyperthermia: focus on superparamagnetic iron oxide nanoparticles. Adv. Colloid Interface Sci. 166, 8–23.

Leary, S.P., Liu, C.Y., Apuzzo, M.L., 2006. Toward the emergence of nanoneurosurgery: Part II—Nanomedicine: diagnostics and imaging at the nanoscale level. Neurosurgery 58, 805–823.

Lee, H.J., Park, J., Yoon, O.J., Kim, H.W., Kim, D.H., Lee, W.B., et al., 2011. Amine-modified single-walled carbon nanotubes protect neurons from injury in a rat stroke model. Nat. Nanotechnol. 6, 121.

Li, C., Mezzenga, R., 2013. The interplay between carbon nanomaterials and amyloid fibrils in bio-nanotechnology. Nanoscale 5, 6207–6218.

Lin, Y., Zhu, N., Yu, P., Su, L., Mao, L., 2009. Physiologically relevant online electrochemical method for continuous and simultaneous monitoring of striatum glucose and lactate following global cerebral ischemia/reperfusion. Anal. Chem. 81, 2067–2074.

Lu, A.H., Salabas, E.L., Schüth, F., 2007. Magnetic nanoparticles: synthesis, protection, functionalization, and application. Angew. Chem. Int. Ed. 46, 1222–1244.

Malarkey, E.B., Parpura, V., 2010. Carbon nanotubes in neuroscience. Acta Neurochir. Suppl. 106, 337–341.

Mieszawska, A.J., Mulder, W.J., Fayad, Z.A., Cormode, D.P., 2013. Multifunctional gold nanoparticles for diagnosis and therapy of disease. Mol. Pharmaceutics 10, 831–847.

Montesinos, R.N., 2017. Liposomal drug delivery to the central nervous system. Liposomes. IntechOpen.

Nagatsu, T., Sawada, M., 2009. L-Dopa therapy for Parkinson's disease: past, present, and future. Parkinsonism Relat. Disord. 15, S3–S8.

Nair, S., Dileep, A., Rajanikant, G., 2012. Nanotechnology based diagnostic and therapeutic strategies for neuroscience with special emphasis on ischemic stroke. Curr. Med. Chem. 19, 744–756.

Nguyen, Q.T., Olson, E.S., Aguilera, T.A., Jiang, T., Scadeng, M., Ellies, L.G., et al., 2010. Surgery with molecular fluorescence imaging using activatable cell-penetrating peptides decreases residual cancer and improves survival. Proc. Natl. Acad. Sci. U.S.A. 107, 4317–4322.

Nicholls, F.J., Rotz, M.W., Ghuman, H., MacRenaris, K.W., Meade, T.J., Modo, M., 2016. DNA–gadolinium–gold nanoparticles for in vivo T1 MR imaging of transplanted human neural stem cells. Biomaterials 77, 291–306.

Niu, S., Zhang, L.K., Zhang, L., Zhuang, S., Zhan, X., Chen, W.Y., et al., 2017. Inhibition by multifunctional magnetic nanoparticles loaded with alpha-synuclein RNAi plasmid in a Parkinson's disease model. Theranostics 7, 344.

Nunes, A., Al-Jamal, K., Nakajima, T., Hariz, M., Kostarelos, K., 2012. Application of carbon nanotubes in neurology: clinical perspectives and toxicological risks. Arch. Toxicol. 86, 1009–1020.

Odom, T.W., Nehl, C.L., 2008. How gold nanoparticles have stayed in the light: the 3M's principle. ACS Nano 2, 612–616.

Pampaloni, N.P., Giugliano, M., Scaini, D., Ballerini, L., Rauti, R., 2018. Advances in nano neuroscience: from nanomaterials to nanotools. Front. Neurosci. 12.

Papasani, M.R., Wang, G., Hill, R.A., 2012. Gold nanoparticles: the importance of physiological principles to devise strategies for targeted drug delivery. Nanomed. Nanotechnol. Biol. Med. 8, 804–814.

Patel, D.A., Henry, J.E., Good, T.A., 2007. Attenuation of beta-amyloid-induced toxicity by sialic-acid-conjugated dendrimers: role of sialic acid attachment. Brain Res 0006-8993, 1161, 95–105. Available from: https://doi.org/10.1016/j.brainres.2007.05.055. 17604005.

Pathak, S., Cao, E., Davidson, M.C., Jin, S., Silva, G.A., 2006. Quantum dot applications to neuroscience: new tools for probing neurons and glia. J. Neurosci. 26, 1893–1895.

Paviolo, C., Haycock, J.W., Yong, J., Yu, A., Stoddart, P.R., McArthur, S.L., 2013. Laser exposure of gold nanorods can increase neuronal cell outgrowth. Biotechnol. Bioeng. 110, 2277–2291.

Paviolo, C., Stoddart, P., 2017. Gold nanoparticles for modulating neuronal behavior. Nanomaterials 7, 92.

Polte, J., Ahner, T.T., Delissen, F., Sokolov, S., Emmerling, F., Thünemann, A.F., et al., 2010. Mechanism of gold nanoparticle formation in the classical citrate synthesis method derived from coupled in situ XANES and SAXS evaluation. J. Am. Chem. Soc. 132, 1296–1301.

Ren, C., Hu, X., Zhou, Q., 2018. Graphene oxide quantum dots reduce oxidative stress and inhibit neurotoxicity in vitro and in vivo through catalase-like activity and metabolic regulation. Adv. Sci. 5, 1700595.

Roman, J.A., Niedzielko, T.L., Haddon, R.C., Parpura, V., Floyd, C.L., 2011. Single-walled carbon nanotubes chemically functionalized with polyethylene glycol promote tissue repair in a rat model of spinal cord injury. J. Neurotrauma 28, 2349–2362.

Ross, C., Taylor, M., Fullwood, N., Allsop, D., 2018. Liposome delivery systems for the treatment of Alzheimer's disease. Int J Nanomedicine 1178-2013, 13, 8507–8522. Available from: https://doi.org/10.2147/IJN.S183117. 30587974.

Saeedi, M., Eslamifar, M., Khezri, K., Dizaj, S.M., 2019. Applications of nanotechnology in drug delivery to the central nervous system. Biomed Pharmacother 1950-6007, 111, 666−675. Available from: https://doi.org/10.1016/j.biopha.2018.12.133. 30611991.

Sanati, M., Khodagholi, F., Aminyavari, S., Ghasemi, F., Gholami, M., Kebriaeezadeh, A., et al., 2019. Impact of gold nanoparticles on amyloid β-induced Alzheimer's disease in a rat animal model: involvement of STIM proteins. ACS Chem. Neurosci. 10.

Shah, S., 2016. The nanomaterial toolkit for neuroengineering. Nano Convergence 3, 25.

Shevtsov, M., Nikolaev, B., Marchenko, Y., Yakovleva, L., Skvortsov, N., Mazur, A., et al., 2018. Targeting experimental orthotopic glioblastoma with chitosan-based superparamagnetic iron oxide nanoparticles (CS-DX-SPIONs). Int. J. Nanomed. 13, 1471.

Singh, A., Garg, G., Sharma, P., 2010. Nanospheres: a novel approach for targeted drug delivery system. Int. J. Pharm. Sci. Rev. Res. 5, 84−88.

Soni, S., Ruhela, R.K., Medhi, B., 2016. Nanomedicine in central nervous system (CNS) disorders: a present and future prospective. Adv. Pharm. Bull. 6, 319.

Tan, C.-C., Yu, J.T., Wang, H.F., Tan, M.S., Meng, X.F., Wang, C., et al., 2014. Efficacy and safety of donepezil, galantamine, rivastigmine, and memantine for the treatment of Alzheimer's disease: a systematic review and meta-analysis. J. Alzheimers Dis. 41, 615−631.

Tang, M., Wang, M., Xing, T., Zeng, J., Wang, H., Ruan, D.-Y., 2008. Mechanisms of unmodified CdSe quantum dot-induced elevation of cytoplasmic calcium levels in primary cultures of rat hippocampal neurons. Biomaterials 29, 4383−4391.

Tang, M., Li, Z., Chen, L., Xing, T., Hu, Y., Yang, B., et al., 2009. The effect of quantum dots on synaptic transmission and plasticity in the hippocampal dentate gyrus area of anesthetized rats. Biomaterials 30, 4948−4955.

Teleanu, D.M., Chircov, C., Grumezescu, A.M., Teleanu, R.I., 2019. Neuronanomedicine: an up-to-date overview. Pharmaceutics 11, 101.

Thomas, S., Grohens, Y., Ninan, N., 2015. Nanotechnology Applications for Tissue Engineering. William Andrew.

Thomsen, L.B., Thomsen, M.S., Moos, T., 2015. Targeted drug delivery to the brain using magnetic nanoparticles. Ther. Delivery 6, 1145−1155.

Torchilin, V.P., 2005. Recent advances with liposomes as pharmaceutical carriers. Nat. Rev. Drug Discovery 4, 145.

Wu, T., Zhang, T., Chen, Y., Tang, M., 2016. Research advances on potential neurotoxicity of quantum dots. J. Appl. Toxicol. 36, 345−351.

Xiang, Y., Wu, Q., Liang, L., Wang, X., Wang, J., Zhang, X., et al., 2012. Chlorotoxin-modified stealth liposomes encapsulating levodopa for the targeting delivery against the Parkinson's disease in the MPTP-induced mice model. J. Drug Target. 20, 67−75.

Xu, L., Zhang, H., Wu, Y., 2013. Dendrimer advances for the central nervous system delivery of therapeutics. ACS Chem. Neurosci. 5, 2−13.

Yang, Z.-Z., Zhang, Y.Q., Wang, Z.-Z., Wu, K., Lou, J.-N., Qi, X.-R., 2013. Enhanced brain distribution and pharmacodynamics of rivastigmine by liposomes following intranasal administration. Int. J. Pharm. 452, 344−354.

Yu, M., Huang, Z., Liu, Z., Chen, J., Liu, Y., Tang, L., et al., 2018. Annealed gold nanoshells with highly-dense hotspots for large-area efficient Raman scattering substrates. Sens. Actuators B Chem. 262, 845−851.

Zaidi, N.A., Giblin, S., Terry, I., Monkman, A., 2004. Room temperature magnetic order in an organic magnet derived from polyaniline. Polymer 45, 5683−5689.

Zhang, F., Magruder, J.T., Lin, Y.A., Crawford, T.C., Grimm, J.C., Sciortino, C.M., et al., 2017. Generation-6 hydroxyl PAMAM dendrimers improve CNS penetration from intravenous administration in a large animal brain injury model. J. Controlled Release 249, 173–182.

Zhao, D., Alizadeh, D., Zhang, L., Liu, W., Farrukh, O., Manuel, E., et al., 2011. Carbon nanotubes enhance CpG uptake and potentiate antiglioma immunity. Clin Cancer Res 1078-0432, 17 (4), 771–782. Available from: https://doi.org/10.1158/1078-0432.CCR-10-2444. 21088258.

CHAPTER

Polymeric nanomaterials for ocular drug delivery

11

Siddarth Raghuvanshi[1], Bridget La Prairie[1,2], Sridaran Rajagopal[1,2,3] and Vikramaditya G. Yadav[1,2]

[1]*Department of Chemical and Biological Engineering, The University of British Columbia, Vancouver, BC, Canada*

[2]*School of Biomedical Engineering, The University of British Columbia, Vancouver, BC, Canada*

[3]*Department of Mechanical Engineering, The University of British Columbia, Vancouver, BC, Canada*

11.1 Introduction

Sight is incredibly important to our quality of life, and as with all organs, the eyes can often develop complications that impact their functions. Due to the importance of sight, a loss of vision is strongly correlated with a decrease in the quality of life as well as increases in diseases such as depression (DiNuzzo et al., 2001; Horowitz, 2003; Horowitz et al., 2005). Ocular impairments are more common in older populations (Alghamdi et al., 2016). In combination with the aging population of most of the first world, this will lead to ocular diseases rising in number in the coming years with the rate of ocular impairment increasing with an estimate of 36 million in 2017 and 115 million in 2050 (Bourne et al., 2017). While there have been significant improvements made in the field of ocular surgery, the eye remains to be relatively impermeable to drug delivery. While physical methods of delivery such as intravitreal injections (an injection into the vitreous humor near the back of the retina) can be used in some cases, they have poor rates of patient compliance. Topical deliveries, mainly eye drops, are commonly used but are inefficient since over 95% of the formulated drug is lost as drops leak out of the eye. The common approach of oral/systemic methods of entry also cannot overcome these barriers for a sufficient bioavailability in the eye without causing toxicity.

The issue with current ocular drug delivery can be traced to the unique anatomy of the eye. This anatomy presents both static (layers of cornea, sclera, and blood–aqueous and blood–retinal barriers) and dynamic (tear dilution and blood flow) barriers. These two barriers can be ascribed to three major hurdles based on anatomical position: the protective features, anterior segment, and the posterior segment. Each of these hurdles has specific barriers that hinder current attempts

Advances in Polymeric Nanomaterials for Biomedical Applications. DOI: https://doi.org/10.1016/B978-0-12-814657-6.00012-4

to deliver drugs to the eye. In this chapter, we will highlight these three anatomical hurdles and address specific issues with current methods of treatments. We will then introduce various nanopolymer case studies that demonstrate how to circumvent the hurdles. Lastly, we will discuss potential avenues to apply nanopolymers toward ocular drug delivery in the future.

11.2 Anatomical hurdles for drug delivery

The unique anatomy of the eye evolved in the way it did to keep out microbial infections (Sack et al., 2001). These defenses range from outer defenses such as the lid, lashes, and the tear layer to inner defenses that include tightly bound epithelial cells (Fig. 11.1). The eye is composed of three layers of tissue—the outer connective, the middle vascular, and the inner neural tissues (Agrahari et al., 2016). For the purpose of drug delivery, it is better to divide the eye into the anterior and posterior segments. The anterior of the eye is composed of the iris, cornea, capillary body, lens, and aqueous humor. The posterior eye is composed of the retina, vitreous humor, sclera, and choroid. In addition to these two segments, the various protective features of the eye also present a significant hurdle.

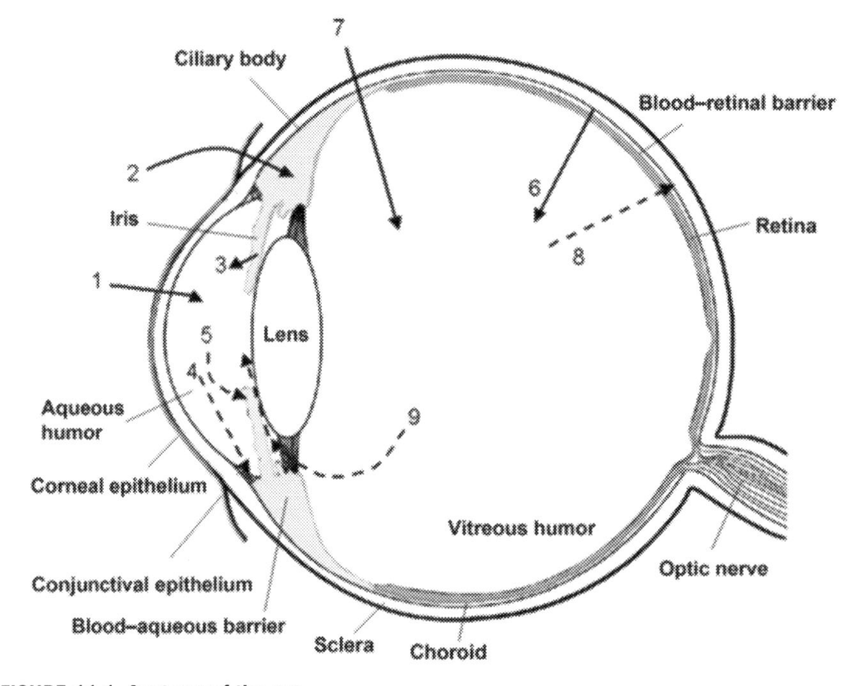

FIGURE 11.1 Anatomy of the eye.

This image labels many of the significant hurdles for the purpose of ocular drug delivery.

Through an in-depth understanding of why the anatomical structure prevents traditional treatment, we can better design nanopolymers to treat ocular diseases.

11.2.1 Protective features of the eye

Tears are one of the eye's major defenses, and the tear film is composed of three different layers: an outer lipid layer, a middle aqueous layer, and a final mucin layer. The volume and turnover rate of tears are one of the major concerns while trying to deliver drugs topically. The conjunctival cul-de-sac, the targeted area during topical delivery, can only accommodate around 7–10 μL of fluid. As typical topically administration is around 25–35 μL, a significant portion of the drop will be drained and not reach the targeted tissue. The low volume also does not allow for the development of a high initial concentration gradient, which is essential for delivery. In addition, as the liquid is removed through the nasolachrymal drainage, it also has the potential to harm the patient if the drug has secondary effects in other tissues. With more than 1000 tear proteins identified (Zhou et al., 2012) the tear's protein content is another hurdle for nanopolymer-based drug delivery. The major components are lysozyme, lactoferrin, and tear-specific lipocalin (TSL), which compose 80% of the total protein concentration. Lactoferrin composes 15%–30% of the reflex tear protein and is also present in significant quantities in saliva. This protein elicits antimicrobial activity by binding of its cationic N-terminal region to bacterial lipopolysaccharides or by chelating and clearing iron, which reduces the iron needed for by bacteria for growth. These antimicrobial properties also extend to yeast and fungi as well as some viruses such as HIV (Swart et al., 1998). Interestingly, it has been shown that certain pathogenic bacteria can use lactoferrin as a source of iron (Vogel, 2012). On the other hand, lysozyme breaks down the polysaccharide layer of bacterial cells and chitin in the fungal cell wall. In addition, lysozyme also prevents HIV transmission in tears and saliva (Lee-Huang et al., 1999). Finally, TSL elicits protective activity by binding to small hydrophobic molecules. Importantly, TSL has a lipid-binding domain that can bind/release lipids for transport into the cell through endocytosis facilitated by the lipocalin interacting membrane receptor. It presents a possible avenue for the purpose of drug delivery for lipid-based nanopolymer drug delivery systems. In addition, unlike lactoferrin and lysozyme, TSL is negatively charged. This is speculated to result in electrostatic interactions between the TSL and lactoferrin or lysozyme leading to an increase in the protective properties of tears (Gasymov et al., 1999).

11.2.2 Anterior structure of the eye

The anterior structure of the eye is composed of the cornea, conjunctiva, iris-ciliary body, the lens, and the aqueous humor. These regions are affected by diseases such as glaucoma and cataracts and are generally targeted by topical treatments, which make up 90% of ophthalmic marketed products (Bachu et al., 2018;

Dawson et al., 2011). The cornea is the initial barrier that spans the anterior structure of the eye above the aqueous humor at around 540–700 μm thick (Dawson et al., 2011). As the outermost layer of the organ, crossing this barrier is imperative for penetration into the eye. The cornea is composed of five different layers: epithelium, Bowman's membrane, stroma, Descemet's membrane, and endothelium (Eghrari et al., 2015). Within the eye the most problematic layers are the epithelium and stroma (Gaudana et al., 2010; Janagam et al., 2017; Lakhani et al., 2018). These two adjacent layers are hydrophobic and lipophobic, respectively, making penetration through both of them challenging. The corneal epithelium is composed of 4–6 layers of cells around 50 μm thick (Dawson et al., 2011). The outermost layer of the ocular system is composed of one or two layers of squamous cells. These outermost cells are a significant barrier to drug delivery because of their tight junctions (zonula occludens) in the intercellular region (Klyce and Crosson, 1985). These junctions limit paracellular transport to drugs that are quite small (<5 kDa) and lipophilic.

The stroma comprises 90% of the thickness of the cornea. This region is incredibly hydrated. This hydrophilic environment presents a significant barrier to a lipophilic drug's passage through the cornea (Gaudana et al., 2010). The stroma is however permeable by both hydrophilic and lipophilic drugs due to the large gaps in the interfibrillar space but does limit the size of the drug which is able to pass through. Current drug delivery technologies can only transport 5%–10% of their drug payloads into the aqueous humor, which illustrates how challenging it is for drugs to permeate the cornea. Most of the dosage is lost either by systemic absorption leading to negative effects or spillage leading to a waste of drug. Due to the above barriers, a drug delivery modality that is capable of penetrating the ocular tissue will have an incredible impact on drug delivery.

Aside from the corneal pathway, the conjunctival–scleral pathway is also an option in the anterior of the eye due to its larger surface area (Ghate and Edelhauser, 2006; Janagam et al., 2017). However, this larger surface also allows for a lot of tear dilution and tear turnover as mentioned earlier. Compared to the cornea, this route is significantly more accessible for larger hydrophilic drugs around the range of 20–40 kDa. In addition, this route contains more permeable tight junctions which lead to better penetration (Dawson et al., 2011) (Fig. 11.2). The conjunctiva is highly vascularized unlike the cornea and therefore a much higher rate of systemic effect for drugs targeting that area (Lakhani et al., 2018). In addition, one of the two blood–ocular barriers, the blood–aqueous barrier is present in the anterior of the eye. The blood–aqueous barrier is located in the uvea and is composed primarily of the ciliary body. In this barrier, transfer from the blood to the eye dominates over transfer from the eye to the blood (Cunha-Vaz, 1979). The majority of aqueous substances that pass this barrier end-up in the aqueous humor. The partition coefficient of drugs between the aqueous humor and the plasma is typically 0.2–0.3, and this number can be even higher for lipid-soluble molecules. The blood–aqueous barrier largely prohibits the transfer of proteins into the aqueous humor from the plasma. All of these hurdles demonstrate why most ocular

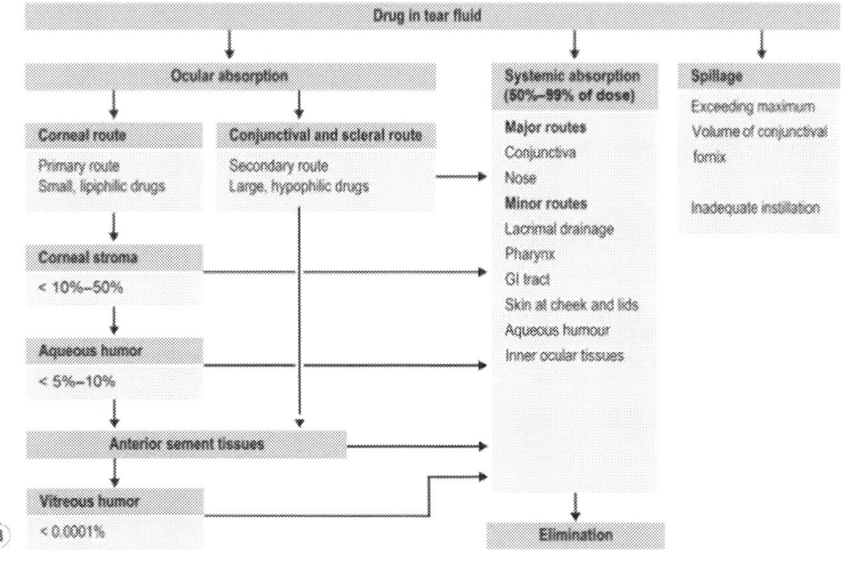

FIGURE 11.2

Distribution of eye drugs within the body and ocular tissue.

Dawson, D.G., Ubels, J.L., Edelhauser, H.F., 2011. Cornea and Sclera. In: Adler's Physiol. Eye, 11th ed., Elsevier, pp. 71–130. https://www-clinicalkey-com.ezproxy.library.ubc.ca/#!/content/book/3-s2.0-B9780323057141000042?scrollTo= %23hl0001068.

drug delivery methods for the eye are so lackluster. The anterior region of the eye is much more targetable when compared to the posterior region of the eye. For example, if the vitreous humor was targeted via topical solution, less than 0.0001% of the solution would be delivered there. Therefore drug delivery modalities including nanopolymers are so vital for the purpose of drug delivery.

11.2.3 Posterior region of the eye

The posterior region of the eye is composed of the sclera, choroid, retinal pigment epithelium, neural retina, the optic nerve, and the vitreous humor. The posterior section of the eye is more available in terms of vascular exchange. For this reason, systemic administration is more effective compared to the anterior region. However, as the eye is a much smaller organ compared to the rest of the body and the presence of the two blood–ocular barriers, systematic administration will not result in a sufficient drug concentration. The posterior region of the blood–ocular barrier contains similar tight junctions to the epithelial cells in the cornea. These cells have zonula occludens which seal in the intercellular space surrounding the endothelial cells of the blood–retinal barrier (Shakib and Cunha-Vaz, 1966). However, unlike the blood–brain barrier, very little is known about the blood–retinal barrier, and significantly more research before it can be targeted using similar approaches as the blood–brain barrier. With the combination of the barriers present in the anterior of the eye, the lack of systemic administration to the eyes, and the presence of the blood–retinal barrier, it is extremely challenging for the delivery of drugs to the posterior region of the eye. To resolve these issues, medicine requires novel methods for ocular drug delivery.

11.3 Applications of liposomes in ocular delivery

Liposomes are a powerful system for drug delivery. These bi-layered, hollow phospholipid spheres have been studied and used for over 50 years (Bangham and Horne, 1964). They are capable of encapsulating small molecules, proteins, and even DNA (Mishra et al., 2011; Patel et al., 2013; Sahoo et al., 2008). For example, the small-molecule drug Vertepofrin has been administered in a liposomal formulation via injection into the bloodstream. This liposomal formulation helps the drug to be taken in by plasma low-density lipoproteins (Allison et al., 1994). These proteins are overexpressed on cells which contribute to CNV (Schmidt-Erfurth and Hasan, 2000). Through the use of this liposomal formulation, we are able to selective target cells and spare cells to avoid off-target damage. In addition to being used as a selective delivery mechanism, liposomes are also able to permeate ocular tissues such as the corneal tissue (Schaeffer and Krohn, 1982). For the permeation of the corneal epithelium the charge and the shape of the liposome play a significant role, with positively charged unilamellar liposomes being the best at penetrating the epithelium. Liposomes also decrease the rate of clearance by the protective features of the eye, allowing the increase of drug availability (Neves et al., 2016; Yamaguchi et al., 2009). In addition to demonstrations for the anterior region of the eye, other researchers have also demonstrated the ability of liposomes to help to target the posterior region of the eye.

Viral infections in ocular tissues such as herpes simplex virus and cytomegalovirus (CMV) can lead to blindness within 4–6 months (Kestelyn and Cunningham, 2001; Shen and Tu, 2007). Ganciclovir (GCV) is a drug that has been shown to be effective at treating CMV due to its antiviral properties (Cantrill et al., 1989). However, GCV is unable to penetrate the ocular tissue and be transported to the posterior region due to its low lipophilicity, which is particularly problematic for transport through the vitreous humor. However, a liposomal formulation allows for GCV to have a concentration on the order of 2–10 times higher in the posterior region of the eye (Shen and Tu, 2007). In both of these examples, liposomes increase both corneal permeation, as well as anterior and posterior bioavailability In addition, liposomes allow the delivery of new modalities such as siRNA-based therapies (Yu-Wai-Man et al., 2016). The "second generation" of liposomes allowed for the composition, size, and charge. An important change in the second generation was the addition of poly(ethylene glycol) (PEG)

(Akbarzadeh et al., 2013; Immordino et al., 2006). These modifications need to be fine-tuned for optimal liposomal drug delivery. In addition, the presence of PEG in the liposome allows for efficient ligand attachment to the liposome. This allows for a much higher degree of specificity of the liposome as the ligand binds and delivers the liposome to a specific cell type based on surface marker (Sapra and Allen, 2003). This ligand bound liposome hold a lot of process in the current cancer trial and are a promising area to limit off-target effects by liposomes in ocular drug delivery.

11.4 Applications of nanomicelles in ocular delivery

Nanomicelles are generated by mixing an amphiphilic molecule such as a surfactant or polymer with a solvent (Chevalier and Zemb, 1990). Nanomicelles typically refer to micelles generated from amphiphilic molecule inside a polar solvent so the hydrophobic ends are bundled inside and the hydrophilic ends are placed outside of the structure (Trivedi and Kompella, 2010) (Fig. 11.3). This regular topology of nanomicelles is used for the delivery of hydrophobic drugs, whereas the reverse topology, which is generated in a nonpolar solvent, is used to transport hydrophilic drugs. While both micelles and liposome share common characteristics, polymeric micelles can be composed of a range of amphiphilic molecules as opposed liposomes, which are by definition made of phospholipids.

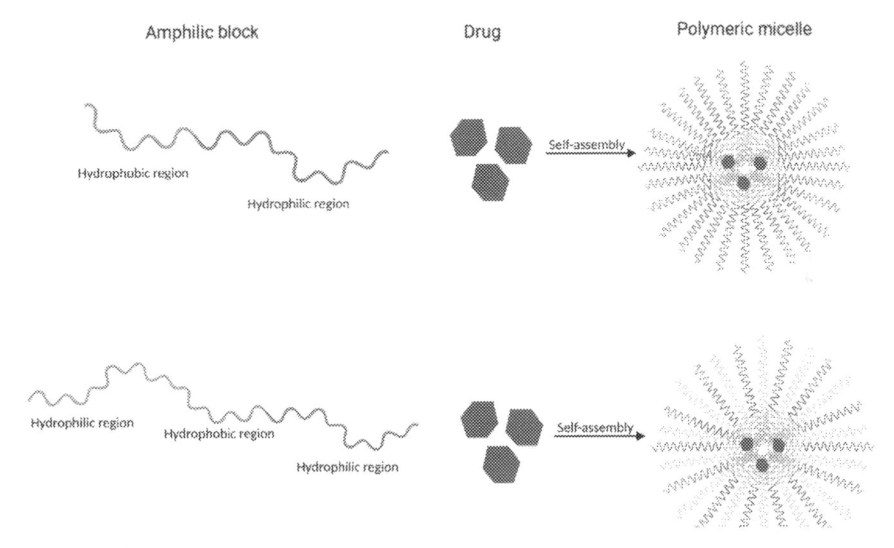

FIGURE 11.3

Use of block copolymers can modulate the physicochemical properties of the micelles, especially transport and biochemical interactions.

Studies of nanomicellar effectiveness have demonstrated an improved ability to permeate the corneal epithelium. Studies have shown over a twofold increase in bioavailability without any damage to the eye compared to an aqueous solution with identical concentration (Giammona et al., 2009; Gupta et al., 2000). These studies demonstrate that nanomicelles can effectively deliver a diverse collection of compounds through the corneal epithelium by simply modulating the copolymer. Other papers have also evaluated the toxicity of nanomicelles, as well as the effect of nanomicelles delivery on drug effect (Di Tommaso et al., 2011; Pepić et al., 2004). The current research points to nanomicelles as a drug delivery method able to better permeate the corneal epithelium in a nontoxic manner and enhance drug effects through greater bioavailability. In addition to nanomicelles permeating the corneal epithelium, they are able to penetrate and maintain their concentration in the posterior region of the eye without systemic effects. Similar to tumors, CNV cells have an increased permeability compared to normal tissues allowing for accumulation of the macromolecule (Kimura et al., 2001; Matsumura and Maeda, 1986). Researchers have used this property to deliver nanomicelles to CNV cells and avoid off-target activity (Ideta et al., 2004). In the study by Ideta et al. the free molecule was shown to have less accumulation in the targeted region 1 h after treatment. In addition, the free molecule caused a higher rate of mortality compared to nanomicelle in the mice, showing the ability of nanomicelles to limit systemic adverse effects. Interestingly, despite eliciting fewer adverse effects, the residence time of the nanomicelles in the blood was much higher—nearly 168 h—compared to the freeform of the molecules. This presents an interesting possibility for diseases where a longer delivery window with slow cell uptake is demanded. The duration of the nanomicelle can also be controlled through the modification of the polymer used to create the nanomicelle.

This is the major advantage when dealing with nanomicelles, unlike liposomes the polymer used can be modified. This changes the properties of the nanomicelle leading to a more efficient method for drug delivery. For example, chitosan, a polymer derived from chiton in shrimp shells, is a cationic polymer that was shown to increase precorneal retention due to its mucoadhesive properties (Felt et al., 1999). In addition, chitosan was also shown to be able to open the tight junctions to allow for paracellular drug penetration (Ilium, 1998). Based on these effective properties for ocular drug delivery, researchers built a chitosan-based nanomicelle. The chitosan-based nanomicelle was shown to be more effective for corneal drug delivery compared to the surfactant control (Pepić et al., 2010).

11.5 Applications of dendrimers in ocular delivery

Dendrimers are branched three-dimensional polymeric structures in which all bonds originate from a central core. These molecules grow outward with each branching unit; these branching units are bonded by attaching themselves to the previous outermost unit. While nanomicelles and liposomes are powerful drug delivery systems,

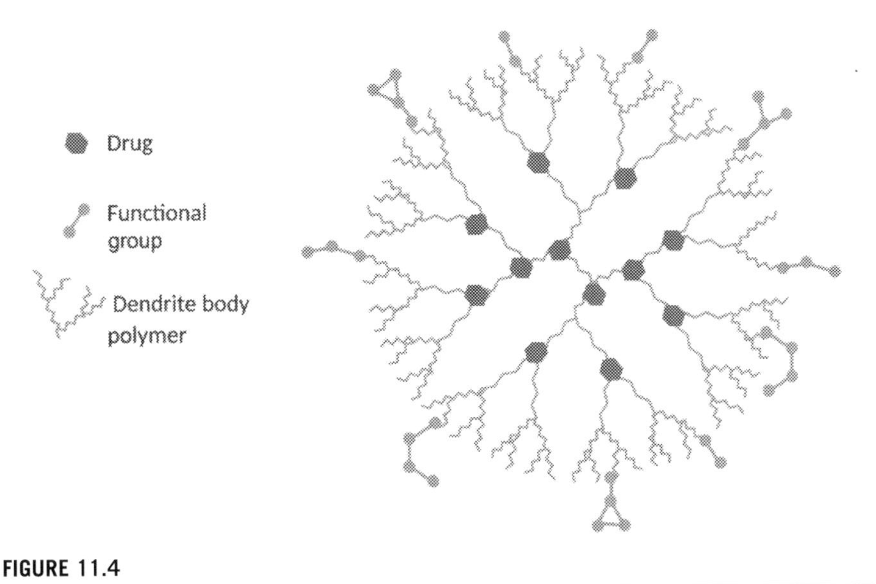

FIGURE 11.4

A schematic of dendrimer-based delivery vehicles.

their nature allows for structural changes in the presence of external stress (Svenson, 2009). However, dendrimers are significantly more uniform and controllable in manufacturing. In addition, dendrimers are able to have multiple functionalities appended to the outermost branches. Polyamidoamine (PAMAM) dendrimers are one of the most wildly used dendrimer scaffolds in biology due to their water soluble and biocompatible nature (Gillies and Fréchet, 2005) (Fig. 11.4).

Due to this, PAMAM dendrimers are commonly used in ocular drug delivery (Omerović and Vranić, 2020). In a study, researchers attempted to use PAMAM dendrimers to increase viscosity and adhesion of the solution to increase corneal residence time (Vandamme and Brobeck, 2005). The current research into dendrimers for ocular drug delivery is limited compared to other nanomaterials such as liposomes or nanoparticles. However, the potential of dendrimers due to their stable and manipulatable structure and functional groups makes them a strong candidate for ocular drug delivery.

11.6 Applications of additional nanoparticles in ocular delivery

There is a large group of nanoparticles used for drug delivery that do not fit into a group or category like those discussed earlier. Based on their assembly, nanoparticles can form nanospheres or nanocapsules (Guterres et al., 2007). In nanospheres, the drug is dispersed throughout the structure of the particles, whereas the drug is located within the cavities of nanocapsules. Similar to nanomicelles, chitosan has been used to increase the residence time of the nanoparticle on the surface of the eye. Unlike nanomicelles, chitosan nanoparticles do not require the addition of another amphiphilic molecule. Similar to chitosan nanomicelles, chitosan nanoparticles are able to enter the ocular tissues and accumulated in the cornea and conjunctiva. In vivo research in rabbits showed that chitosan nanoparticles had a low toxicity and irritation (De Campos et al., 2001; de Campos et al., 2004; Salamanca et al., 2006).

Dexamethasone, an autoinflammatory agent, has been used as a therapy for chronic posterior diseases such as uveitis (Muñoz-Fernández and Martín-Mola, 2006). As mentioned, the posterior region is capable of rapidly clearing free molecules from the vitreous humor. Dexamethasone, which has a pharmacokinetic half-life of 3 h, necessitates repeated intravitreal injections. The high concentration and frequency of dosing lead to numerous side effects such as cataracts, retinal detachment, and vitreous hemorrhage as well as poor patient compliance (Yasukawa et al., 2005). Instead, nanoparticles are able to sidestep the issue of rapid clearance showing their promise as a tool for the posterior region of the eye. Research have shown that dexamethasone-loaded nanoparticles are able to continuously release the drug at a relatively constant level for around 50 days (Zhang et al., 2009). The drug concentration was sufficient to suppress inflammation for more than a month with just a single injection. In addition, the dexamethasone stayed within the vitreous tissue and had a low systemic concentration, which significantly diminished off-target effects. Lipid nanoparticles are also being used a drug delivery method to ocular tissue. While similar in composition to liposomes, lipid nanoparticles are assembled using different methods and are solid at body temperature and do not have a lipid bilayer (Müller et al., 2002). This leads to lipid nanoparticles being easier to assemble at-scale. Moreover, lipid nanoparticles are less likely to leak their cargo (Mehnert and Mäder, 2012). There are two types of lipid nanoparticles: the first generation of solid lipid nanoparticles and the second generation of nanostructured lipid carriers (Müller et al., 2002). The second generation of particles has a higher loading capacity, lower water content, and minimize potential active compound loss. Both generations of lipid nanoparticles have been used in ocular delivery. Similar to other nanoparticles, lipid nanoparticles have been used to increase bioavailability in the posterior of the eye and permeability across the cornea (Araújo et al., 2011; Gökçe et al., 2009; Kumar and Sinha, 2016; Shen et al., 2009). Interestingly, research has also focused on improving ocular attachment of lipid nanoparticles through the use of mucoadhesive polymers such as chitosan (Liu et al., 2016).

11.7 Future outlook

Nanomicelles, liposomes, and dendrimers can successfully overcome the anatomical challenges discussed in this chapter. Nevertheless, each of these modalities faces multiple challenges such as stability and drug uptake in the posterior section of the eye. The stability and residence time of ocular carriers could be improved by increasing the viscosity of the formulation, which will directly improve the mucoadhesive nature of the treatment. Polymers such as poloxamers have thermoreversible properties and could meet this requirement. The storage moduli of poloxamers increase from less than 1000 to more than 5000 Pa as the polymer crosses the transition threshold temperature (Fakhari et al., 2017). This classifies poloxamers as smart polymeric drug carriers, as they activate under appropriate physiological conditions. The transitive property of poloxamers can also be adapted with other parameters such as pH, location of action, and presence of biological markers (Alsaggar and Liu, 2018; Lynch et al., 2020). Another area of active advancement is the use of noninvasive liposomal ocular drug carriers. Current liposomal carriers are generally administered to the patient through methods such as intravitreal injections, prolonged topical application, or systemic delivery. To this end, i-arginylglycylaspartic acid (iRGD)-modified liposomal carriers have been shown to interact with corneal epithelial cells, where after the iRGD can be cleaved by proteases. This phenomenon does not occur for conventional RGD. The cleaved iRGD then binds to neuropilin-1, which activates the endocytic transport pathway, which is a very effective method for ocular drug delivery (Huang et al., 2020).

Similar to nanomicelles and liposomal drug carriers, dendrimers have also attracted interest as noninvasive drug carriers. Similar to liposomal delivery, dendrimer complexes modified with RGD hexapeptide have proven to penetrate the anatomical barriers of the conjunctiva (Yang et al., 2019). Hyaluronic acid polymers are also being explored for ocular drug delivery. Hyaluronic acid is a natural polysaccharide abundant in extracellular matrix and has been widely used in skin care and wound healing (Wang et al., 2014) Hyaluronic acid polymers are particularly useful in ocular drug delivery because they are a component in the vitreous humor and have ligands for several receptors such as CD-44 that are found in many retinal cells (Lynch et al., 2020). Currently, the US FDA has approved several implantable ocular drug delivery devices. Ozurdex, a biodegradable polymer implant, is used to treat macular edema that causes vision loss in diabetic patients (Clemente-Tomás et al., 2017). The implant is therapeutically active for 6 months, after which it is absorbed by the patient's body. nVISTA, another device of this type, uses a silicon nanochannel membrane for prolonged drug delivery to posterior section of the eye via diffusion (Trani et al., 2019). The silicon membrane architecture provides mechanical stability to the device and provides enough resistance for sustained zero-order drug release in the vitreous humor. This particular mechanism can work without pumps, actuation, or clinician intervention and has a therapeutic active period of 2 years (Trani et al., 2019). Cyclodextrins are another potential carrier of lipophilic drugs across the corneal barrier. Cyclodextrins are cyclic oligosaccharides with α-(1,4)-linked α-D-glucopyranose units. The external surface of these molecules is hydrophilic owing to the hydroxyl group, which allows the molecule to form hydrogen bonds with the hydrated lachrymal layer of the eye. The inner cavity of cyclodextrin is hydrophobic, which allows the formation of inclusion complex with lipophilic agents either by hydrogen bonding, van der Waals forces, or charge–transfer interactions. In the aqueous solution, dynamic equilibrium is created between the free cyclodextrin and drug molecules and the complex (Bíró and Aigner, 2019). After application on the eye surface, only the free lipophilic molecule can penetrate through the cornea, the hydrophilic cyclodextrin remains and is eventually eliminated through the nasolacrimal pathway (Bíró and Aigner, 2019).

References

Agrahari, V., Mandal, A., Agrahari, V., Trinh, H.M., Joseph, M., Ray, A., et al., 2016. A comprehensive insight on ocular pharmacokinetics. Drug Delivery Transl. Res. 6 (6), 735–754. Available from: https://doi.org/10.1007/s13346-016-0339-2.

Akbarzadeh, A., Rezaei-Sadabady, R., Davaran, S., Joo, S.W., Zarghami, N., Hanifehpour, Y., et al., 2013. Liposome: classification, preparation, and applications. Nanoscale Res. Lett. 8 (1), 102. Available from: https://doi.org/10.1186/1556-276X-8-102.

Alghamdi, Y.A., Mercado, C., McClellan, A.L., et al., 2016. Epidemiology of meibomian gland dysfunction in an elderly population. Cornea 35, 731–735.

Allison, B.A., Pritchard, P.H., Levy, J.G., 1994. Evidence for low-density lipoprotein receptor-mediated uptake of benzoporphyrin derivative. Br. J. Cancer 69 (5), 833–839. Available from: https://doi.org/10.1038/bjc.1994.162.

Alsaggar, M., Liu, D., 2018. Organ-based drug delivery. J. Drug Target. 26 (5–6), 385–397.

Araújo, J., Nikolic, S., Egea, M.A., Souto, E.B., Garcia, M.L., 2011. Nanostructured lipid carriers for triamcinolone acetonide delivery to the posterior segment of the eye. Colloids Surf. B Biointerfaces 88 (1), 150–157. Available from: https://doi.org/10.1016/j.colsurfb.2011.06.025.

Bachu, R.D., Chowdhury, P., Al-Saedi, Z.H.F., Karla, P.K., Boddu, S.H.S., 2018. Ocular drug delivery barriers-role of nanocarriers in the treatment of anterior segment ocular diseases. Pharmaceutics 10 (1). Available from: https://doi.org/10.3390/pharmaceutics10010028.

Bangham, A.D., Horne, R.W., 1964. Negative staining of phospholipids and their structural modification by surface-active agents as observed in the electron microscope. J. Mol. Biol. 8 (5), 660–668. Available from: https://doi.org/10.1016/S0022-2836(64)80115-7.

Bíró, Aigner, 2019. Current approaches to use cyclodextrins and mucoadhesive polymers in ocular drug delivery—a mini-review. Sci. Pharm. 87 (3), 15.

Bourne, R.R.A., Flaxman, S.R., Braithwaite, T., Cicinelli, M.V., Das, A., Jonas, J.B., et al., 2017. Magnitude, temporal trends, and projections of the global prevalence of blindness and distance and near vision impairment: a systematic review and meta-analysis. Lancet Global Health 5 (9), e888–e897. Available from: https://doi.org/10.1016/S2214-109X(17)30293-0.

Cantrill, H.L., Henry, K., Melroe, N.H., Knobloch, W.H., Ramsay, R.C., Balfour, H.H., 1989. Treatment of cytomegalovirus retinitis with intravitreal ganciclovir: long-term results. Ophthalmology 96 (3), 367–374. Available from: https://doi.org/10.1016/S0161-6420(89)32900-9.

Chevalier, Y., Zemb, T., 1990. The structure of micelles and microemulsions. Rep. Prog. Phys. 53 (3), 279–371. Available from: https://doi.org/10.1088/0034-4885/53/3/002.

Clemente-Tomás, R., Hernández-Pérez, D., Neira-Ibáñez, P., Farías-Rozas, F., Torrecillas-Picazo, R., Osorio-Alayo, V., et al., 2017. Intracrystalline Ozurdex®: therapeutic effect maintained for 18 months. Int. Ophthalmol. 39 (1), 207–211.

Cunha-Vaz, J., 1979. The blood-ocular barriers. Surv. Ophthalmol. 23 (5), 279–296. Available from: https://doi.org/10.1016/0039-6257(79)90158-9.

Dawson, D.G., Ubels, J.L., Edelhauser, H.F., 2011. Cornea and sclera. In: Adler's Physiol. Eye, 11th ed. Elsevier, pp. 71–130. Available from: https://www-clinicalkey-com.ezproxy.library.ubc.ca/#!/content/book/3-s2.0-B9780323057141000042?scrollTo = %23hl0001068.

de Campos, A.M., Diebold, Y., Carvalho, E.L.S., Sánchez, A., José Alonso, M., 2004. Chitosan nanoparticles as new ocular drug delivery systems: in vitro stability, in vivo fate, and cellular toxicity. Pharm. Res. 21 (5), 803–810. Available from: https://doi.org/10.1023/B:PHAM.0000026432.75781.cb.

De Campos, A.M., Sánchez, A., Alonso, M.J., 2001. Chitosan nanoparticles: a new vehicle for the improvement of the delivery of drugs to the ocular surface. Application to cyclosporin A. Int. J. Pharm. 224 (1), 159–168. Available from: https://doi.org/10.1016/S0378-5173(01)00760-8.

Di Tommaso, C., Torriglia, A., Furrer, P., Behar-Cohen, F., Gurny, R., Möller, M., 2011. Ocular biocompatibility of novel cyclosporin A formulations based on methoxy poly (ethylene glycol)-hexylsubstituted poly(lactide) micelle carriers. Int. J. Pharm. 416 (2), 515–524. Available from: https://doi.org/10.1016/j.ijpharm.2011.01.004.

DiNuzzo, A.R., Black, S.A., Lichtenstein, M.J., Markides, K.S., 2001. Prevalence of functional blindness, visual impairment, and related functional deficits among elderly Mexican Americans. J. Gerontol. Ser. A 56 (9), M548–M551. Available from: https://doi.org/10.1093/gerona/56.9.M548.

Eghrari, A.O., Riazuddin, S.A., Gottsch, J.D., 2015. Chapter Two—Overview of the cornea: structure, function, and development. In: Hejtmancik, J.F., Nickerson, J.M. (Eds.), Progress in Molecular Biology and Translational Science, vol. 134. Academic Press, pp. 7–23. Available from: https://doi.org/10.1016/bs.pmbts.2015.04.001.

Fakhari, A., Corcoran, M., Schwarz, A., 2017. Thermogelling properties of purified poloxamer 407. Heliyon 3 (8).

Felt, O., Furrer, P., Mayer, J.M., Plazonnet, B., Buri, P., Gurny, R., 1999. Topical use of chitosan in ophthalmology: tolerance assessment and evaluation of precorneal retention. Int. J. Pharm. 180 (2), 185–193. Available from: https://doi.org/10.1016/S0378-5173(99)00003-4.

Gasymov, O.K., Abduragimov, A.R., Yusifov, T.N., Glasgow, B.J., 1999. Interaction of tear lipocalin with lysozyme and lactoferrin. Biochem. Biophys. Res. Commun. 265 (2), 322–325. Available from: https://doi.org/10.1006/bbrc.1999.1668.

Gaudana, R., Ananthula, H.K., Parenky, A., Mitra, A.K., 2010. Ocular drug delivery. AAPS J. 12 (3), 348–360. Available from: https://doi.org/10.1208/s12248-010-9183-3.

Ghate, D., Edelhauser, H.F., 2006. Ocular drug delivery. Expert Opin. Drug Delivery 3 (2), 275–287. Available from: https://doi.org/10.1517/17425247.3.2.275.

Giammona, G., Cavallaro, G., Licciardi, M., Civiale, C., Paladino, G.M., Mazzone, M.G., 2009. Ophthalmic Pharmaceutical Composition Containing Amphiphilic Polyaspartamide Copolymers (United States Patent No. US20090221545A1). Available from: https://patents.google.com/patent/US20090221545A1/en.

Gillies, E.R., Fréchet, J.M.J., 2005. Dendrimers and dendritic polymers in drug delivery. Drug Discovery Today 10 (1), 35–43. Available from: https://doi.org/10.1016/S1359-6446(04)03276-3.

Gökçe, E.H., Sandri, G., Eğrilmez, S., Bonferoni, M.C., Güneri, T., Caramella, C., 2009. Cyclosporine A-loaded solid lipid nanoparticles: ocular tolerance and in vivo drug release in rabbit eyes. Curr. Eye Res. 34 (11), 996–1003. Available from: https://doi.org/10.3109/02713680903261405.

Gupta, A.K., Madan, S., Majumdar, D.K., Maitra, A., 2000. Ketorolac entrapped in polymeric micelles: preparation, characterisation and ocular anti-inflammatory studies. Int. J. Pharm. 209 (1), 1–14. Available from: https://doi.org/10.1016/S0378-5173(00)00508-1.

Guterres, S.S., Alves, M.P., Pohlmann, A.R., 2007. Polymeric nanoparticles, nanospheres and nanocapsules, for cutaneous applications. Drug Target. Insights 2, 147–157.

Horowitz, A., 2003. Depression and vision and hearing impairments in later life [Text]. Available from: https://www.ingentaconnect.com/content/asag/gen/2003/00000027/00000001/art00007.

Horowitz, A., Reinhardt, J.P., Kennedy, G.J., 2005. Major and subthreshold depression among older adults seeking vision rehabilitation services. Am. J. Geriatr. Psychiatry 13 (3), 180–187. Available from: https://doi.org/10.1097/00019442-200503000-00002.

Huang, H., Yang, X., Li, H., Lu, H., Oswald, J., Liu, Y., et al., 2020. iRGD decorated liposomes: a novel actively penetrating topical ocular drug delivery strategy. Nano Res. 13 (11), 3105–3109.

Ideta, R., Yanagi, Y., Tamaki, Y., Tasaka, F., Harada, A., Kataoka, K., 2004. Effective accumulation of polyion complex micelle to experimental choroidal neovascularization in rats. FEBS Lett. 557 (1–3), 21–25. Available from: https://doi.org/10.1016/S0014-5793(03)01315-2.

Ilium, L., 1998. Chitosan and its use as a pharmaceutical excipient. Pharm. Res. 15 (9), 1326–1331. Available from: https://doi.org/10.1023/A:1011929016601.

Immordino, M.L., Dosio, F., Cattel, L., 2006. Stealth liposomes: review of the basic science, rationale, and clinical applications, existing and potential. Int. J. Nanomed. 1 (3), 297–315.

Janagam, D.R., Wu, L., Lowe, T.L., 2017. Nanoparticles for drug delivery to the anterior segment of the eye. Adv. Drug Delivery Rev. 122, 31–64. Available from: https://doi.org/10.1016/j.addr.2017.04.001.

Kestelyn, P.G., Cunningham Jr, E.T., 2001. HIV/AIDS and blindness. Bull. World Health Organ. 79, 208–213. Available from: https://doi.org/10.1590/S0042-96862001000300008.

Kimura, H., Yasukawa, T., Tabata, Y., Ogura, Y., 2001. Drug targeting to choroidal neovascularization. Adv. Drug Delivery Rev. 52 (1), 79–91. Available from: https://doi.org/10.1016/S0169-409X(01)00190-9.

Klyce, S.D., Crosson, C.E., 1985. Transport processes across the rabbit corneal epithelium: a review. Curr. Eye Res. 4 (4), 323–331. Available from: https://doi.org/10.3109/02713688509025145.

Kumar, R., Sinha, V.R., 2016. Solid lipid nanoparticle: an efficient carrier for improved ocular permeation of voriconazole. Drug Dev. Ind. Pharm. 42 (12), 1956–1967. Available from: https://doi.org/10.1080/03639045.2016.1185437.

Lakhani, P., Patil, A., Majumdar, S., 2018. Recent advances in topical nano drug-delivery systems for the anterior ocular segment. Ther. Delivery 9 (2), 137–153. Available from: https://doi.org/10.4155/tde-2017-0088.

Lee-Huang, S., Huang, P.L., Sun, Y., Huang, P.L., Kung, H., Blithe, D.L., et al., 1999. Lysozyme and RNases as anti-HIV components in β-core preparations of human chorionic gonadotropin. Proc. Natl. Acad. Sci. U.S.A. 96 (6), 2678–2681. Available from: https://doi.org/10.1073/pnas.96.6.2678.

Liu, D., Li, J., Pan, H., He, F., Liu, Z., Wu, Q., et al., 2016. Potential advantages of a novel chitosan-*N*-acetylcysteine surface modified nanostructured lipid carrier on the performance of ophthalmic delivery of curcumin. Sci. Rep. 6 (1), 1–14. Available from: https://doi.org/10.1038/srep28796.

Lynch, C.R., Kondiah, P.P.D., Choonara, Y.E., Toit, L.C.D., Ally, N., Pillay, V., 2020. Hydrogel biomaterials for application in ocular drug delivery. Front. Bioeng. Biotechnol. 8.

Matsumura, Y., Maeda, H., 1986. A new concept for macromolecular therapeutics in cancer chemotherapy: mechanism of tumoritropic accumulation of proteins and the antitumor agent smancs. Cancer Res. 46 (12 Pt 1), 6387–6392.

Mehnert, W., Mäder, K., 2012. Solid lipid nanoparticles: production, characterization and applications. Adv. Drug Delivery Rev. 64, 83–101. Available from: https://doi.org/10.1016/j.addr.2012.09.021.

Mishra, G.P., Bagui, M., Tamboli, V., Mitra, A.K., 2011. Recent applications of liposomes in ophthalmic drug delivery. J. Drug Delivery 2011, 1–14. Available from: https://doi.org/10.1155/2011/863734.

Müller, R.H., Radtke, M., Wissing, S.A., 2002. Solid lipid nanoparticles (SLN) and nanostructured lipid carriers (NLC) in cosmetic and dermatological preparations. Adv. Drug Delivery Rev. 54, S131–S155. Available from: https://doi.org/10.1016/S0169-409X(02)00118-7.

Muñoz-Fernández, S., Martín-Mola, E., 2006. Uveitis. Best practice & research. Clin. Rheumatol. 20 (3), 487–505. Available from: https://doi.org/10.1016/j.berh.2006.03.008.

Neves, L.F.F., Duan, J., Voelker, A., Khanal, A., McNally, L., Steinbach-Rankins, J.M., et al., 2016. Preparation and optimization of anionic liposomes for delivery of small peptides and cDNA to human corneal epithelial cells. J. Microencapsulation 33 (4), 391–399. Available from: https://doi.org/10.1080/02652048.2016.1202343.

Omerović, N., Vranić, E., 2020. Application of nanoparticles in ocular drug delivery systems. Health Technol. 10 (1), 61–78. Available from: https://doi.org/10.1007/s12553-019-00381-w.

Patel, A., Cholkar, K., Agrahari, V., Mitra, A.K., 2013. Ocular drug delivery systems: an overview. World J. Pharmacol. 2 (2), 47–64. Available from: https://doi.org/10.5497/wjp.v2.i2.47.

Pepić, I., Hafner, A., Lovrić, J., Pirkić, B., Filipović-Grčić, J., 2010. A nonionic surfactant/chitosan micelle system in an innovative eye drop formulation. J. Pharm. Sci. 99 (10), 4317–4325. Available from: https://doi.org/10.1002/jps.22137.

Pepić, I., Jalsenjak, N., Jalsenjak, I., 2004. Micellar solutions of triblock copolymer surfactants with pilocarpine. Int. J. Pharm. 272 (1–2), 57–64. Available from: https://doi.org/10.1016/j.ijpharm.2003.11.032.

Sack, R.A., Nunes, I., Beaton, A., Morris, C., 2001. Host-defense mechanism of the ocular surfaces. Biosci. Rep. 21 (4), 463–480. Available from: https://doi.org/10.1023/A:1017943826684.

Sahoo, S.K., Dilnawaz, F., Krishnakumar, S., 2008. Nanotechnology in ocular drug delivery. Drug Discovery Today 13 (3), 144–151. Available from: https://doi.org/10.1016/j.drudis.2007.10.021.

Salamanca, A.E., de, Diebold, Y., Calonge, M., García-Vazquez, C., Callejo, S., Vila, A., et al., 2006. Chitosan nanoparticles as a potential drug delivery system for the ocular surface: toxicity, uptake mechanism and in vivo tolerance. Invest. Ophthalmol. Vis. Sci. 47 (4), 1416–1425. Available from: https://doi.org/10.1167/iovs.05-0495.

Sapra, P., Allen, T.M., 2003. Ligand-targeted liposomal anticancer drugs. Prog. Lipid Res. 42 (5), 439–462. Available from: https://doi.org/10.1016/S0163-7827(03)00032-8.

Schaeffer, H.E., Krohn, D.L., 1982. Liposomes in topical drug delivery. Invest. Ophthalmol. Vis. Sci. 22 (2), 220–227.

Schmidt-Erfurth, U., Hasan, T., 2000. Mechanisms of action of photodynamic therapy with verteporfin for the treatment of age-related macular degeneration. Surv. Ophthalmol. 45 (3), 195–214. Available from: https://doi.org/10.1016/S0039-6257(00)00158-2.

Shakib, M., Cunha-Vaz, J.G., 1966. Studies on the permeability of the blood-retinal barrier. IV. Junctional complexes of the retinal vessels and their role in the permeability of the blood-retinal barrier. Exp. Eye Res. 5 (3), 229–234. Available from: https://doi.org/10.1016/s0014-4835(66)80011-8.

Shen, J., Wang, Y., Ping, Q., Xiao, Y., Huang, X., 2009. Mucoadhesive effect of thiolated PEG stearate and its modified NLC for ocular drug delivery. J. Controlled Release 137 (3), 217–223. Available from: https://doi.org/10.1016/j.jconrel.2009.04.021.

Shen, Y., Tu, J., 2007. Preparation and ocular pharmacokinetics of ganciclovir liposomes. AAPS J. 9 (3), E371. Available from: https://doi.org/10.1208/aapsj0903044.

Svenson, S., 2009. Dendrimers as versatile platform in drug delivery applications. Eur. J. Pharm. Biopharm. 71 (3), 445–462. Available from: https://doi.org/10.1016/j.ejpb.2008.09.023.

Swart, P.J., Kuipers, E.M., Smit, C., Van Der Strate, B.W.A., Harmsen, M.C., Meijer, D.K. F., 1998. Lactoferrin. In: Spik, G., Legrand, D., Mazurier, J., Pierce, A., Perraudin, J.-P. (Eds.), Advances in Lactoferrin Research. Springer, pp. 205–213. Available from: https://doi.org/10.1007/978-1-4757-9068-9_24.

Trani, N.D., Jain, P., Chua, C.Y.X., Ho, J.S., Bruno, G., Susnjar, A., et al., 2019. Nanofluidic microsystem for sustained intraocular delivery of therapeutics. Nanomed. Nanotechnol. Biol. Med. 16, 1–9.

Trivedi, R., Kompella, U.B., 2010. Nanomicellar formulations for sustained drug delivery: Strategies and underlying principles. Nanomedicine 5 (3), 485. Gale OneFile: Health and Medicine.

Vandamme, Th. F., Brobeck, L., 2005. Poly(amidoamine) dendrimers as ophthalmic vehicles for ocular delivery of pilocarpine nitrate and tropicamide. J. Controlled Release 102 (1), 23–38. Available from: https://doi.org/10.1016/j.jconrel.2004.09.015.

Vogel, H.J., 2012. Lactoferrin, a bird's eye view. Biochem. Cell Biol. 90 (3), 233–244. Available from: https://doi.org/10.1139/o2012-016.

Wang, H., Sun, H., Wei, H., Xi, P., Nie, S., Ren, Q., 2014. Biocompatible hyaluronic acid polymer-coated quantum dots for CD44 + cancer cell-targeted imaging. J. Nanopart. Res. 16 (10).

Yamaguchi, M., Ueda, K., Isowaki, A., Ohtori, A., Takeuchi, H., Ohguro, N., et al., 2009. Mucoadhesive properties of chitosan-coated ophthalmic lipid emulsion containing indomethacin in tear fluid. Biol. Pharm. Bull. 32 (7), 1266–1271. Available from: https://doi.org/10.1248/bpb.32.1266.

Yang, X., Wang, L., Li, L., Han, M., Tang, S., Wang, T., et al., 2019. A novel dendrimer-based complex co-modified with cyclic RGD hexapeptide and penetratin for noninvasive targeting and penetration of the ocular posterior segment. Drug Delivery 26 (1), 989–1001.

Yasukawa, T., Ogura, Y., Sakurai, E., Tabata, Y., Kimura, H., 2005. Intraocular sustained drug delivery using implantable polymeric devices. Adv. Drug Delivery Rev. 57 (14), 2033–2046. Available from: https://doi.org/10.1016/j.addr.2005.09.005.

Yu-Wai-Man, C., Tagalakis, A.D., Manunta, M.D., Hart, S.L., Khaw, P.T., 2016. Receptor-targeted liposome-peptide-siRNA nanoparticles represent an efficient delivery system for MRTF silencing in conjunctival fibrosis. Sci. Rep. 6 (1), 1–11. Available from: https://doi.org/10.1038/srep21881.

Zhang, L., Li, Y., Zhang, C., Wang, Y., Song, C., 2009. Pharmacokinetics and tolerance study of intravitreal injection of dexamethasone-loaded nanoparticles in rabbits. Int. J. Nanomed. 4, 175–183.

Zhou, L., Zhao, S.Z., Koh, S.K., Chen, L., Vaz, C., Tanavde, V., et al., 2012. In-depth analysis of the human tear proteome. J. Proteomics 75 (13), 3877–3885. Available from: https://doi.org/10.1016/j.jprot.2012.04.053.

CHAPTER

12 Current and future challenges in polymeric nanomaterials for biomedical applications

Gokcen B. Demirel[1], Aydan Dag[2], Gulsah Albayrak[3] and Zeynep Cimen[1]

[1]*Department of Chemistry, Polatlı Faculty of Arts and Sciences, Ankara Hacı Bayram Veli University, Ankara, Turkey*

[2]*Department of Pharmaceutical Chemistry, Faculty of Pharmacy, Bezmialem Vakıf University, İstanbul, Turkey*

[3]*Department of Medical Biology, Faculty of Medicine, Ufuk University, Ankara, Turkey*

12.1 Introduction

Multifunctional nanocarriers have a very promising potential to develop personalized therapeutic nanocarriers. Early detection of diseases, targeted drug delivery, and drug tracking in the blood circulation are desired properties of a multifunctional nanocarrier (Daglar et al., 2014; Kurtay et al., 2017). For this purpose, scientists are trying to combine diagnosis/tracking and treatment properties into one system which is called all-in-one nanocarrier system. Various nanoparticles such as inorganic, metallic, core/shell, and polymeric nanoparticles have been synthesized for developing efficient personal therapeutic nanocarriers (Duan and Li, 2013). Among these therapeutic nanocarriers, polymeric nanoparticles have significant potential due to their easily controllable chemical and physical properties. Their controllable properties allow the synthesis of desired molecular architectures for biomedical and pharmaceutical applications. So far, different forms of polymeric nanocarriers including nanoparticles, nanocomposites, dendrimers, micelles, and core/shell systems have been synthesized using a variety of methods for using in biomedical applications (Daglar et al., 2014; Elsabahy and Wooley, 2012; Banik et al., 2016). Developed nanocarriers generally exhibited excellent outstanding performance for in vitro applications. However, in clinical trials, most of them have failed because there are many challenges and biological barriers in vivo applications which are needed to be overcome to reach the targeted site. Therefore scientists have started to investigate these challenges and have tried to find new solutions to overcome them. Every study about the engineering of polymeric nanocarriers is important to identify the mysterious journey of nanocarriers in the human body. Scientists have learned more information about the

Advances in Polymeric Nanomaterials for Biomedical Applications. DOI: https://doi.org/10.1016/B978-0-12-814657-6.00003-3

challenges that are faced in blood circulation before reaching the targeted site, and they have developed new strategies and methods (Petros and DeSimone, 2010; He et al., 2010b; Kulkarni and Feng, 2013; Banik et al., 2016). Hence, it can be clearly said that the following physicochemical properties such as stability, size, shape, biocompatibility, surface charge, mechanical properties, and also bioimaging properties of therapeutic polymeric nanoparticles are very important in clinical applications. In this chapter, we will focus on the current limitations of physicochemical and bioimaging properties of polymeric nanoparticles on their therapeutic efficiencies. Moreover, we will discuss besides the current challenges and also improving strategies which have important to develop personal nanomedicine in future.

12.2 Physicochemical properties of polymeric nanoparticles

Various types of polymeric nanoparticles have been developed as a therapeutic biomaterial. However, only a few of them have successfully reached the targeted site in the bloodstream in clinical trials. Because, the bloodstream has a very complex structure, and it has many therapeutical and toxicological limitations (Allen and Cullis, 2004; Daglar et al., 2014). When the polymeric nanoparticles enter into the blood circulation, the body's clearing mechanism which is called reticuloendothelial system (RES) is activated (Daglar et al., 2014; Aderem and Underhill, 1999; Elsabahy and Wooley, 2012). If RES defines the polymeric nanocarriers as foreign entities, the body tries to remove them via different kinds of clearance routes. At this point, the physicochemical properties such as particle size, morphology, charge, and composition of nanoparticles play a very significant role in the fabrication of ideal polymeric nanocarriers. Because, researchers have shown that they directly affect the blood stability, cellular uptake, biodistribution, endocytic pathway, intracellular distribution, and bioavailability of nanoparticles (Elsabahy and Wooley, 2012). Thus it can be said that the optimization of the physicochemical properties of particles is necessary for improving the therapeutic efficacy of nanocarriers. However, there are many challenges need to be resolved to get an efficient therapeutic efficiency from the particles. In this section, we will give a brief overview about the current challenges caused by the physicochemical properties of polymeric nanoparticles, and we will also discuss the new strategies for future prospects.

12.2.1 Size

The size of nanocarriers is a very important for circulation time, clearance, selective tissue distribution, uptake mechanisms, degradation, and the toxicity of the nanoparticles (Kulkarni and Feng, 2013; Mitragotri and Lahann, 2009). Various size of particles in the range of nanometers to a few microns have been investigated for intravenous applications (Juliano and Stamp, 1975; Ilium et al., 1982; Muro et al., 2008; Davis et al., 2008; Duan and Li, 2013). The researchers exhibited that large-sized (> 1 μm) particles have a tendency to accumulate in the liver and spleen due to the possible aggregation and capillary occlusion (Davis et al., 2008; Duan and Li, 2013; Elsabahy and Wooley, 2012). Small nanoparticles that are smaller than 5 nm are filtered rapidly from the blood via extravasation or renal clearance (Davis et al., 2008; Duan and Li, 2013; Choi et al., 2007; Elsabahy and Wooley, 2012). The medium sizes (20–100 nm) of nanoparticles have the highest potential for in vivo applications. Because their circulation time is longer than the other different size of particles into the bloodstream. Moreover, the medium size of nanoparticles is also large enough to escape from kidney's filtration, and they are small enough to avoid opsonization. In addition, the recent studies indicate that intermediated sized polymeric nanoparticles can be uptake easily by cells due to the more effective interaction and adhesion with biological cells in comparison to the smaller or larger particles (Iversen et al., 2011; Elsabahy and Wooley, 2012). He et al. (2010a,b) investigated the effects of particle size and surface charge on cellular uptake and biodistribution using fluorescent dye-labeled functionalized chitosan nanoparticles. They investigated in vivo biodistribution of dye-labeled chitosan nanoparticles. Their experimental results showed that approximately 150 nm size of polymeric nanoparticles was selectively taken up by targeted cancer cells. Moreover, these polymeric nanoparticles delivered the cargo molecules to the desired site with an effective therapeutic efficacy and also created minor side effects. They concluded that cellular uptake decreased with an increase in particle size. Cabral et al. (2011) investigated the comparison of the accumulation of different sizes of drug-loaded polymeric micelles in both highly and poorly permeable tumors. They reported that the polymer micelles which their size in the range of 30–100 nm successfully penetrated to the highly permeable tumors in mice. On the other hand, they reported that the penetration efficiency of particles for poorly permeable tumors is size dependent. They reported that only 30 nm micelles showed antitumor effect because they could penetrate into the poorly permeable pancreatic tumors. Cabral et al. (2011) enhanced the penetration efficiency of the larger micelles using a transforming growth factor-b (TGF-β) inhibitor. They demonstrated that sub-100 nm micellar nanomedicines showed no size-dependent restrictions on extravasation and penetration in tumors, whereas the nanomedicine smaller than 50 nm can only penetrate to the poorly permeable hypovascular tumors as seen in Fig. 12.1.

Kulkarni and Feng (Kulkarni and Feng, 2013) investigated the size effect of TPGS-modified polystyrene particles in the size range of 25–500 nm on the transport efficiencies across both GastroIntestinal (GI) and the Blood–Brain Barrier (BBB) for imaging and therapy of brain cancer (Fig. 12.2). They reported that TPGS-modified particles of 100 and 200 nm sized have potential to deliver the drug across the GI barrier and the BBB. Kulkarni and Feng concluded that particle size and surface coating are two important parameters which can dramatically influence the nanoparticles biodistribution after intravenous administration.

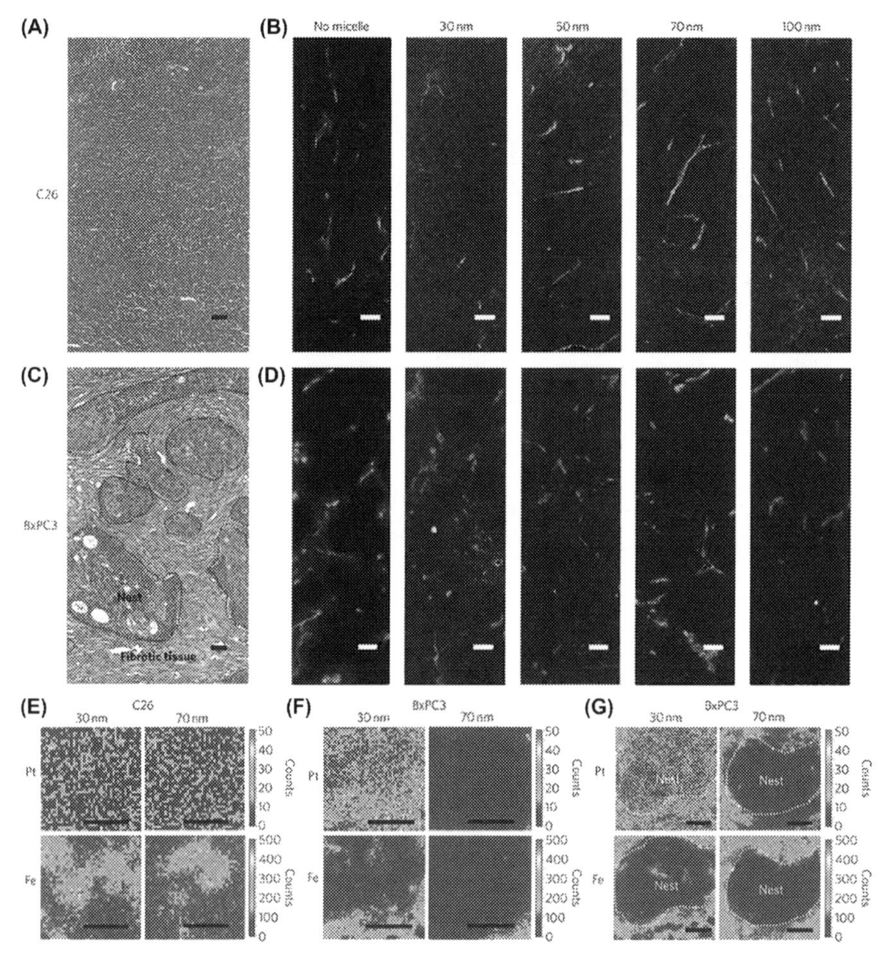

FIGURE 12.1

Microdistribution of fluorescently labeled polymeric nanoparticles of varying sizes in tumors. Scale bars, 50 mm.

Reprinted from Cabral, H., Matsumoto, Y., Mizuno, K., Chen, Q., Murakami, M., Kimura, M., et al., (2011). Accumulation of sub-100 nm polymeric micelles in poorly permeable tumours depends on size. Nat. Nanotechnol. 6 (12), 815–823 with permission from Springer Nature 2011.

Tran et al. (2014) have synthesized self-assembled polymeric nanoparticles composed of polynorbornene-cholesterol/poly(ethylene glycol) [P(NBCh9-*b*-NBPEG)] as anticancer drug (DOX) carrier. They reported that below 200 nm-size of P(NBCh9-*b*-NBPEG) nanoparticles exhibited an efficient cellular uptake and dose-dependent cytotoxicity in HeLa cells. Dehaini et al. (2016) synthesized ultra-small lipid–coated polymeric nanoparticles under 25 nm in size to investigate the toxicity of the particles in tumors. They reported that these lipids coated

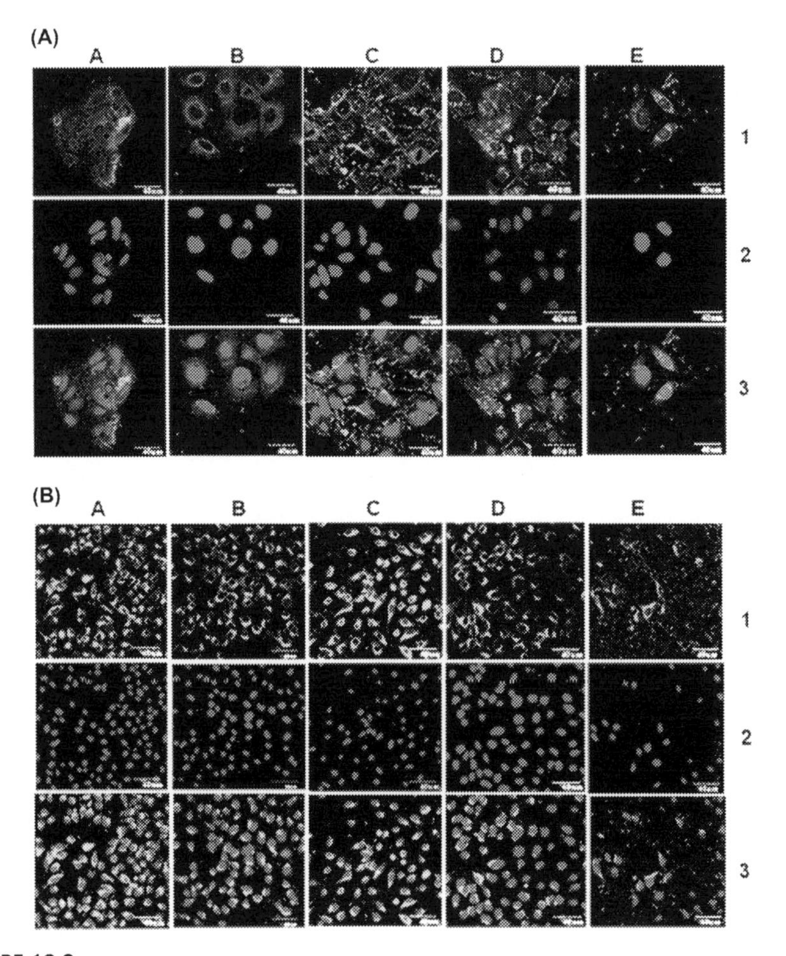

FIGURE 12.2

Confocal laser scanning microscopy images of Caco-2 (A) and MDCK (B) cells with the fluorescent TPGS coated PS NPs. Column *A*, *B*, *C*, *D*, and *E* are for the 25, 50, 100, 200, and 500 nm sized PS-TPGS NPs formulations, respectively. Scale bar = 40 μm.

Reprinted from Kulkarni, S.A., Feng, S.S., (2013). Effects of particle size and surface modification on cellular uptake and biodistribution of polymeric nanoparticles for drug delivery. Pharm. Res. 30 (10), 2512–2522 with permission from Springer Nature 2013.

ultra-small polymeric nanoparticles effectively accumulated at the desired tumors and released effectively the chemotherapeutic drug, docetaxel. Dehaini et al. (2016) demonstrated that these targeted ultra-small polymeric nanoparticles are able to outperform than the clinically used formulation of the drug. Bruni et al. (2017) synthesized ultra-small polymeric nanoparticles consist of a hydrophobic poly-ε-caprolactone core and a brush-like polyethylene glycol (PEG) hydrophilic

Table 12.1 Polymeric particles size for therapeutic applications.

Size of the spherical polymeric particles	Applications	References
<10 nm	Kidney filtration	Elsabahy and Wooley (2012)
10–20 nm	Imaging to cross blood–brain barrier (BBB)	Petros and DeSimone (2010)
20–100 nm	Therapeutic applications (suitable size to escape physiological barriers and filtration by liver and spleen)	Elsabahy and Wooley (2012); Moghimi et al. (2005); Swami et al. (2012)
100–200 nm	Therapeutic applications (suitable size for prolonged circulation)	Petros and DeSimone (2010)
200 nm–1 μm	Generally filtrated by the spleen	Swami et al. (2012)
>1 μm	Larger particles aim to accumulate in liver and spleen. Generally removed from circulation immediately	Elsabahy and Wooley (2012); Petros and DeSimone (2010)

Reproduced from Banik, B.L., Fattahi, P., Brown, J.L., (2016). Polymeric nanoparticles: the future of nanomedicine. Wiley Interdiscip. Rev. Nanomed. Nanobiotechnol. 8 (2), 271–299 with permission from Wiley 2016.

shell with a tuneable size in the range of 5–30 nm. They observed that these ultra-small core/shell polymeric nanoparticles were able to cross the glomerular filtration barrier and accumulated in the kidney glomerulus. According to the literature, it can be concluded that polymeric nanoparticles which smaller than 100 nm are removed by RES which reduce the uptake efficiency due to the reduced circulation time. Moderate size which are 100–200 nm particles are taken up by receptor-mediated endocytosis, whereas larger particles are internalized by phagocytosis (Kulkarni and Feng, 2013). On the other hand, several studies have shown that the size of polymeric nanoparticles is not the only parameter for specific cellular uptake for therapeutic applications but the shape, surface chemistry, and mechanical properties of nanoparticles are also crucial parameters (Tang et al., 2014; Banik et al., 2016). Therefore, the optimum size definition for an ideal polymeric nanocarrier is not completely possible but the following table (Table 12.1) might be useful in enlightening the effects of nanoparticles size for therapeutic applications.

12.2.2 Morphology

In recent years, the researchers discovered that the morphology of nanoparticles is also an important parameter besides particle size for therapeutic applications (Tan et al., 2013; Banik et al., 2016; Demirel et al., 2020). Many researchers reported that the shape affects the circulation time, biodistribution, and cellular uptake mechanism of the particles (Dasgupta et al., 2014; Truong et al., 2014,

Arnida et al., 2011; Demirel et al., 2020). Therefore, it can be said that the therapeutic performance of the nanoparticles might be improved by controlling of their morphology. Spherical morphology can be defined as traditional morphology because of being the most common shape of the nanoparticles. Recently, researchers are working on the nonspherical polymeric nanoparticles to be able to use their advantage of geometric structures (Champion et al., 2007; Park et al., 2010). Recent studies showed that the nonspherical shaped nanoparticles might be the key to overcome biological barriers due to their geometric features and different physical and chemical properties compared to the spherical particles (Park et al., 2010; Doshi et al., 2009). The anisotropic-shaped nanoparticles exhibit excellent interactions with biological systems in adhesion, cellular uptake, cargo delivery, and in vivo circulation time (Doshi et al., 2009; He et al., 2012; Banik et al., 2016). Geng and coworkers (Geng et al., 2007) have fabricated highly stable polymer filomicelles consist of biodegradable PEG-*b*-poly(ε-caprolactone) and nonbiodegradable PEG-*b*-polyethylethylene to compare the transportation properties with spheres of similar chemistry. They observed that the filomicelles exhibited ten times longer circulation time than their spherical counterparts due to the reducing rate of clearance by the mononuclear phagocytic system. The clearance of filomicelles occurred upon the persistent decrease in length, which was more significant for the biodegradable poly(ε-caprolactone) than the nondegradable polyethylethylene due to the hydrolysis of poly(ε-caprolactone) over time. They also reported that the filomicelles demonstrated an effective drug release profile and they caused the shrinking of human-derived tumors in mice. Gratton et al. (2008a) have demonstrated that the particle shape is an important parameter and affects significantly the mechanism of cellular uptake of polymeric nanoparticles. They fabricated various shapes of PEG-based hydrogel particles using top-down particle fabrication technique. They investigated the mechanism of nonspherical particle internalization by HeLa cells using transmission electron microscopy. According to their investigation, it was found that the internalization rates of high aspect ratio rod-like particles were almost four times faster than more symmetric cylindrical low aspect ratio particles. In a recent study, Li et al. (2015) have performed a theoretical simulation to reveal the shape effect of PEGylated nanoparticles on the cellular internalization efficiency by large-scale dissipative particle dynamics simulations. They have studied various shapes of PEGylated nanoparticles containing sphere, rod, cube, and disk, and they observed that the spherical PEGlayted nanoparticles showed the fastest internalization rate, followed by the cubic NPs, then rod- and disk-like nanoparticles (Li et al., 2015). Kumar et al. (2015) fabricated different shapes of ovalbumin conjugated-polystyrene particles (Fig. 12.3) to reveal the morphological effect of over immune cells and response.

They reported that smaller spherical particles generated stronger Th1 and Th2 immune responses compared to the other type of particles. On the other hand, larger rod-shaped particles produced a Th2-biased response against ovalbumin. Moreover, they investigated the internalization of different shape particles by

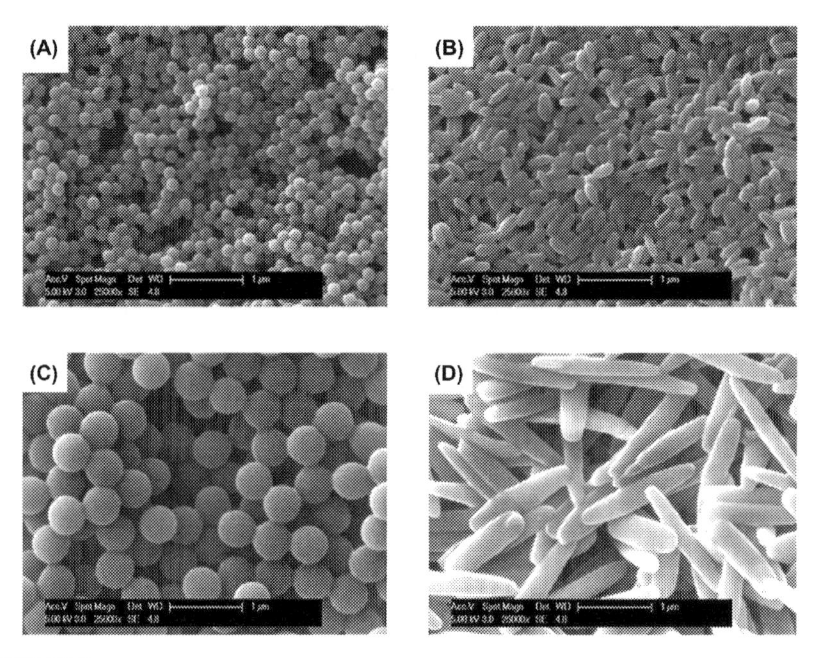

FIGURE 12.3

SEM images of different shape ovalbumin (Ova) conjugated-polystyrene particles (A) Spheres-193 nm, (B) Rods-376 nm, (C) Spheres-521 nm, and (D) Rods-1530 nm. Scale bars = 1 μm.

Reprinted from Kumar, S., Anselmo, A.C., Banerjee, A., Zakrewsky, M., Mitragotri, S., (2015). Shape and size-dependent immune response to antigen-carrying nanoparticles. J. Control. Release 220 (Pt A), 141–148 with permission from Elsevier 2015.

dendritic cells. Small-sized spherical ova-conjugated particles and large-sized rod ova-conjugated particles were internalized by dendritic cells and successfully delivered ovalbumin. These results exhibited that both size and shape are important factors for immune responses. In recently, an interesting study has been performed by He and Park (2016) for the understanding of the shape effect of the polymeric particles on cellular uptake. They fabricated keyboard character shaped poly(lactic-*co*-glycolic acid) (PLGA) microparticles that differ from traditionally shaped particles such as a rod, spherical, etc. They examined the impacts of the unusual shaped PLGA microparticles on cellular uptake by LnCAP cells. They observed that rod-like PLGA microparticles such as letter l, number 1, and arrow key were successfully internalized by cancer cells as expected. On the other hand, the letter O and number 0 which have no sharp features could not penetrate the cells at all. According to their experiments, they concluded that rod-like and sharp features of PLGA microparticles were successfully internalized by the cancer cells. Hinde et al. (2017) have synthesized four different shapes (worms, micelles, rods, and vesicles) of polymeric particles consisting of poly(oligoethylene glycol methacrylate)-*b*-poly(styrene-*co*-vinylbenzaldehyde) P(OEGMA)-*b*-P(ST-*co*-PVBA) block copolymer to compare the cellular uptake efficiencies of the nanoparticles that changes with particle geometry. They reported that rods-like and worms-like polymeric nanoparticles successfully entered the nucleus but micelles and vesicles did not achieve the nucleus by passive diffusion.

As a consequence of aforementioned researches, it can be concluded that the particle geometry is a key factor to enhance the cellular adhesion and also internalization. However, to obtain optimal geometry is not enough to overcome the biological barriers and to prolong blood circulation. In this case, both size and geometry should be at optimal values for desired therapeutic applications.

12.2.3 Surface chemistry

Surface chemistry plays an important role to organize the charge, biodistribution, hydrophilicity, immunogenicity, intracellular bioavailability properties of the polymeric nanoparticles. Hence, polymeric nanoparticles are desired to be biocompatible and biodegradable for biomedical applications. For the biocompatibility of the particles, the components and used material in the synthesis such as the polymer, monomer, and solvent is very crucial. Polymeric particles can be formulated using two different types of polymers as to be synthetic and natural components (Xiao et al., 2011). Natural polymers are very promising materials for the fabrication of therapeutic nanoparticles due to their desired biocompatibility and biodegradability properties. The most used natural polymeric materials can be listed as sodium alginate, chitin, gelatin, hyaluronic acid (HA), cellulose, and polyhydroxyalkanoates (Xiao et al., 2011). In general, natural polymers are to be used together with synthetic polymers such as PEG, PLGA, polyvinyl alcohol, etc. to enhance their mechanical properties, biostabilities, and therapeutic efficiencies. Choi et al. (2012) established theranostic nanocarriers to early tumor detection and targeted-treatment using PEG-conjugated HA nanoparticles. PEG-conjugated HA nanoparticles exhibited remarkable tumor targeting ability and significant suppression of tumor growth with a reduced systemic toxicity. The surface engineering of polymeric particles might provide control over cellular distribution (Gref et al., 1995; Phillips et al., 2012; Nance et al., 2012; Mastorakos et al., 2015). Song et al. (2017) prepared poly(lactic acid) (PLA) nanoparticles to investigate their bioadhesive and internalization properties with changing the surface chemistry of nanoparticles. They fabricated PLA, PEG-conjugated PLA, hyperbranched glycerol (HPG)-conjugated PLA, and aldehyde groups containing PLA–HPG–CHO nanoparticles to investigate the interaction of different surface decorated nanoparticles with cells in the context of the brain/tumor cellular microenvironment. According to experiments, PLA–HPG nanoparticles exhibited more "stealth" effect than PLA–PEG nanoparticles. They reported that all "stealth" nanoparticles were uptake by all types of cells. However, they showed that the internalization and therapeutic efficacy of the particles did not always correlate with each other. It is known that the surface charge of the particles plays an important role for blood stability, physical stability, cellular uptake, mucus penetration, and endocytosis of the nanoparticles. The type of charge and also the quantity of charge on the particle surface is a very critical issue in blood circulation. The excess of positive charge might cause the aggregation and clearance of particles by possible blood vessels. It is known that the cellular uptake increase by increasing zeta-potential of the particles due to the negatively charged proteoglycans on the cell surface (Gratton et al., 2008b). He et al. (2010a,b) synthesized fluorescent dye-labeled carboxymethyl chitosan grafted nanoparticles to investigate the effects of size and surface charges on the biodistribution of the particles. They observed that cationic particles having zeta-potential of +15 mV exhibited more efficient accumulation at the tumor site when compared to more negative particles. Generally, cationic particles are preferred for therapeutic application due to their efficient interactions between cationic particles with the negative cell membrane. However, researchers observed that the excessive quantity of positive charge on the particles surface might cause toxicity (Elsabahy and Wooley, 2012). Therefore, the quantity of particles charge and size must be in a balanced manner. For instance, Xiao et al. (2011) demonstrated that optimal surface charge of polymeric nanocarriers for cancer treatment should be slightly negative due to the decreased the undesirable elimination of particles from the blood circulation. In general, it is accepted that cationic particles can easily uptake by cells but also can cause undesired interaction with any cell types (Elsabahy and Wooley, 2012). Negatively charged particles have longer circulation in blood but it is observed that they do not accumulate at the desired site when compared to positively charged particles.

According to these findings, it is explicit that to obtain optimum surface charge is still challenging. The next generation of nanomedicine might be designed with charge switchable properties. For instance, firstly particles are prepared with negatively charged for obtaining longer circulation time in order to effectively reach the desired site within the body. When the particles reached the desired site, they might change their surface charge from negative to positive to attach the cell membrane, and as a result, more efficient delivery can be obtained. Therefore it can be said that new generation particles which have both long circulation half-life in blood and more effective interactions with targeted cells should be designed.

12.2.4 Toxicity

Toxicity can be defined as undesired interactions between nanoparticles and biological tissues. Several physicochemical factors such as size, morphology, chemical components, surface charge, aggregation, and solubility might cause the toxicity of the particles (Shin et al., 2015; Banik et al., 2016; Shao et al., 2015). Researchers are working on new synthesis methods to minimize these undesired interactions. As mentioned before, particle size and surface chemistry are very important parameters, and they significantly influence cellular delivery mechanism and in vivo biodistribution of particles. Therefore, it can be said that size and chemical composition of polymeric nanoparticles are the main factors in assessing a nanomaterial's toxicity. Evaluation of the toxicity response of polymeric nanoparticles with in vitro and in vivo studies is also a problem for the nanoparticles. In order to determine the toxicity of polymeric nanoparticles, firstly a detailed database should be composed of in vitro and in vivo studies depending on the relationship between physicochemical properties of particles and their toxicity effects on the biological tissues. In this regard, more accurate testing models are required in order to make better predictions about toxicity (Banik et al., 2016; Elsabahy and Wooley, 2012). For instance, Gilkey et al. (2015) described a physiologically based pharmacokinetics (PBPK) model to determine polymeric nanoparticles biodistribution in mice. PBPK-based models are very useful pharmacological tools to simulate the distribution of nanoparticles in the human body. To understand the relationship between the drug distribution and physicochemical properties of nanoparticles is very important for improving future nanomedicine (Moss and Siccardi, 2014). At this point, PBPK-based modeling helps to gain foresight because this tool integrates system data that describes a population of interest with drug/nanoparticle in vitro data through a mathematical description of absorption, distribution, metabolism, and elimination (Moss and Siccardi, 2014). However, there are still many problems need to be solved because a large amount of input systems is required for these models to be able to report a predictive response of risks and benefits. There are also some incoherencies in the literature regarding the technical and experimental complexities. Generally, limitations about the toxicity analyses of nanoparticles are related with instruments, nanoparticles, biological, and physiological variations (Li et al., 2010). For instance, many studies about the toxicity of nanoparticles have been conducted in mice and rats. However, their usage in this setting is limited by their long developmental cycle and ethical concerns (Brohi et al., 2017). The underlying reason to prefer rats and mice is due to their relatively low cost and shorter lifespan. Their shorter lifespan enables researchers to perform follow-up studies after nanomaterial applications. But these studies might also not reflect the human responses due to the anatomical and systemic differences (Park and Lakes, 2007). More in vivo researches are needed in order to get a more relevant picture of the toxicity. In vitro cell culture experiments seem technically suitable in detecting the effects of oxidative stress and early inflammatory processes, whereas they are mostly unable to reflect the bio-kinetic aspects of these effects. However, in vitro studies might not always correlate with in vivo studies (Landsiedel et al., 2014; Voigt et al., 2014). It can be said that fundamental associations between nanoparticles size, composition, morphology, reactivity, and aggregation are needed further investigation in order to enlighten their molecular toxicity mechanism and to find the solutions for the toxicity of these systems (Buzea et al., 2007). Hence, it can be said that new methods and modeling programs are still needed to be developed to be able to predict these limitations and find better solutions for the toxicity of the system.

12.2.5 Biological barriers

The main aim of the fabricating nanomedicine is the effective transportation of therapeutic drugs and to provide the efficient concentration of drug at the targeted site. The surface of polymeric nanocarriers can be functionalized with peptides, antibodies, folic acid, sugar molecules, etc. to direct the nanocarriers to the desired cells, tumors, or organs. The nanocarriers meet many biological barriers throughout their journey which are defined as body's defence system. If these biological barriers identify the nanocarriers as a threat, they try to eliminate them from the body. For this purpose, the properties of these biological barriers should be defined properly and polymeric nanocarriers must be designed to be able to pass them. Barua and Mitragotri (2014) classified these defence systems of the body as the endothelial barrier, cellular barrier, and skin and mucosal barrier. The size, shape, charge, surface functionalization, and mechanical properties of polymeric nanoparticles play a very critical role to overcome these whole barriers and reach the goal site. The BBB is a kind of endothelial barrier that tightly controls the transport of particles between the blood and the brain to control the internal environment of the brain (Wong et al., 2013; Löscher and Potschka, 2005; Wong et al., 2012; Dube et al., 2017). It is known that most of the central nervous system drugs are not successful in clinical trials due to poor brain penetration (Pardridge, 2005). However, it is observed that nonpermissive epithelium give permission for transportation of particles under certain pathological conditions (Barua and Mitragotri, 2014). He et al. (2017) synthesized BBB-penetrating amphiphilic polymer nanoparticles for the treatment of brain metastasis of triple negative breast cancer (Fig. 12.4A). They demonstrated that the amphiphilic polymeric nanoparticles crossed the BBB via systemic administration in healthy mice and in a brain metastasis of breast cancer mouse model as seen in Fig. 12.4B.

Many polymeric nanoparticles have been developed for targeted and controllable delivery of therapeutic agents (Dube et al., 2017). The polymeric nanoparticles are tried to direct transportation along with cell-mediated drug delivery to overcome the challenges of mass transport across barriers. For this purpose, the surface of the nanoparticles is functionalized with receptor-targeting ligands, peptides, sugar molecules, and so forth. Banga et al. (2017) have been synthesized small-sized polymeric nanoparticles for ovarian cancer treatment. They functionalized the particle surface with oligonucleotide molecules to enhance the colloidal stability and cellular uptake of the particles. They exhibited that functionalized small-sized oligonucleotide polymeric nanoparticles exhibited an efficient cellular uptake, which manifests in a cytotoxicity that is comparable to the free drug. Wadajkar and coworkers (Wadajkar et al., 2017) have developed receptor-targeted and biodegradable polymeric nanocarriers to decrease nonspecific adhesivity and to improve cellular uptake of particles in brain tumor cells. These receptor-targeting polymeric nanoparticles improved brain tissue dispersion, tumor cell uptake, and tumor retention in vitro, ex vivo, and in vivo tests.

(A)

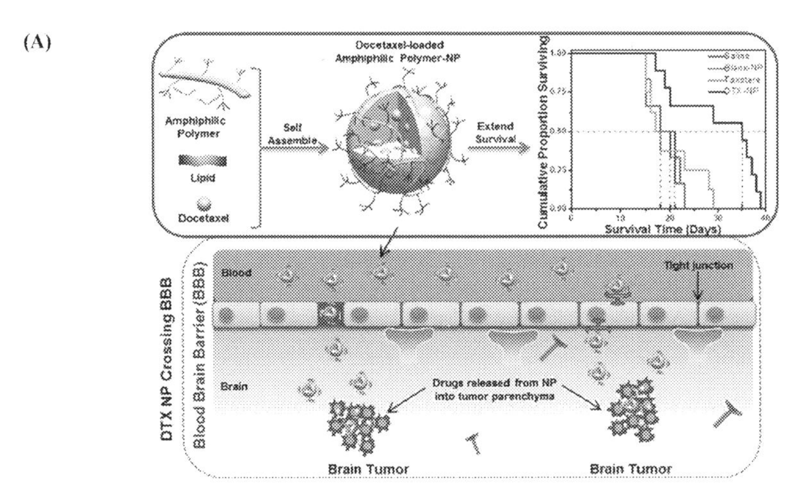

(B)

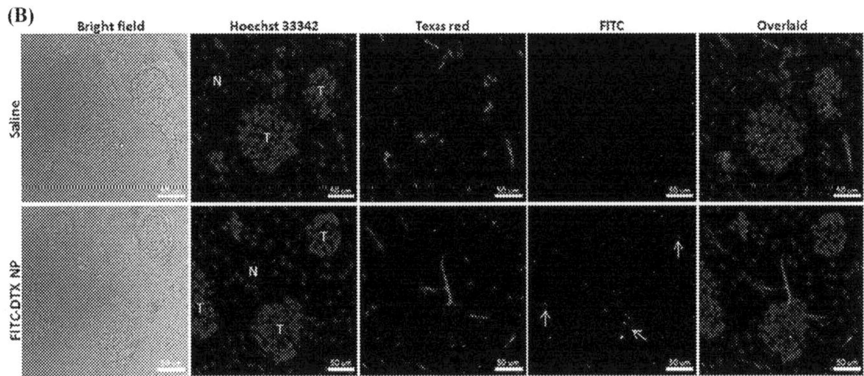

FIGURE 12.4

(A) Schematic illustration of fabrication of amphiphilic polymeric nanoparticles and proposed enhanced permeability and retention (EPR)/transcytosis mechanism for overcoming the BBB. (B) Confocal microscopic images of brain sections taken from mice-bearing brain metastases 2 h after injection of saline (top panel) or targeted amphiphilic polymeric nanoparticles. Arrows point to representative nanoparticles away from blood vessels and accumulated into microscopic tumor lesions. Scale = 50 μm for all images. *BBB*, blood–brain barrier.

Reordered from He, C., Cai, P., Li, J., Zhang, T., Lin L., Abbasi, A.Z., et al., (2017). Blood-brain barrier-penetrating amphiphilic polymer nanoparticles deliver docetaxel for the treatment of brain metastases of triple negative breast cancer. J. Control. Release 246, 98–109 with permission from Elsevier 2017.

Skin structure and diffusion limitation is also an important barrier for transdermal transportation of therapeutic agents. Polymeric nanocarriers have a promising potential for the transdermal delivery due to their efficient skin penetration ability. Biodegradable synthetic and also natural polymers are used for transdermal drug delivery (Santander-Ortega et al., 2010). Mittal et al. (2013) prepared biocompatible and biodegradable chitosan-coated PLGA (Chit-PLGA) nanoparticles for transfollicular delivery. They showed that Chit-PLGA nanoparticles exhibited an efficient delivery to the hair follicles on excised pig ears. Raza et al. (2013) reported that the skin penetration of tretinoin increased compared to commercial creams when using nanocarriers systems such as liposomes, solid lipid nanoparticles, and lipid nanoparticles. Singka et al. (2010) examined the permeation of 100 nm nanogels with sodium carbonate-mediated release of methotrexate, and an increase in methotrexate permeation across porcine skin was observed. Romero et al. (2016) investigated the penetration of cyclosporine A (CyA) through barrier defected porcine skin via polymeric nanoparticles. They observed that CyA-loaded polymeric nanoparticle exhibited better penetration through skin barrier defected than bulk cyclosporine A. Therefore they reported that drug-loaded nanocarriers have a promising potential to enhance penetration of the drug into the skin. However, many studies are performed in vitro conditions but these studies are not enough to test the penetration efficiency of nanocarriers through the skin barriers. Therefore more in vivo studies should be performed to translate the knowledge for potential human usage.

Mucosa is a membrane that lines into the various cavities such as nasal cavities, oral cavities in the body and covers the surface of internal organs such as eyes and stomach. The mission of mucosa is to protect the inside of the body from pathogens, dirt, viruses, and bacteria. On the other hand, drug-loaded nanocarriers or drugs can be absorbed via mucosal routes. This seems to be a very important advantage for controlled drug delivery. Unfortunately, the mucosa might be defined as a biological barrier due to having a limited bioavailability of mucosal delivery (Gonzalez-Paredes et al., 2017; Niu et al., 2017). For this purpose, new nanocarriers have been developed to increase the mucosal delivery efficiency (Wu et al., 2018). In this case, the surface properties of nanoparticles are the most important parameter to increase the mucus penetration of the particles. Maisel et al. (2016) fabricated PEG-coated PS nanoparticles with changing molecular weight of PEG to investigate the interactions of nanoparticles with mucins. Their results showed that the molecular weight of the PEG affected the interactions of nanoparticles with mucin and higher molecular weight PEG-coated PS nanoparticles exhibited an efficient and rapid transportation through human cervicovaginal mucus ex vivo and vaginal epithelium in vivo. Researchers demonstrated that the cationic charged particles show higher internalization into the cells but positively charged nanoparticles interact with mucin fibers, and as a consequence, the particles cannot transport to the underlying epithelium (Wu et al., 2018). Therefore the researchers are trying to design the surface charge changeable particles which have the ability to change their surface charge from negative to positive during penetrating the mucus layer (Perera et al., 2015; Bonengel et al., 2015; Netsomboon and Bernkop-Schnürch, 2016). The research indicates that the surface modulation of polymeric nanocarriers is very important for increasing mucus penetration. It can be said that while mucosa is a very promising delivery site for numerous diseases but still have limits to need to be overcome for efficient therapy.

12.3 Polymeric nanoparticles for bioimaging

Bioimaging techniques as well as bioimaging probes prospect to open an amazing section in the biomedical field (Vadivambal and Jayas, 2015). The ability to image will be critical in diagnosing and ultimately understanding the disease or disorder. There are many bioimaging modalities with different principles and equipments used to understand biological processes at the molecular, cellular, and clinical level, for example, magnetic resonance imaging (MRI) and functional magnetic resonance imaging (fMRI), X-ray, computed tomography (CT), positron emission tomography (PET), single-photon emission computed tomography (SPECT), optical imaging, sonography, and photoacoustic imaging (Dhawan et al., 2008). Each imaging modality poses its own benefits and drawbacks, which should be taken into consideration to select the most appropriate technique for the best outcome. As an example, MRI does not use radiation but rather radio waves, and it provides higher spatial, temporal resolution, and soft tissue penetration as compared with other imaging modalities, that is, radioactive-labeling imaging techniques. On the other hand, the major drawbacks of MRI technique are time-consuming and also high cost needed. PET/SPECT are the other most commonly used imaging modalities in the clinic and also exhibit high sensitivity with unlimited tissue penetration. As compared to PET/SPECT, an optical imaging technique (bioluminescence or fluorescence imaging) is simple to manage, and the contrast agent used for bioimaging modalities are less impractical to dispose of than those consisting radionucleotide techniques. Additionally, optical imaging technique offers multicolors of light in order to screen and measure many different properties of an organ or tissue along with high sensitivity but it has many inherent drawbacks such as low tissue penetration depth, long-term stability, photobleaching, and spatial resolution compared with electron or X-ray microscopy (Yi et al., 2014). Ultrasound imaging takes advantage of high resolution at much lower cost than MRI or PET/SPECT, but has lower penetration depth. Consequently, in order to achieve better performance, combining two or more imaging modalities seems essential. An advanced platform for future clinical applications relating to accurate functional and structural information obtained from what are necessarily include multiple imaging modalities are required for subsequent efficient treatment. In recent years, tremendous efforts have been heavily focused on improving bioimaging techniques and/or creating most effective bioprobes to help a clinician for precise early diagnosing, or examining, or characterizing diseases and then utilizing a certain known therapy to treat the disease by monitoring body response. However, there are still some research areas that need to be addressed. For example, there has been no efficient technique developed in bioimaging yet that quantitatively tells a medical specialist by how much a tumor cell growth or shrinks after standard therapy regimen. Likewise, bioimaging techniques cannot always distinguish accurately the differences between cancerous and noncancerous lesions. As an example, MRI cannot always detect microcalcifications, which might indicate breast cancer at the primary stages. Similarly, many of the most image processing, segmentation, and acquisition methods are also other important parts of bioimaging that need to be improved but they will not be discussed herein.

Polymeric nanomaterials have been extensively explored in medical research for diagnosis, therapy, imaging-guided therapy (theranostic), tissue/organ repair, and regeneration due to their desirable biocompatibility, biodegradability, and designability. Tremendous effort has been made for developing polymer-based nanocarriers system and eventually polymers; for example, PEG (Harris and Chess, 2003), poly(D, L-glycolic acid), poly(D, L-lactic acid) (Makadia and Siegel, 2011), and poly(ε-caprolactone) (Ulery et al., 2011) have been approved by FDA (Food and Drug Administration) for clinical usage (Bobo et al., 2016). More recently, interest has shifted more toward combining clinically used imaging techniques with therapeutic nanoparticles.

So far, many polymer-based nano-sized imaging structures have been studied for diagnostic applications. For example, polymeric chains have been covered onto gold, silver, iron oxide, and lanthanides (Huang et al., 2007; Sotiriou and Pratsinis, 2011; Laurent et al., 2010; Mader et al., 2010). Quantum dots (QDs) with their potential fluorescence properties have also been conjugated with polymers. Carbon-based nanomaterials (carbon nanotubes, graphene, etc.) (Bhunia et al., 2013), and more recently transition metal dichalcogenides (MoS_2, WSe_2, WS_2,) (Manzeli et al., 2017) another widely studied inorganic materials, have also been presented as an outstanding candidate for appropriate optical and photoacoustic imaging (Xu and Wang, 2016). While these systems have demonstrated promising results in vitro and in vivo imaging platform, their metallic or organic/inorganic nature has gained concerns about poor aqueous stability, biocompatibility, immunogenicity, and high toxicity which need to be investigated in detail before clinical application. On the other hand, fluorescent dyes are most frequently used to tag biological molecules, and they also have some similar limitations in cellular imaging such as ultrasensitivity, high cytotoxicity, poor aqueous stability, and photostability.

In this section, we will give recent and future challenges in polymeric nanomaterial systems with a particular emphasize on their applications in the bioimaging field. As mentioned above, a variety of bioimaging modalities are used. However, the content of this section is more selective, focusing on in vitro and in vivo optical imaging techniques in combination with other bioimaging modalities. We also give some examples of polymeric nanomaterials combined with contrast agents for MRI, nano/microbubbles for ultrasound imaging, radioactive agents for PET and SPECT, and carbon derivatives for photoacoustic imaging. Optical bioimaging probe must have some necessities, for example, it must show the absence of nonspecific cellular interactions, high quantum efficiency, high resistance to photo-bleaching, colloidal stability, low toxicity and being small, biocompatible, water dispersible, and total excretion from the body. On the note of optical bioimaging, further probe architectures and evaluation of these nanoparticles for clinical bioimaging applications is still needed.

12.3.1 Photostability

Photostability is one of the most important parameters for fluorophores. Almost all of the fluorophores suffer from their low photostability. The fluorescence intensity decays rapidly upon continuous illumination of light (Lakowicz, 2006). This phenomenon is also termed photo-bleaching, and this obstacle limits the utility of employing fluorescence spectroscopy or microscopy for capturing and investigating long-term biological activities. Photo-bleaching is consistently a big concern in real time bioimaging applications of fluorescent/luminescent probes. Moreover, many fluorophores are very unstable in cellular medium, which results in changing their photophysical, photochemical properties, and their spectral behavior. Improvement is a general strategy for achieving highly fluorescent/luminescent, nonphototoxic, and photostable probes for long-term tracking of biological tissue/organ is still greatly required for optical imaging (Brovko, 2010). Comparably enhanced photostability has been reported (Bruchez et al., 1998; Chan and Nie, 1998; Wu et al., 2003; Liu et al., 2013; Osminkina et al., 2012) in a variety of different fluorophores, such as organic dye–based nanoparticles, inorganic QDs (Burns et al., 2006) organic and polymeric (Qin et al., 2013) fluorescent dots, and some fluorescent proteins (Shaner et al., 2008).

It has been shown that physical or chemical encapsulation of an organic dye into the polymeric system just reduces its photobleaching under continuous illumination of light as compared to free organic dyes (Guo et al., 2014). This is because such some polymeric nanoparticles with hydrophobic core have further interactions with an organic dye, resulting in protection of dye from decomposition, photooxidation, and photodegradation. As an example to this strategy, more recently polymer-based nanoparticles consist of di(thiophene-2-yl)-diketopyrrolopyrrole that exhibit little cytotoxicity toward tumor cells and desirable photostability as compared to known QDs or physical blends of organic dye/polymer complexes have confirmed by Huang et al. (2015). They demonstrated that di(thiophene-2-yl)-diketopyrrolopyrrole can be covalently linked to the poly(ε-caprolactone) hydrophobic core of the polymeric nanoparticles to form fluorescent bioprobe (PCL-DPP-PCL) nanostructures, which show enhanced photostability in cell imaging and long-term tracing. In another study, poly(ethylene glycol)-*block*-poly(ε-caprolactone) (PEG − PCL) polymeric nanoparticles loaded with silicon naphthalocyanine (SiNc) was found to reveal strong near-infrared (NIR) absorption in aqueous media as seen in Fig. 12.5A. Its extinction coefficient was found $2.8 \times 10^5\ M^{-1}\ cm^{-1}$ which is almost three times higher than when compared to that of FDA approved clinical imaging agent ICG ($1.0 \times 10^5\ M^{-1}\ cm^{-1}$) (Taratula et al., 2015). After excitation with NIR light for 30 min, the SiNc-loaded polymeric nanoparticles did not show a noticeable alteration of SiNc absorption intensity or fluorescence emission as shown in Fig. 12.5B.

Most of the organic fluorescent dyes are not soluble in aqueous media, and this aggregation usually causes the emission of the dye to be quenched in water. This is called as aggregation-caused quenching (ACQ) effect (Yuan et al., 2010).

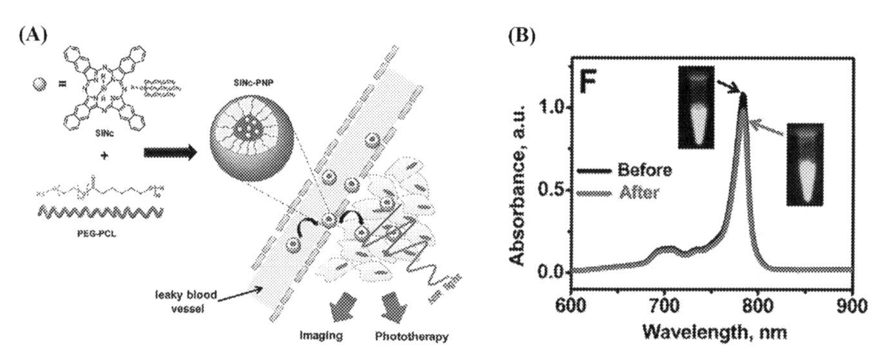

FIGURE 12.5

(A) Schematic presentation of the design of a single-agent based theranostic nanoplatform (SiNc-PNP); (B) absorption spectra and fluorescence images (insets) of SiNc-PNP aqueous solution before and after irradiation with NIR light. *NIR*, near-infrared.

Readapted with permission from Taratula, O., Doddapaneni, B.S., Schumann, C., Li, X., Bracha, S., Milovancev M., et al., (2015). Naphthalocyanine-based biodegradable polymeric nanoparticles for image-guided combinatorial phototherapy. Chem. Mater. 27 (17), 6155–6165. Copyright (2015) American Chemical Society.

On the contrary to ACQ molecules, many of the aggregation-induced emission (AIE) molecules are highly emissive in the aggregated or solid state but nonemissive in their dissolved state. As an example of this strategy, two different AIE-active dyes were incorporated into the hyperbranched polymeric system, constructing ratiometric sensors for pH sensing and imaging as seen in Fig. 12.6A (Bao et al., 2015). In this case, hyperbranched polylactite-PEG polymers were functionalized with two AIE fluoropores and used to visualize pH mapping in vitro. They demonstrated and monitored that the emission wavelength can be changed with regards to pH values in the cell compartments. Lower pH values lead to green emission as seen in Fig. 12.6C. According to fluorescence image of HeLa cells, the pH values of spots 1 and 2 were founded to be 6.0 ± 0.2 and 5.2 ± 0.2. These values belonged to endosomes and lysosomes, respectively.

QDs has become promising alternatives to organic fluorescent dyes as imaging probes due to their high quantum efficiency, long wavelength emission spectra, and resistance to photobleaching (Qu and Peng, 2002). However, the usefulness of QD can be limited because of their several challenges including poor resistance to enzymatic degradation, hydrolysis, and toxicity (Tsoi et al., 2013). For instance, CdSe and CdTe display severe toxicity to biological systems. As an alternative to QDs, conjugated polymers (CP) have attracted significant interest in biomedical imaging field because of their unique optical and chemical properties including excellent photostability, high emission band, brightness, and comparably low toxicity (Zhu et al., 2016). In addition to their good photophysical properties, the supramolecular organization of CP offers an opportunity to produce nanostructures and can also be used to promote specific fluorescent imaging

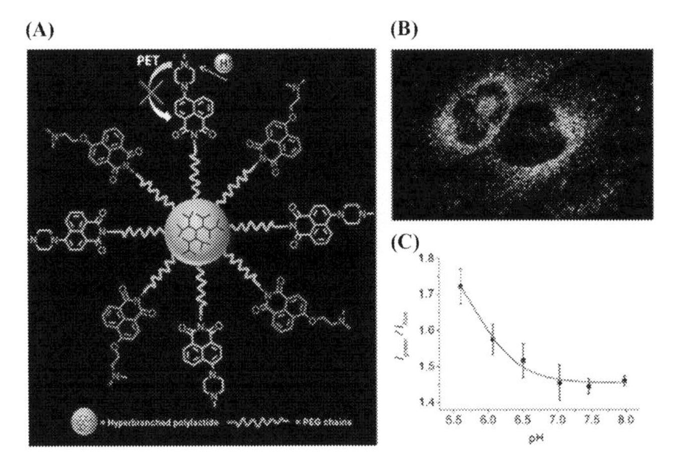

FIGURE 12.6

(A) Hyperbranched polylactide-PEG nanoparticles functionalized with a green emissive AIE fluorophore as pH-sensitive probe and a blue emissive AIE fluorophore. (B) The calibration curve about the relation between Igreen/Iblue and pH obtained using nigericin; (C) the pH map for untreated HeLa cells based on the curve in (B). *PEG*, poly(ethylene glycol); *AIE*, aggregation-induced emission.

Reprinted with permission from Bao, Y., Keersmaecker, H.D., Corneillie, S., Yu, F., Mizuno, H., Zhang, G., et al., (2015). Tunable ratiometric fluorescence sensing of intracellular pH by aggregation-induced emission-active hyperbranched polymer nanoparticles, Chem. Mater. 27 (9), 3450–3455. Copyright (2015) American Chemical Society.

probes (Li and Liu, 2012; Wu et al., 2008; Li et al., 2009; Wu et al., 2011). Miniemulsion, nanoprecipitation, and encapsulation methods are used for the preparation of conjugated polymeric nanoparticles (CPNPs). Similarly, CPNPs has exhibited potential not only for diagnosis but also therapy or both (Pecher and Mecking, 2010; Li and Liu, 2012). For example, Wu et al. (2008) created various CPNPs which showed unprecedented brightness, great emission rates even in small particle diameters. In another work, optical properties of poly[1-phenyl-2-(*p*-trimethylsilyl)phenylacetylene] (PDPA-C1) in water were compared with other CP such as PDPA-C18 and poly[2-(ethylhexyloxy)-5-methoxy]-1,4-phenylenevinylene (MEH-PPV) and some commercial polymers (Kim et al., 2014). They were reported that PDPA-C1 is one of the most feasible polymers for tremendously photostable and fluorescent CPNP in bioimaging applications. The fluorescence quantum yield (Φ_F) value of PDPA-C1 (1.50×10^{-9}) was found quite low. This evidenced that Φ_F value of PDPA-C1 was lower that of the other commercial polymers ($\sim 10^{-8}$), indicating with higher photostability. In another work, Zhu et al. investigated the bioimaging potential of multilayered CPNPs in cells, lymph node tracking and in vivo tumor imaging in zebrafish and mice (Zhu et al., 2016). In that case, four different multilayered CPNPs were synthesized and covered with silica and an outer PEG in order to increase NIR fluorescence intensity. They showed that the fluorescence intensity is almost 100 times higher as compared to that for the counterpart silica-coated CPNPs. Because of the inherent characteristic structures of CPs, they have much higher photostabilities as compared to other fluorescent compounds such as organic dyes (De Jong and Vissenberg, 1998; Yu et al., 2000; Park et al., 2004) and green fluorescent proteins (Eggeling et al., 1998) in practical bioimaging applications. On the other hand, they also pose some challenges such as low ionization potentials. Photobleaching of CP is attributed to the formation of charge-transfer complexes in aqueous media (Golding and Cox, 2004; Park et al., 2004). To address this challenge, the preparation of biocompatible and biodegradable CPs with desired optical properties for clinical bioimaging applications is still a top priority. The gold nanoparticles with different size and shape were embedded in PLGA matrix via an electrohydrodynamic cojetting procedure to produce a hybrid material. This method was reported as a new route to prepare multicompartment fibers, cylinders, and microgels. The obtained hybrid materials revealed high photostability and offered new possibilities for long-term screening by surface-enhanced Raman scattering microscopy (Strozyk et al., 2017).

12.3.2 Size

Nanoparticle size plays a key role in bioimaging applications. By changing the size and composition of metal nanoparticles including QDs, upconverting nanophosphors, Au, Ag, and Pt the emission wavelength can be tuned from the ultraviolet, visible, and NIR region allowing for further specific applications. Metal nanoparticles consisting of Au, Ag, and Pt are not fluorescent, though somewhat scatter light very efficiently. As compared to other metallic nanoparticles, a major drawback of QDs is their smaller size below the limits of renal clearance (Choi et al., 2007). The other issues are to think about their metallic nature. As mentioned above, this can be prevented by immobilizing biocompatible and biodegradable molecules to form the nanostructure. Actually, in vitro and in vivo bioimaging might need different requirements. As mentioned above, for in vitro imaging, the particle size should be smaller to be taken up by the cells. However, for in vivo imaging, the particle size should be higher than 6–8 nm for preventing renal clearance and similarly lower than 200 nm for avoiding accumulating in tissues/organs. It is important to screen nanoparticles before the lysosome trapping. Apparently, uptake of noble metal nanoparticles into cell compartments and endocytosis mechanism of these nanoparticles involve a range of problems, and their mechanisms are still being discussed. As an illustrative example, Nabiev et al. (2007) prepared two different sizes CdTe QDs probes to show the size specific penetration into cellular organelles. The red-emitting 3.4 nm of the probe is localized in the cytoplasm. On the other hand, green-emitting optical probe with the size of 2 nm can easily enter to the cell nucleus. It is important to note that the intracellular uptaking not only depends on particle sizes but also their surface charge. Because the cell membranes are negatively charged, it is known that positively charged compounds covered on the surface of QDs assist the progress of their uptake by cells as a result of electrostatic interaction with the cell membrane. QDs decorated with peptides (Liu et al., 2011; Rozenzhak et al., 2005; Smith et al., 2008), phospholipids (Wen et al., 2013), dendrimers (Derfus et al., 2004), and positively charged polymers, such as poly(*N*-isopropylacrylamide) (Kim et al., 2010) and chitosan (Geng et al., 2013), were used to investigate their intracellular uptake behavior. As an alternative to QDs, the CPNs are self-assembled in aqueous solution and the nanostructures can be obtained with different size by a nanoprecipitation process. For example, poly[9,9-di((*S*)-2-methylbutyl)fluorene]-*co*-bis(difluoroboron)1,2-bis((1*H*-pyrrol-2yl)methylene) hydrazine-15-*co*-4,7-di(thiophen-2-yl)-2,1,3-benzothiadiazole (PFBOPHYDBT) polymeric nanoparticles were prepared with three different sizes consisting of 80, 120, and 190 nm. UV-Vis and fluorescence results evidenced that increasing the diameters of CPNs showed a red shift (Dai et al., 2015). The polymeric nanoparticles with the size of 80 nm were applied for in vitro cell imaging due to their far-red/NIR fluorescence emission, low cytotoxicity, and desirable photostability. It can be said that, optical properties of the dye-loaded fluorescent polymeric nanoparticles ultimately depend on their size. This is because of the different packing of compounds resulting in variation of spectral behavior. There are not many works published searching the size effect on (pre-) clinical practice.

12.3.3 Brightness

For optical imaging, brightness is quite important to use a contrast agent at lower dosages with high sensitivity. Reducing the dosage of the contrast agent is also important to reduce undesirable side effects. One of the other important parameters in many biological applications is to provide the possible highest brightness even in the smallest particle size. Therefore one of the important parameters is that the brightness per volume of a particular fluorescent material is independent of the particle size. The brightness of a fluorescent molecule is determined by the quantum yield and the extinction coefficient ($\varepsilon \times \Phi_F$) (Lavis and Raines, 2008). Thus sensitivity and resolution are defined by means of the signal obtained from a single molecule. For most organic fluorophores, the ε is lower than $10^2\ mM^{-1}\ cm^{-1}$, and therefore, even when the quantum-yielding is close to 1, it approaches that value (Thapaliya et al., 2017). As an example, the brightness of an ICG is only $11\ mM^{-1}\ cm^{-1}$ (Schaafsma et al., 2011). Strategies to increase brightness in nanoparticles are based on two general approaches. The first one is to use doping agents to prevent ACQ. The second one is to control the distribution of fluorescent molecule in the nanoparticles with avoiding aggregation. Fluorescent nanoparticles have been formed by encapsulating identical chromophores into the same polymer assemblies to increase the brightness approaching $10^4\ mM^{-1}\ cm^{-1}$ (He et al. (2010a,b); Luo et al., 2011; Altinoglu and Adair, 2010; Yi et al., 2014). Such brightness values are of a great magnitude that can be achieved with individual organic fluorophores and extend beyond the semiconductor QDs (Wagh et al., 2012; Jin et al., 2011). An AIE polymeric nanoparticle system with particle sizes in the range of 50–90 nm was synthesized by miniemulsion polymerization of methyl methacrylate (MMA) following with 1-allyl-1-methyl-2,3,4,5-tetraphenylsilole (AMTPS) (Cao et al., 2016). The prepared poly (MMA-*co*-AMTPS) nanoparticles emitted blue green fluorescence and showed high brightness and Φ_F values. In another work, borondipyrromethene (BODIPY) fluorophores incorporated AIE polymeric NPs were microinjected into nematodes, where they maintain their inherent brightness values and provide the visualization of the nematodes with signal-to-noise ratios higher than those accessible with the monomer model (Thapaliya et al., 2017).

12.3.4 Color

Optical techniques can allow different imaging colors of cellular and intracellular components in terms of using appropriate probes. In most cases, diagnostic probes are especially architecture to target biological tissues such as receptors, proteins, membranes ion channels, etc. They are also suitable for screening cell viability, cell proliferation, endocytosis and exocytosis, drug release, multicolor gene expression experiments, and multiple-labeling studies. As compared to other fluorescent materials, QDs show greater flexibility (Gao et al., 2004). QDs have a wavelength of less than 655 nm, although the emission bands are sharp. This makes them suitable for use in multicolor applications because of their wide absorption spectra. When QDs are excited by a single light source, they can emit various color fluorescence. As an example, the multicolor capability of QD imaging in live animals was examined by using CdSe-ZnS QDs probes. In that case, QDs were protected by both a coordinating ligand, tri-*n*-octylphosphine oxide, and an amphiphilic ABC type triblock copolymer coating (Zhang and Yang, 2013). Depending on their nanostructure design, QDs showed different colors under the same illumination source. Another example for tunable fluorescence emission is for biodegradable photoluminescent polymers. They can be classified into a range of different emission colors from 475 nm (cyan) to 649 nm (far-red). They offer advantages over the traditional fluorescent organic dyes and QDs because of their biocompatibility, low toxicity, controlled degradability, and high quantum yields (Zhang and Yang, 2013; Yang et al., 2009; Zhang et al., 2013). In CPN the absorption and emission bands are generally wide. To sharpen the emission peak, conventional dyes such as BODIPY, or cyanines are integrated into the nanoparticulate system (Rong et al., 2013). In addition to these examples, NIR dyes especially cyanines and upconversion nanoparticles (UCNPs) have also been used as multicolor optical probes. There is a growing interest in the application of far-red and NIR region because of minimum auto-fluorescence and greater penetration depth (Dong et al., 2015; González-Béjar et al., 2016). For UCNPs, tuning the amount of both sensitizer and activator can offer to distinctive spectral profiles as seen in Fig. 12.7 (Wei et al., 2014).

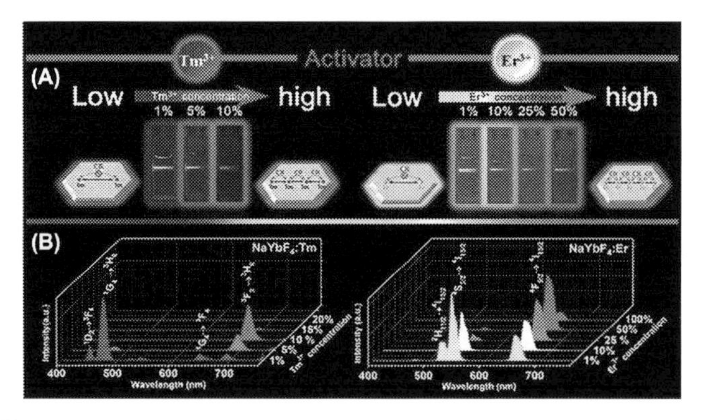

FIGURE 12.7

Modulating multicolor upconversion emissions by controlling the doping concentration of activators. (A) The fluorescence photographs of $NaYbF_4$:Tm and $NaYbF_4$:Er UCNPs with the concentration of the activator varying from low to high. (B) UC emission spectra of 1, 5, 10, 15, and 20 mol.% Tm^{3+} ions doped $NaYbF_4$:Tm and 1, 10, 25, 50, and 100 mol.% Er^{3+} ions doped $NaYbF_4$:Er UCNPs. *UCNPs*, upconversion nanoparticles.

Reproduced with permission from Wei, W., Zhang, Y., Chen, R., Goggi, J., Ren, N., Huang, L., et al., (2014). Cross relaxation, induced pure red upconversion in activator- and sensitizer-rich lanthanide nanoparticles. Chem. Mater. 26 (18), 5183–5186. Copyright (2014) American Chemical Society.

Hilderbrand et al. (2009) employed UCNPs to monitor them in the blood vessels. They used red-upconverting Y_2O_3:Yb, Er UCNPs, as the inorganic emitting core, and further covered them to PAA loading, PEG conjugation, and cyanine dye conjugation. This multicolor nanoconjugate system was intravenously administrated into the mouse through tail vein injection. Then, the mouse ear lobe was imaged and discriminated that both the upconversion and NIR fluorescence signals, with high signal-to-background ratio, were monitored in the bloodstream of the mouse ear (Hilderbrand et al., 2009).

12.4 Conclusions and future prospects

There is an urgent need for the fast and precise diagnosis with effective personalized therapy all over the world. Recent advances in materials science and nanotechnology have made nanomaterials important for improving human health. The main purpose of nanomedicine is to create the most sensitive and specific diagnostic tools and therapy regimens for clinical implementation. In this regard, polymeric nanoparticles hold great promise for developing personalized nanomedicine because of having many fabrication advantages such as size, shape, morphology, charge, and composition which are easily controlled. This chemically and physically controllable nature of polymers is very important to secure their current and future development and success of polymeric nanocarriers. However, the fabrication of the polymeric nanoparticles has some limitations such as the batch-to-batch variation, the possible toxicity, immunological reactions, and the complexity of both the nanoparticles and available technologies for physical, chemical, and biological evaluations. The size and morphology of the polymeric nanoparticles are very important to enhance cell permeability, in vivo, in vitro stability, accumulation at the targeted sites, prolong the circulation time, and the biodistribution of the particles. On the other hand, the surface charge and chemistry of the particles play an important role in the interactions between the nanoparticles and cells. It is known that positively charged polymeric particles are very effective in attaching on the negatively charged cell membranes. However, many studies indicate that the zeta-potential values of particles are very critical because over a certain value, the particles exhibit toxicity for biomedical applications. Moreover, polymeric nanoparticles face with several biological barriers into the blood circulation. These biological barriers can be defined as the defense system of the human body to protect the body from the foreign materials. Polymeric nanoparticles must hide from these defense systems. In this regard, they must be compatible with the biological tissues in terms of size, shape, charge, and surface chemistry.

On the other hand, polymeric nanocarriers are one of the most important examples of nanomedicine that have enormous potential in imaging techniques because of their unique adaptable properties. Novel diagnostic probe architectures and nanomaterials, fluorescent polymeric nanoparticles, dyes, and proteins push the limits of sensing, labeling, specificity, and filling the gap between the living tissues and bioengineered tools. Basically, the usage of polymeric nanocarriers might change the application limits of biotechnology and medicine. Optical imaging techniques depend on fluorescence, and light scattering phenomena are getting more popular, especially for bio-sensing and bioimaging. This is results from their simplicity in the detection systems. Fluorescent polymeric systems with advanced optical properties (e.g., high photostability, high Φ_F), good biocompatibility, suitable size have been synthesized through sophisticated molecular designs and advanced synthetic technologies. In addition to this, contrast agents might be integrated into nanoparticle systems offering dual/multimodal imaging modalities such as MRI, X-ray CT, and photoacoustic imaging through nanostructure construction and surface modification. However, in order to use the full potential of fluorescent polymeric nanocarriers, detailed experimental evidence is needed. Despite recent progress, there are still challenges associated with using fluorescent probes for both in vitro and in vivo bioimaging applications. For example, optimizing the optical properties of fluorescent polymers in biological environment is highly desired. To conclude, appropriate sized, monodisperse, preciously bright, highly photostable, far-red/NIR fluorescent biocompatible polymeric system with high colloidal and chemical stability are required especially for in vivo bioimaging applications. Actually, it is expected and anticipated that automated image characterization strategies can be improved for labeling and accurate identification of disease through their macroscopic or nanoscopic images.

In conclusion, it is very complicated to combine both diagnosis and treatment properties into one nanoparticle system. Researchers are still working hard on developing all-in-one polymeric nanoparticles system which is able to overcome all mentioned challenges. For this purpose, new synthesis methods with the cutting-edge approaches and also biological and theoretical evaluations are needed to be developed. We believe that when all of the aforementioned limitations are overcome, the future polymeric nanoparticles will change and collaborate to improve the diagnosis, imaging/tracking, and treatment of many diseases.

References

Aderem, A., Underhill, D., 1999. Mechanisms of phagocytosis in macrophages. Annu. Rev. Immunol. 17 (1), 593–623.

Allen, T.M., Cullis, P.R., 2004. Drug delivery systems: entering the mainstream. Science 303 (5665), 1818–1822.

Altinoglu, E.I., Adair, J.H., 2010. Near-infrared imaging with nanoparticles. Wiley Interdiscipl. Rev. Nanomed. Nanobiotechnol 2 (5), 461–477.

Arnida, N.V., Janát-Amsbury, M.M., Ray, A., Peterson, C.M., Ghandehari, H., 2011. Geometry and surface characteristics of gold nanoparticles influence their biodistribution and uptake by macrophages. Eur. J. Pharm. Biopharm. 77 (3), 417–423.

Banga, R.J., Krovi, S.A., Narayan, S.P., Sprangers, A.J., Liu, G., Mirkin, C.A., et al., 2017. Drug-loaded polymeric spherical nucleic acids: enhancing colloidal stability and cellular uptake of polymeric nanoparticles through dna surface-functionalization. Biomacromolecules 18 (2), 483–489.

Banik, B.L., Fattahi, P., Brown, J.L., 2016. Polymeric nanoparticles: the future of nanomedicine. Wiley Interdiscip. Rev. Nanomed. Nanobiotechnol. 8 (2), 271–299.

Bao, Y., Keersmaecker, H.D., Corneillie, S., Yu, F., Mizuno, H., Zhang, G., et al., 2015. Tunable ratiometric fluorescence sensing of intracellular pH by aggregation-induced emission-active hyperbranched polymer nanoparticles. Chem. Mater. 27 (9), 3450–3455.

Barua, S., Mitragotri, S., 2014. Challenges associated with penetration of nanoparticles across cell and tissue barriers: a review of current status and future prospects. Nano Today 9 (2), 223–243.

Bhunia, S.K., Saha, A., Maity, A.R., Ray, S.C., Jana, N.R., 2013. Carbon nanoparticle-based fluorescent bioimaging probes. Sci. Rep. 3, 1473.

Bobo, D., Robinson, K.J., Islam, J., Thurecht, K.J., Corrie, S.R., 2016. Nanoparticle-based medicines: a review of FDA-approved materials and clinical trials to date. Pharm. Res. 33 (10), 2373–2387.

Bonengel, S., Prüfert, F., Perera, G., Schauer, J., Bernkop-Schnürch, A., 2015. Polyethylene imine-6-phosphogluconic acid nanoparticles—a novel zeta potential changing system. Int. J. Pharm. 483 (1-2), 19–25.

Brohi, R.D., Wang, L., Talpur, H.S., Wu, D., Khan, F.A., Bhattarai, D., et al., 2017. Toxicity of nanoparticles on the reproductive system in animal models: a review. Front. Pharmacol. 5 (8), 606.

Brovko, L., 2010. Bioluminescence and Fluorescence for In Vivo Imaging. SPIE Press, Bellingham.

Bruchez, M., Moronne, M., Gin, P., Weiss, S., Alivisatos, A.P., 1998. Semiconductor nanocrystals as fluorescent biological labels. Science 281 (5385), 2013–2016.

Bruni, R., Possenti, P., Bordignon, C., Li, M., Ordanini, S., Messa, P., et al., 2017. Ultrasmall polymeric nanocarriers for drug delivery to podocytes in kidney glomerulus. J. Control. Release 255, 94–107.

Burns, A., Ow, H., Wiesner, U., 2006. Fluorescent core-shell silica nanoparticles: towards "Lab on a Particle" architectures for nanobiotechnology. Chem. Soc. Rev. 35 (11), 1028–1042.

Buzea, C., Pacheco, I.I., Robbie, K., 2007. Nanomaterials and nanoparticles: sources and toxicity. Biointerphases 2 (4), MR17–MR71.

Cabral, H., Matsumoto, Y., Mizuno, K., Chen, Q., Murakami, M., Kimura, M., et al., 2011. Accumulation of sub-100 nm polymeric micelles in poorly permeable tumours depends on size. Nat. Nanotechnol. 6 (12), 815–823.

Cao, Z., Liang, X., Chen, H., Gao, M., Zhao, Z., Chen, X., et al., 2016. Bright and biocompatible AIE polymeric nanoparticles prepared from miniemulsion for fluorescence cell imaging. Polym. Chem. 7 (35), 5571–5578.

Champion, J.A., Katare, Y.K., Mitragotri, S., 2007. Making polymeric micro- and nanoparticles of complex shapes. Proc. Natl. Acad. Sci. U. S. A. 104 (29), 11901–11904.

Chan, W.C., Nie, S., 1998. Quantum dot bioconjugates for ultrasensitive nonisotopic detection. Science 281 (5385), 2016–2018.

Choi, H.S., Liu, W., Misra, P., Tanaka, E., Zimmer, J.P., Ipe, B.I., et al., 2007. Renal clearance of quantum dots. Nat. Biotechnol. 25 (10), 1165–1170.

Choi, K.Y., Jeon, E.J., Yoon, H.Y., Lee, B.S., Na, J.H., Min, K.H., et al., 2012. Theranostic nanoparticles based on PEGylated hyaluronic acid for the diagnosis, therapy and monitoring of colon cancer. Biomaterials 33 (26), 6186–6193.

Daglar, B., Ozgur, E., Corman, M.E., Uzun, L., Demirel, G.B., 2014. Polymeric nanocarriers for expected nanomedicine: current challenges and future prospects. RSC Adv. 4, 48639–48659.

Dai, C., Yang, D., Zhang, W., Bao, B., Cheng, Y., Wang, L., 2015. Far-red/near-infrared fluorescent conjugated polymer nanoparticles with size-dependent chirality and cell imaging applications. Polym. Chem. 6 (21), 3962–3969.

Dasgupta, S., Auth, T., Gompper, G., 2014. Shape and orientation matter for the cellular uptake of nonspherical particles. Nano Lett. 14 (2), 687–693.

Davis, M.E., Chen, Z.G., Shin, D.M., 2008. Nanoparticle therapeutics: an emerging treatment modality for cancer. Nat. Rev. Drug. Discov. 7 (9), 771–782.

De Jong, M.J.M., Vissenberg, M.C.J.M., 1998. Theory of luminescence quenching and photobleaching in conjugated polymers. Philips J. Res. 51 (4), 495–510.

Dehaini, D., Fang, R.H., Luk, B.T., Pang, Z., Hu, C.M.J., Kroll, A.V., et al., 2016. Ultrasmall lipid-polymer hybrid nanoparticles for tumor- penetrating drug delivery. Nanoscale 8 (30), 14411–14419.

Demirel, G.B., Aygul, E., Dag, A., Atasoy, S., Cimen, Z., Cetin, B., 2020. Folic Acid-Conjugated pH and Redox-Sensitive Ellipsoidal Hybrid Magnetic Nanoparticles for Dual-Triggered Drug Release. ACS Appl. Bio Mater. 3 (8), 4949–4961.

Derfus, A.M., Chan, W.C.W., Bhatia, S.N., 2004. Intracellular delivery of quantum dots for live cell labeling and organelle tracking. Adv. Mater. 16 (12), 961–966.

Dhawan, A.P., Huang, H.K., Kim, D.-S., 2008. Principles and Advanced Methods in Medical Imaging and Image Analysis. World Scientific Publishing Company, Boston, USA, ISBN: 978-981-281-480-7.

Dong, H., Du, S.-R., Zheng, X.-Y., Lyu, G.-M., Sun, L.-D., Li, L.-D., et al., 2015. Lanthanide nanoparticles: from design toward bioimaging and therapy. Chem. Rev. 115 (19), 10725–10815.

Doshi, N., Zahr, A.S., Bhaskar, S., Lahann, J., Mitragotri, S., 2009. Red blood cell-mimicking synthetic biomaterial particles. Proc. Natl. Acad. Sci. U. S. A. 106 (51), 21495–21499.

Duan, X., Li, Y., 2013. Physicochemical characteristics of nanoparticles affect circulation, biodistribution, cellular internalization, and trafficking. Small 9 (9-10), 1521–1532.

Dube, T., Chibh, S., Mishra, J., Panda, J.J., 2017. Receptor targeted polymeric nanostructures capable of navigating across the blood-brain barrier for effective delivery of neural therapeutics. ACS Chem. Neurosci. 8 (10), 2105–2117.

Eggeling, C., Widengren, J., Rigler, R., Seidel, C.A.M., 1998. Photobleaching of fluorescent dyes under conditions used for single-molecule detection: evidence of two-step photolysis. Anal. Chem. 70 (13), 2651–2659.

Elsabahy, M., Wooley, K.L., 2012. Design of polymeric nanoparticles for biomedical delivery applications. Chem. Soc. Rev. 41 (7), 2545–2561.

Gao, X., Cui, Y., Levenson, R.M., Chung, L.W., Nie, S., 2004. In vivo cancer targeting and imaging with semiconductor quantum dots. Nat. Biotechnol. 22 (8), 969–976.

Geng, Y., Dalhaimer, P., Cai, S., Tsai, R., Tewari, M., Minko, T., et al., 2007. Shape effects of filaments versus spherical particles in flow and drug delivery. Nat. Nanotechnol. 2 (4), 249–255.

Geng, Y., Lin, D., Shao, L., Yan, F., Ju, H., 2013. Cellular delivery of quantum dot-bound hybridization probe for detection of intracellular pre-microRNA using chitosan/poly (γ-glutamic acid) complex as a carrier. PLoS One 8 (6), e65540.

Gilkey, M.J., Krishnan, V., Scheetz, L., Jia, X., Rajasekaran, A.K., Dhurjati, P.S., 2015. Physiologically based pharmacokinetic modeling of fluorescently labeled block copolymer nanoparticles for controlled drug delivery in leukemia therapy. CPT Pharmacomet. Syst. Pharmacol. 4 (3), 167–174.

Golding, I., Cox, E.C., 2004. RNA dynamics in live *Escherichia coli* cells. Proc. Natl Acad. Sci. U. S. A. 101 (31), 11310–11315.

González-Béjar, M., Francés-Soriano, L., Pérez-Prieto, J., 2016. Upconversion nanoparticles for bioimaging and regenerative medicine. Front. Bioeng. Biotechnol. 4, 47.

Gonzalez-Paredes, A., Torres, D., Alonso, M.J., 2017. Polyarginine nanocapsules: a versatile nanocarrier with potential in transmucosal drug delivery. Int. J. Pharm. 529 (1-2), 474–485.

Gratton, S.E., Napier, M.E., Ropp, P.A., Tian, S., DeSimone, J.M., 2008a. Microfabricated particles for engineered drug therapies: elucidation into the mechanisms of cellular internalization of PRINT particles. Pharm. Res. 25 (12), 2845–2852.

Gratton, S.E., Ropp, P.A., Pohlhaus, P.D., Luft, J.C., Madden, V.J., Napier, M.E., et al., 2008b. The effect of particle design on cellular internalization pathways. Proc. Natl Acad. Sci. U. S. A. 105 (33), 11613–11618.

Gref, R., Domb, A., Quellec, P., Blunk, T., Müller, R.H., Verbavatz, J.M., et al., 1995. The controlled intravenous delivery of drugs using PEG-coated sterically stabilized nanospheres. Adv. Drug. Deliv. Rev. 16 (2-3), 215–233.

Guo, M., Mao, H., Li, Y., Zhu, A., He, H., Yang, H., et al., 2014. Dual imaging-guided photothermal/photodynamic therapy using micelles. Biomaterials 35 (16), 4656–4666.

Harris, J.M., Chess, R.B., 2003. Effect of pegylation on pharmaceuticals. Nat. Rev. Drug. Discov. 2 (3), 214–221.

He, Y., Park, K., 2016. Effects of the microparticle shape on cellular uptake. Mol. Pharm. 13 (7), 2164–2171.

He, X., Wang, K., Cheng, Z., 2010a. In vivo near-infrared fluorescence imaging of cancer with nanoparticle-based probes. Wiley Interdiscipl. Rev. Nanomed. Nanobiotechnol 2 (4), 349–366.

He, C., Hu, Y., Yin, L., Tang, C., Yin, C., 2010b. Effects of particle size and surface charge on cellular uptake and biodistribution of polymeric nanoparticles. Biomaterials 31 (13), 3657–3666.

He, J., Perez, M.T., Zhang, P., Liu, Y., Babu, T., Gong, J., et al., 2012. A general approach to synthesize asymmetric hybrid nanoparticles by interfacial reactions. J. Am. Chem. Soc. 134 (8), 3639–3642.

He, C., Cai, P., Li, J., Zhang, T., Lin, L., Abbasi, A.Z., et al., 2017. Blood-brain barrier-penetrating amphiphilic polymer nanoparticles deliver docetaxel for the treatment of brain metastases of triple negative breast cancer. J. Control. Release 246, 98–109.

Hilderbrand, S.A., Shao, F., Salthouse, C., Mahmood, U., Weissleder, R., 2009. Upconverting luminescent nanomaterials: application to in vivo bioimaging. Chem. Commun. 0 (28), 4188–4190.

Hinde, E., Thammasiraphop, K., Duong, H.T.T., Yeow, J., Karagoz, B., Boyer, C., et al., 2017. Pair correlation microscopy reveals the role of nanoparticle shape in intracellular transport and site of drug release. Nat. Nanotechnol. 12 (1), 81–89.

Huang, X., Jain, P.K., El-Sayed, I.H., El-Sayed, M.A., 2007. Gold nanoparticles: interesting optical properties and recent applications in cancer diagnostics and therapy. Nanomedicine (Lond.) 2 (5), 681–693.

Huang, S., Liu, S., Wang, K., Yang, C., Luo, Y., Zhang, Y., et al., 2015. Highly fluorescent and bioresorbable polymeric nanoparticles with enhanced photostability for cell imaging. Nanoscale 7 (3), 889–895.

Ilium, L., Davis, S.S., Wilson, C.G., Thomas, N.W., Frier, M., Hardy, J.G., 1982. Blood clearance and organ deposition of intravenously administered colloidal particles. the effects of particle size, nature and shape. Int. J. Pharm. 12 (2–3), 135–146.

Iversen, T.G., Skotland, T., Sandvig, K., 2011. Endocytosis and intracellular transport of nanoparticles: present knowledge and need for future studies. Nano Today 6 (2), 176–185.

Jin, Y., Ye, F., Zeigler, M., Wu, C.F., Chiu, D.T., 2011. Near-infrared fluorescent dye-doped semiconducting polymer dots. ACS Nano 5 (2), 1468–1475.

Juliano, R., Stamp, D., 1975. The effect of particle size and charge on the clearance rates of liposomes and liposome encapsulated drugs. Biochem. Biophys. Res. Commun. 63 (3), 651–658.

Kim, C., Lee, Y., Kim, J.S., Jeong, J.H., Park, T.G., 2010. Thermally triggered cellular uptake of quantum dots immobilized with poly(N-isopropylacrylamide) and cell penetrating peptide. Langmuir 26 (18), 14965–14969.

Kim, B.S.-I., Jin, Y.-J., Lee, W.-E., Byun, D.J., Yu, R., Park, S.-J., et al., 2014. Highly fluorescent, photostable, conjugated polymer dots with amorphous, glassy-state, coarsened structure for bioimaging. Adv. Optical Mater. 3 (1), 78–86.

Kulkarni, S.A., Feng, S.S., 2013. Effects of particle size and surface modification on cellular uptake and biodistribution of polymeric nanoparticles for drug delivery. Pharm. Res. 30 (10), 2512–2522.

Kumar, S., Anselmo, A.C., Banerjee, A., Zakrewsky, M., Mitragotri, S., 2015. Shape and size-dependent immune response to antigen-carrying nanoparticles. J. Control. Release 220 (Pt A), 141–148.

Kurtay, G., Yılmaz, M., Kuralay, F., Demirel, G.B., 2017. Chapter 15: Multifunctional therapeutic hybrid nanocarriers for targeted and triggered drug delivery: recent trends and future prospects. Nanostructures for Drug Delivery, A Volume in Micro and Nano Technologies. Elsevier, pp. 461−493.

Lakowicz, J.R., 2006. Principles of Fluorescence Spectroscopy. Springer, US.

Landsiedel, R., Sauer, U.G., Ma-Hock, L., Schnekenburger, J., Wiemann, M., 2014. Pulmonary toxicity of nanomaterials: a critical comparison of published in vitro assays and in vivo inhalation or instillation studies. Nanomedicine 9 (16), 2557−2585.

Laurent, S., Bridot, J.-L., Elst, L.V., Muller, R.N., 2010. Magnetic iron oxide nanoparticles for biomedical applications. Future Med. Chem. 2 (3), 427−449.

Lavis, L.D., Raines, R.T., 2008. Bright ideas for chemical biology. ACS Chem. Biol. 3 (3), 142−155.

Li, K., Liu, B., 2012. Polymer encapsulated conjugated polymer nanoparticles for fluorescence bioimaging. J. Mater. Chem. 22 (4), 1257−1264.

Li, K., Pan, J., Feng, S.-S., Wu, A.W., Pu, K.-Y., Liu, Y., et al., 2009. Generic strategy of preparing fluorescent conjugated-polymer-l oaded poly(DL-lactide-co-glycolide) nanoparticles for targeted cell imaging. Adv. Funct. Mater. 19 (22), 3535−3542.

Li, M., Al-Jamal, K.T., Kostarelos, K., Reineke, J., 2010. Physiologically based pharmacokinetic modeling of nanoparticles. ACS Nano 4 (11), 6303−6317.

Li, Y., Kröger, M., Liu, W.K., 2015. Shape effect in cellular uptake of PEGylated nanoparticles: comparison between sphere, rod, cube and disk. Nanoscale 7 (40), 16631−16646.

Liu, B.R., Huang, Y.W., Winiarz, J.G., Chiang, H.J., Lee, H.J., 2011. Intracellular delivery of quantum dots mediated by a histidine- and arginine-rich HR9 cell-penetrating peptide through the direct membrane translocation mechanism. Biomaterials 32 (13), 3520−3537.

Liu, Q., Guo, B., Rao, Z., Zhang, B., Gong, J.R., 2013. Strong two-photon-induced fluorescence from photostable, biocompatible nitrogen-doped graphene quantum dots for cellular and deep-tissue imaging. Nano Lett. 13 (6), 2436−2441.

Löscher, W., Potschka, H., 2005. Blood-brain barrier active efflux transporters: ATP-binding cassette gene family. NeuroRx 2 (1), 86−98.

Luo, S., Zhang, E., Su, Y., Cheng, T., Shi, C., 2011. A review of NIR dyes in cancer targeting and imaging. Biomaterials 32 (29), 7127−7138.

Mader, H.S., Kele, P., Saleh, S.M., Wolfbeis, O.S., 2010. Upconverting luminescent nanoparticles for use in bioconjugation and bioimaging. Curr. Opin. Chem. Biol. 14 (5), 582−596.

Maisel, K., Reddy, M., Xu, Q., Chattopadhyay, S., Cone, R., Ensign, L.M., et al., 2016. Nanoparticles coated with high molecular weight PEG penetrate mucus and provide uniform vaginal and colorectal distribution in vivo. Nanomedicine (Lond.) 11 (11), 1337−1343.

Makadia, H.K., Siegel, S.J., 2011. Poly lactic-co-glycolic acid (PLGA) as biodegradable controlled drug delivery carrier. Polymers 3 (3), 1377−1397.

Manzeli, S., Ovchinnikov, D., Pasquier, D., Yazyev, O.V., Kis, A., 2017. 2D transition metal dichalcogenides. Nat. Rev. Mater. 2, 17033.

Mastorakos, P., Zhang, C., Berry, S., Oh, Y., Lee, S., Eberhart, C.G., et al., 2015. Highly PEGYlated DNA nanoparticles provide uniform and widespread gene transfer in the brain. Adv. Healthc. Mater. 4 (7), 1023−1033.

Mitragotri, S., Lahann, J., 2009. Physical approaches to biomaterial design. Nat. Mater. 8 (1), 15−23.

Mittal, A., Raber, A.S., Schaefer, U.F., Weissmann, S., Ebensen, T., Schulze, K., et al., 2013. Non-invasive delivery of nanoparticles to hair follicles: a perspective for transcutaneous immunization. Vaccine 31 (34), 3442–3451.

Moghimi, S.M., Hunter, A.C., Murray, J.C., 2005. Nanomedicine: current status and future prospects. FASEB J. 19 (3), 311–330.

Moss, D.M., Siccardi, M., 2014. Optimizing nanomedicine pharmacokinetics using physiologically based pharmacokinetics modelling. Br. J. Pharmacol. 171 (17), 3963–3979.

Muro, S., Garnacho, C., Champion, J.A., Leferovich, J., Gajewski, C., Schuchman, E.H., et al., 2008. Control of endothelial targeting and intracellular delivery of therapeutic enzymes by modulating the size and shape of ICAM-1-targeted carriers. Mol. Ther. 16 (8), 1450–1458.

Nabiev, I., Mitchell, S., Davies, A., Williams, Y., Kelleher, D., Moore, R., et al., 2007. Nonfunctionalized nanocrystals can exploit a cell's active transport machinery delivering them to specific nuclear and cytoplasmic compartments. Nano Lett. 7 (11), 3452–3461.

Nance, E.A., Woodworth, G.F., Sailor, K.A., Shih, T.Y., Xu, Q., Swaminathan, G., et al., 2012. A dense poly(ethylene glycol) coating improves penetration of large polymeric nanoparticles within brain tissue. Sci. Transl. Med. 4 (149), 149ra119.

Netsomboon, K., Bernkop-Schnürch, A., 2016. Mucoadhesive vs. mucopenetrating particulate drug delivery. Eur. J. Pharm. Biopharm. 98, 76–89.

Niu, Z., Tedesco, E., Benetti, F., Mabondzo, A., Montagner, I.M., Marigo, I., et al., 2017. Rational design of polyarginine nanocapsules intended to help peptides overcoming intestinal barriers. J. Control. Release 263, 4–17.

Osminkina, L.A., Tamarov, K.P., Sviridov, A.P., Galkin, R.A., Gongalsky, M.B., Solovyev, V.V., et al., 2012. Photoluminescent biocompatible silicon nanoparticles for cancer theranostic applications. J. Biophotonics 5 (7), 529–535.

Pardridge, W.M., 2005. The blood-brain barrier: bottleneck in brain drug development. NeuroRx 2 (1), 3–14.

Park, J., Lakes, R.S., 2007. Biomaterials: An Introduction. Springer-Verlag, New York.

Park, S.-J., Gesquiere, A.J., Yu, J., Barbara, P.F., 2004. Charge injection and photooxidation of single conjugated polymer molecules. J. Am. Chem. Soc. 126 (13), 4116–4117.

Park, J.G., Forster, J.D., Dufresne, E.R., 2010. High-yield synthesis of monodisperse dumbbell-shaped polymer nanoparticles. J. Am. Chem. Soc. 132 (17), 5960–5961.

Pecher, J., Mecking, S., 2010. Nanoparticles of conjugated polymers. Chem. Rev. 110 (10), 6260–6279.

Perera, G., Zipser, M., Bonengel, S., Salvenmoser, W., Bernkop-Schnürch, A., 2015. Development of phosphorylated nanoparticles as zeta potential inverting systems. Eur. J. Pharm. Biopharm. 97 (Pt A), 250–256.

Petros, R.A., DeSimone, J.M., 2010. Strategies in the design of nanoparticles for therapeutic applications. Nat. Rev. Drug. Discov. 9 (8), 615–627.

Phillips, W.T., Goins, B., Bao, A., Vargas, D., Guttierez, J.E., Trevino, A., et al., 2012. Rhenium-186 liposomes as convection-enhanced nanoparticle brachytherapy for treatment of glioblastoma. Neuro-Oncology 14 (4), 416–425.

Qin, W., Li, K., Feng, G., Li, M., Yang, Z., Liu, B., 2013. Bright and photostable organic fluorescent dots with aggregation-induced emission characteristics for noninvasive long-term cell imaging. Adv. Funct. Mater. 24 (5), 635–643.

Qu, L., Peng, X., 2002. Control of photoluminescence properties of CdSe nanocrystals in growth. J. Am. Chem. Soc. 124 (9), 2049–2055.

Raza, K., Singh, B., Lohan, S., Sharma, G., Negi, P., Yachha, Y., et al., 2013. Nano-lipoidal carriers of tretinoin with enhanced percutaneous absorption, photostability, biocompatibility and anti-psoriatic activity. Int. J. Pharm. 456 (1), 65–72.

Romero, G.B., Arntjen, A., Keck, C.M., Muller, R.H., 2016. Amorphous cyclosporin a nanoparticles for enhanced dermal bioavailability. Int. J. Pharm. 498 (1-2), 217–224.

Rong, Y., Wu, C., Yu, J., Zhang, X., Ye, F., Zeigler, M., et al., 2013. Multicolor fluorescent semiconducting polymer dots with narrow emissions and high brightness. ACS Nano 7 (1), 376–384.

Rozenzhak, S.M., Kadakia, M.P., Caserta, T.M., Westbrook, T.R., Stone, M.O., Naik, R.R., 2005. Cellular internalization and targeting of semiconductor quantum dots. Chem. Commun. 0 (17), 2217–2219.

Santander-Ortega, M.J., Stauner, T., Loretz, B., Ortega-Vinuesa, J.L., Bastos-González, D., Wenz, G., et al., 2010. Nanoparticles made from novel starch derivatives for transdermal drug delivery. J. Control. Release 141 (1), 85–92.

Schaafsma, B.E., Mieog, J.S., Hutteman, M., van der Vorst, J.R., Kuppen, P.J., Löwik, C.W., et al., 2011. The clinical use of indocyanine green as a near-infrared fluorescent contrast agent for image- guided oncologic surgery. J. Surg. Oncol. 104 (3), 323–332.

Shaner, N.C., Lin, M.Z., McKeown, M.R., Steinbach, P.A., Hazelwood, K.L., Davidson, M.W., et al., 2008. Improving the photostability of bright monomeric orange and red fluorescent proteins. Nat. Methods 5 (6), 545–551.

Shao, X.R., Wei, X.Q., Song, X., Hao, L.Y., Cai, X.X., Zhang, Z.R., et al., 2015. Independent effect of polymeric nanoparticle zeta potential/surface charge, on their cytotoxicity and affinity to cells. Cell Prolif. 48 (4), 465–474.

Shin, S.W., Song, I.H., Um, S.H., 2015. Role of physicochemical properties in nanoparticle toxicity. Nanomaterials 5 (3), 1351–1365.

Singka, G.S., Samah, N.A., Zulfakar, M.H., Yurdasiper, A., Heard, C.M., 2010. Enhanced topical delivery and anti-inflammatory activity of methotrexate from an activated nanogel. Eur. J. Pharm. Biopharm. 76 (2), 275–281.

Smith, B.R., Cheng, Z., De, A., Koh, A.L., Sinclair, R., Gambhir, S.S., 2008. Real-time intravital, imaging of RGD-quantum dot binding to luminal endothelium in mouse tumor neovasculature. Nano Lett. 8 (9), 2599–2606.

Song, E., Gaudin, A., King, A.R., Seo, Y.-E., Suh, H.-W., Deng, Y., et al., 2017. Surface chemistry governs cellular tropism of nanoparticles in the brain. Nat. Commun. 8, 15322.

Sotiriou, G.A., Pratsinis, S.E., 2011. Engineering nanosilver as an antibacterial, biosensor and bioimaging material. Curr. Opin. Chem. Eng. 1 (1), 3–10.

Strozyk, M.S., de Aberasturi, D.J., Gregory, J.V., Brust, M., Lahann, J., Liz-Marzán, L.M., 2017. Spatial analysis of metal–PLGA hybrid microstructures using 3D SERS imaging. Adv. Funct. Mater. 27 (33), 1701626.

Swami, A., Shi, J., Gadde, S., Votruba, A.R., Kolishetti, N., Farokhzad, O.C., 2012. Nanoparticles for targeted and temporally controlled drug delivery. In: Svenson, S., Prud'homme, R.K. (Eds.), Multifunctional Nanoparticles for Drug Delivery Applications: Imaging, Targeting, and Delivery. Springer, US, pp. 9–29.

Tan, J., Shah, S., Thomas, A., Ou-Yang, H.D., Liu, Y., 2013. The influence of size, shape and vessel geometry on nanoparticle distribution. Microfluid. Nanofluid. 14 (1-2), 77–87.

Tang, L., Yang, X., Yin, Q., Cai, K., Wang, H., Chaudhury, I., et al., 2014. Investigating the optimal size of anticancer nanomedicine. Proc. Natl. Acad. Sci. U. S. A. 111 (43), 15344–15349.

Taratula, O., Doddapaneni, B.S., Schumann, C., Li, X., Bracha, S., Milovancev, M., et al., 2015. Naphthalocyanine-based biodegradable polymeric nanoparticles for image-guided combinatorial phototherapy. Chem. Mater. 27 (17), 6155–6165.

Thapaliya, E.R., Zhang, Y., Dhakal, P., Brown, A.S., Wilson, J.N., Collins, K.M., et al., 2017. Bioimaging with macromolecular probes incorporating multiple BODIPY fluorophores. Bioconjug. Chem. 28 (5), 1519–1528.

Tran, T.-H., Nguyen, C.T., Gonzalez-Fajardo, L., Hargrove, D., Song, D., Deshmukh, P., et al., 2014. Long circulating self-assembled nanoparticles from cholesterol containing brush-like block copolymers for improved drug delivery to tumors. Biomacromolecules 15 (11), 4363–4375.

Truong, N.P., Whittaker, M.R., Mak, C.W., Davis, T.P., 2014. The importance of nanoparticle shape in cancer drug delivery. Expert. Opin. Drug. Deliv. 12 (1), 129–142.

Tsoi, K.M., Dai, Q., Alman, B.A., Chan, W.C., 2013. Are quantum dots toxic? Exploring the discrepancy between cell culture and animal studies. Acc. Chem. Res. 46 (3), 662–671.

Ulery, B.D., Nair, L.S., Laurencin, C.T., 2011. Biomedical applications of biodegradable polymers. J. Polym. Sci. B Polym. Phys. 49 (12), 832–864.

Vadivambal, R., Jayas, D.S., 2015. Bio-Imaging: Principles, Techniques, and Applications. CRC Press, Boca Raton.

Voigt, N., Henrich-Noack, P., Kockentiedt, S., Hintz, W., Tomas, J., Sabel, B.A., 2014. Toxicity of polymeric nanoparticles in vivo and in vitro. J. Nanopart. Res. 16 (6), 2379.

Wadajkar, A.S., Dancy, J.G., Roberts, N.B., Connolly, N.P., Strickland, D.K., Winkles, J.A., et al., 2017. Decreased non-specific adhesivity, receptor targeted (DART) nanoparticles exhibit improved dispersion, cellular uptake, and tumor retention in invasive gliomas. J. Control. Release 267, 144–153.

Wagh, A., Qian, S.Y., Law, B., 2012. Development of biocompatible polymeric nanoparticles for in vivo NIR and FRET imaging. Bioconjug. Chem. 23 (5), 981–992.

Wei, W., Zhang, Y., Chen, R., Goggi, J., Ren, N., Huang, L., et al., 2014. Cross relaxation, induced pure red upconversion in activator- and sensitizer-rich lanthanide nanoparticles. Chem. Mater. 26 (18), 5183–5186.

Wen, C.-J., Sung, C.T., Aljuffali, I.A., Huang, Y.-J., Fang, J.-Y., 2013. Nanocomposite liposomes containing quantum dots and anticancer drugs for bioimaging and therapeutic delivery: a comparison of cationic, PEGylated and deformable liposomes. Nanotechnology 24 (32), 325101.

Wong, H.L., Wu, X.Y., Bendayan, R., 2012. Nanotechnological advances for the delivery of CNS therapeutics. Adv. Drug. Deliv. Rev. 64 (7), 686–700.

Wong, A.D., Ye, M., Levy, A.F., Rothstein, J.D., Bergles, D.E., Searson, P.C., 2013. The blood-brain barrier: an engineering perspective. Front. Neuroeng. 6, 7. Available from: https://doi.org/10.3389/fneng.2013.00007.

Wu, X., Liu, H., Liu, J., Haley, K.N., Treadway, J.A., Larson, J.P., et al., 2003. Immunofluorescent labeling of cancer marker Her2 and other cellular targets with semiconductor quantum dots. Nat. Biotechnol. 21 (1), 41–46.

Wu, C., Bull, B., Szymanski, C., Christensen, K., McNeill, J., 2008. Multicolor conjugated polymer dots for biological fluorescence imaging. ACS Nano 2 (11), 2415–2423.

Wu, C., Hansen, S.J., Hou, Q., Yu, J., Zeigler, M., Jin, Y., et al., 2011. Design of highly emissive polymer dot bioconjugates for in vivo tumor targeting. Angew. Chem. Int. Ed., Engl. 50 (15), 3430–3434.

Wu, L., Shan, W., Zhang, Z., Huang, Y., 2018. Engineering nanomaterials to overcome the mucosal barrier by modulating surface properties. Adv. Drug. Deliv. Rev. 124, 150–163.

Xiao, K., Li, Y., Luo, J., Lee, J.S., Xiao, W., Gonik, A.M., et al., 2011. The effect of surface charge on in vivo biodistribution of PEG-oligocholic acid based micellar nanoparticles. Biomaterials 32 (13), 3435–3446.

Xu, M., Wang, L.V., 2016. Photoacoustic imaging in biomedicine. Rev. Sci. Instrum. 77 (4), 041101.

Yang, J., Zhang, Y., Gautam, S., Liu, L., Dey, J., Chen, W., et al., 2009. Development of aliphatic biodegradable photoluminescent polymers. Proc. Natl. Acad. Sci. U. S. A. 106 (25), 10086–10091.

Yi, X., Wang, F., Qin, W., Yang, X., Yuan, J., 2014. Near- infrared fluorescent probes in cancer imaging and therapy: an emerging field. Int. J. Nanomed. 9 (1), 1347–1365.

Yu, J., Hu, D.H., Barbara, P.F., 2000. Unmasking electronic energy transfer of conjugated polymers by suppression of O_2 quenching. Science 289 (5483), 1327–1330.

Yuan, W.Z., Lu, P., Chen, S., Lam, J.W., Wang, Z., Liu, Y., et al., 2010. Changing the behavior of chromophores from aggregation-caused quenching to aggregation-induced emission: development of highly efficient light emitters in the solid state. Adv. Mater. 22 (19), 2159–2163.

Zhang, Y., Yang, J., 2013. Design strategies for fluorescent biodegradable polymeric biomaterials. J. Mater. Chem. B 1 (2), 132–148.

Zhang, Y., Tran, R.T., Qattan, I.S., Tsai, Y.T., Tang, L., Liu, C., et al., 2013. Fluorescence imaging enabled urethane-doped citrate-based biodegradable elastomers. Biomaterials 34 (16), 4048–4056.

Zhu, H., Fang, Y., Zhen, X., Wei, N., Gao, Y., Luo, K.Q., et al., 2016. Multilayered semiconducting polymer nanoparticles with enhanced NIR fluorescence for molecular imaging in cells, zebrafish and mice. Chem. Sci. 7 (8), 5118–5125.

Index

Note: Page numbers followed by "*f*" and "*t*" refer to figures and tables, respectively.

E

F

G

H

I

K

L

M

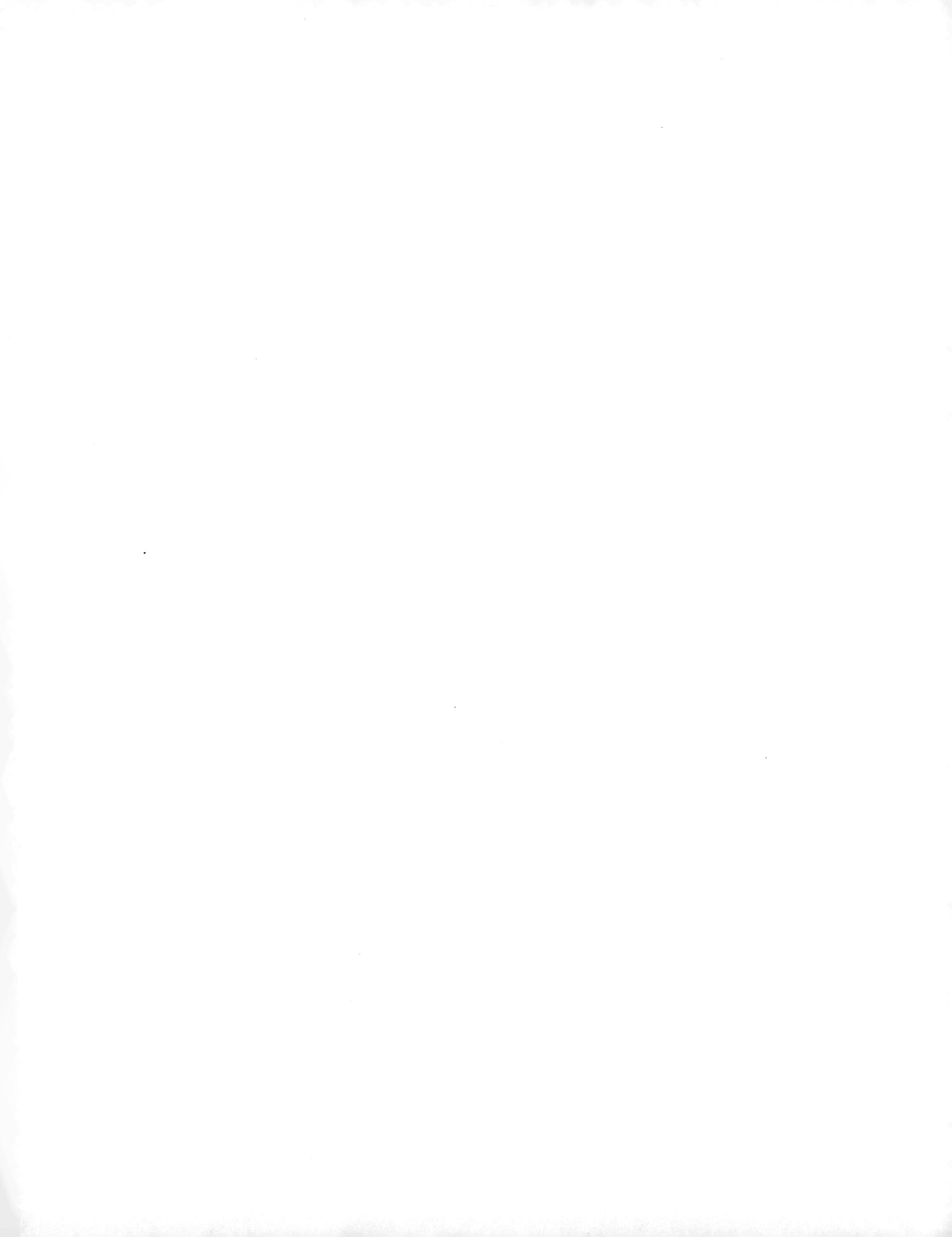

Printed in the United States
by Baker & Taylor Publisher Services